THE LEARNING HEALTHCARE SYSTEM SERIES

IOM ROUNDTABLE ON EVIDENCE-BASED MEDICINE

LEADERSHIP COMMITMENTS TO IMPROVE VALUE IN HEALTH CARE
Finding Common Ground

Workshop Summary

LeighAnne Olsen, W. Alexander Goolsby, and J. Michael McGinnis

Roundtable on Evidence-Based Medicine

INSTITUTE OF MEDICINE
OF THE NATIONAL ACADEMIES

THE NATIONAL ACADEMIES PRESS
Washington, D.C.
www.nap.edu

THE NATIONAL ACADEMIES PRESS   500 Fifth Street, N.W.   Washington, DC 20001

NOTICE: The project that is the subject of this report was approved by the Governing Board of the National Research Council, whose members are drawn from the councils of the National Academy of Sciences, the National Academy of Engineering, and the Institute of Medicine.

This project was supported by the Agency for Healthcare Research and Quality, America's Health Insurance Plans, AstraZeneca, Blue Shield of California Foundation, Burroughs Wellcome Fund, California Health Care Foundation, Centers for Medicare and Medicaid Services, Charina Endowment Fund, Food and Drug Administration, Johnson & Johnson, sanofi-aventis, Stryker, and U.S. Department of Veterans Affairs. Any opinions, findings, conclusions, or recommendations expressed in this publication are those of the author(s) and do not necessarily reflect the view of the organizations or agencies that provided support for this project.

International Standard Book Number-13: 978-0-309-11053-2
International Standard Book Number-10: 0-309-11053-X

Additional copies of this report are available from the National Academies Press, 500 Fifth Street, N.W., Lockbox 285, Washington, DC 20055; (800) 624-6242 or (202) 334-3313 (in the Washington metropolitan area); Internet, http://www.nap.edu.

For more information about the Institute of Medicine, visit the IOM home page at: www.iom.edu.

The serpent has been a symbol of long life, healing, and knowledge among almost all cultures and religions since the beginning of recorded history. The serpent adopted as a logotype by the Institute of Medicine is a relief carving from ancient Greece, now held by the Staatliche Museen in Berlin.

Suggested citation: IOM (Institute of Medicine). 2009. *Leadership Commitments to Improve Value in Health Care: Finding Common Ground: Workshop Summary.* Washington, DC: The National Academies Press.

"Knowing is not enough; we must apply.
Willing is not enough; we must do."

—Goethe

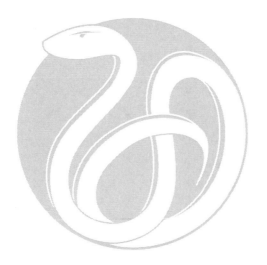

INSTITUTE OF MEDICINE
OF THE NATIONAL ACADEMIES

Advising the Nation. Improving Health.

THE NATIONAL ACADEMIES
Advisers to the Nation on Science, Engineering, and Medicine

The **National Academy of Sciences** is a private, nonprofit, self-perpetuating society of distinguished scholars engaged in scientific and engineering research, dedicated to the furtherance of science and technology and to their use for the general welfare. Upon the authority of the charter granted to it by the Congress in 1863, the Academy has a mandate that requires it to advise the federal government on scientific and technical matters. Dr. Ralph J. Cicerone is president of the National Academy of Sciences.

The **National Academy of Engineering** was established in 1964, under the charter of the National Academy of Sciences, as a parallel organization of outstanding engineers. It is autonomous in its administration and in the selection of its members, sharing with the National Academy of Sciences the responsibility for advising the federal government. The National Academy of Engineering also sponsors engineering programs aimed at meeting national needs, encourages education and research, and recognizes the superior achievements of engineers. Dr. Charles M. Vest is president of the National Academy of Engineering.

The **Institute of Medicine** was established in 1970 by the National Academy of Sciences to secure the services of eminent members of appropriate professions in the examination of policy matters pertaining to the health of the public. The Institute acts under the responsibility given to the National Academy of Sciences by its congressional charter to be an adviser to the federal government and, upon its own initiative, to identify issues of medical care, research, and education. Dr. Harvey V. Fineberg is president of the Institute of Medicine.

The **National Research Council** was organized by the National Academy of Sciences in 1916 to associate the broad community of science and technology with the Academy's purposes of furthering knowledge and advising the federal government. Functioning in accordance with general policies determined by the Academy, the Council has become the principal operating agency of both the National Academy of Sciences and the National Academy of Engineering in providing services to the government, the public, and the scientific and engineering communities. The Council is administered jointly by both Academies and the Institute of Medicine. Dr. Ralph J. Cicerone and Dr. Charles M. Vest are chair and vice chair, respectively, of the National Research Council.

www.national-academies.org

ROUNDTABLE ON EVIDENCE-BASED MEDICINE[1]

Denis A. Cortese (*Chair*), President and Chief Executive Officer, Mayo Clinic

Bruce G. Bodaken, Chairman, President, and Chief Executive Officer, Blue Shield of California

Adam Bosworth, Founder, President and Chief Executive Officer, Keas, Inc.

David R. Brennan, Chief Executive Officer, AstraZeneca PLC

Carolyn M. Clancy, Director, Agency for Healthcare Research and Quality

Michael J. Critelli, Former Executive Chairman, Pitney Bowes, Inc.

Helen Darling, President, National Business Group on Health

James A. Guest, President, Consumers Union

George C. Halvorson, Chairman and Chief Executive Officer, Kaiser Permanente

Carmen Hooker Odom, President, Milbank Memorial Fund

Michael M. E. Johns, Chancellor, Emory University

Cato T. Laurencin, Vice President for Health Affairs, Dean of the School of Medicine, University of Connecticut

Stephen P. MacMillan, President and Chief Executive Officer, Stryker

Mark B. McClellan, Director, Engelberg Center for Healthcare Reform, Brookings Institution

Elizabeth G. Nabel, Director, National Heart, Lung, and Blood Institute

Mary D. Naylor, Professor and Director of Center for Transitions in Health, University of Pennsylvania

Peter Neupert, Corporate Vice President, Health Solutions Group, Microsoft Corporation

Nancy H. Nielsen, President-Elect, American Medical Association

Jonathan B. Perlin, Chief Medical Officer and President, Clinical Services, HCA, Inc.

Richard Platt, Professor and Chair, Harvard Medical School and Harvard Pilgrim Health Care

John C. Rother, Group Executive Officer, AARP

Tim Rothwell, Chairman, Sanofi-Aventis U.S.

John W. Rowe, Professor, Mailman School of Public Health, Columbia University

Donald M. Steinwachs, Professor, Bloomberg School of Public Health, Johns Hopkins University

Andrew L. Stern, President, Service Employees International Union

---

[1]IOM forums and roundtables do not issue, review, or approve individual documents. The responsibility for the published workshop summary rests with the workshop rapporteur and the institution.

v

I. **Steven Udvarhelyi,** Senior Vice President and Chief Medical Officer, Independence Blue Cross

Frances M. Visco, President, National Breast Cancer Coalition

William C. Weldon, Chairman and Chief Executive Officer, Johnson & Johnson

Janet Woodcock, Deputy Commissioner and Chief Medical Officer, Food and Drug Administration

Acting Administrator (ex officio), Centers for Medicare and Medicaid Services

Undersecretary for Health (ex officio), U.S. Department of Veterans Affairs

Roundtable Staff

Katharine Bothner, Senior Program Assistant (through July 2008)
Andrea Cohen, Financial Associate (through December 2008)
Patrick Burke, Financial Associate
W. Alexander Goolsby, Program Officer (through August 2008)
Kiran Gupta, Research Assistant
J. Michael McGinnis, Senior Scholar and Executive Director
LeighAnne Olsen, Program Officer
Daniel O'Neill, Research Associate (through January 2009)
Stephen Pelletier, Consultant
Ruth Strommen, Intern
Pierre Yong, Program Officer
Catherine Zweig, Senior Program Assistant

Reviewers

This report has been reviewed in draft form by individuals chosen for their diverse perspectives and technical expertise, in accordance with procedures approved by the National Research Council's Report Review Committee. The purpose of this independent review is to provide candid and critical comments that will assist the institution in making its published report as sound as possible and to ensure that the report meets institutional standards for objectivity, evidence, and responsiveness to the study charge. The review comments and draft manuscript remain confidential to protect the integrity of the deliberative process. We wish to thank the following individuals for their review of this report:

Patricia Flatley Brennan, University of Wisconsin-Madison School of Nursing
Lynda Bryant-Comstock, GlaxoSmithKline
Julianne Howell, Centers for Medicare and Medicaid Services
Diana B. Petitti, University of Southern California School of Medicine

Although the reviewers listed above have provided many constructive comments and suggestions, they were not asked to endorse the final draft of the report before its release. The review of this report was overseen by **Nancy S. Sung,** Burroughs Wellcome Fund. Appointed by the National Research Council and the Institute of Medicine, she was responsible for making certain that an independent examination of this report was carried out in accordance with institutional procedures and that all review comments were carefully considered. Responsibility for the final content of this report rests entirely with the editors and the institution.

Institute of Medicine
Roundtable on Evidence-Based Medicine
Charter and Vision Statement

The Institute of Medicine's Roundtable on Evidence-Based Medicine has been convened to help transform the way evidence on clinical effectiveness is generated and used to improve health and health care. Participants have set a goal that, by the year 2020, 90 percent of clinical decisions will be supported by accurate, timely, and up-to-date clinical information, and will reflect the best available evidence. Roundtable members will work with their colleagues to identify the issues not being adequately addressed, the nature of the barriers and possible solutions, and the priorities for action, and will marshal the resources of the sectors represented on the Roundtable to work for sustained public–private cooperation for change.

* *

The Institute of Medicine's Roundtable on Evidence-Based Medicine has been convened to help transform the way evidence on clinical effectiveness is generated and used to improve health and health care. We seek the development of a *learning healthcare system* that is designed to generate and apply the best evidence for the collaborative healthcare choices of each patient and provider; to drive the process of discovery as a natural outgrowth of patient care; and to ensure innovation, quality, safety, and value in health care.

Vision: Our vision is for a healthcare system that draws on the best evidence to provide the care most appropriate to each patient, emphasizes prevention and health promotion, delivers the most value, adds to learning throughout the delivery of care, and leads to improvements in the nation's health.

Goal: By the year 2020, 90 percent of clinical decisions will be supported by accurate, timely, and up-to-date clinical information, and will reflect the best available evidence. We feel that this presents a tangible focus for progress toward our vision, that Americans ought to expect at least this level of performance, that it should be feasible with existing resources and emerging tools, and that measures can be developed to track and stimulate progress.

Context: As unprecedented developments in the diagnosis, treatment, and long-term management of disease bring Americans closer than ever to the promise of personalized health care, we are faced with similarly unprecedented challenges to identify and deliver the care most appropriate for individual needs and conditions. Care that is important is often not delivered. Care that is delivered is often not important. In part, this is due to our failure to apply the evidence we have about the medical care that is most effective—a failure related to shortfalls in provider knowledge and accountability, inadequate care coordination and support, lack of insurance, poorly aligned payment incentives, and misplaced patient expectations. Increasingly, it is also a result of our limited capacity for timely generation of evidence on the relative effectiveness, efficiency, and safety of available and emerging interventions. Improving the value of the return on our healthcare investment is a vital imperative that will require much greater capacity to evaluate high-priority clinical interventions, stronger links between clinical research and practice, and reorientation of the incentives to apply new insights. We must quicken our efforts to position evidence development and application as natural outgrowths of clinical care—to foster health care that learns.

Approach: The IOM Roundtable on Evidence-Based Medicine serves as a forum to facilitate the collaborative assessment and action around issues central to achieving the vision and goal stated. The challenges are myriad and include issues that must be addressed to improve evidence development, evidence application, and the capacity to advance progress on both dimensions. To address these challenges, as leaders in their fields, Roundtable members will work with their colleagues to identify the issues not being adequately addressed, the nature of the barriers and possible solutions, and the priorities for action, and will marshal the resources of the sectors represented on the Roundtable to work for sustained public–private cooperation for change.

Activities include collaborative exploration of new and expedited approaches to assessing the effectiveness of diagnostic and treatment interventions, better use of the patient care experience to generate evidence on effectiveness, identification of assessment priorities, and communication strategies to enhance provider and patient understanding and support for interventions proven to work best and deliver value in health care.

Core concepts and principles: For the purpose of the Roundtable activities, we define evidence-based medicine broadly to mean that, *to the greatest extent possible, the decisions that shape the health and health care of Americans—by patients, providers, payers, and policy makers alike—will be grounded on a reliable evidence base, will account appropriately for individual variation in patient needs, and will support the generation of new insights on clinical effectiveness.* Evidence is generally considered to be information from clinical experience that has met some established test of validity, and the appropriate standard is determined according to the requirements of the intervention and clinical circumstance. Processes that involve the development and use of evidence should be accessible and transparent to all stakeholders.

A common commitment to certain principles and priorities guides the activities of the Roundtable and its members, including the commitment to the right health care for each person; putting the best evidence into practice; establishing the effectiveness, efficiency, and safety of medical care delivered; building constant measurement into our healthcare investments; the establishment of healthcare data as a public good; shared responsibility distributed equitably across stakeholders, both public and private; collaborative stakeholder involvement in priority setting; transparency in the execution of activities and reporting of results; and subjugation of individual political or stakeholder perspectives in favor of the common good.

Foreword

In its role as adviser to the nation to improve health, the Institute of Medicine (IOM) endeavors to bring individuals with the best scientific expertise together for discussion and deliberation on issues of national importance. Driving change often requires that scientific consensus be linked with leadership and a shared commitment to action. This spirit is embodied in the work of the IOM's Roundtable on Evidence-Based Medicine. Convened in 2006, the Roundtable comprises senior private- and public-sector leaders representing the key stakeholders shaping health care for Americans. It provides a neutral venue for discussion and collaborative action to transform how evidence is generated and applied to improve the nation's health. Together, Roundtable members have outlined their vision for a learning healthcare system, as expressed in their charter statement, and a goal by which to mark progress—that by 2020, 90 percent of clinical decisions will be supported by accurate, timely, and up-to-date clinical information and will reflect the best available evidence. Through a series of workshops and publications, the Roundtable works to explore the issues and barriers and to identify the key opportunities for collaborative work toward the development of a learning healthcare system.

This publication represents the third in the Learning Healthcare System series and is the result of work by each sector represented on the Roundtable—patients, healthcare professionals, healthcare delivery organizations, healthcare product developers, clinical investigators-evaluators, regulators, insurers, employers-employees, and information technology—to identify the key opportunities for individual and collaborative work to foster progress toward the Roundtable's goal. The results of the work of the

Roundtable members were presented at a 2-day workshop entitled, Leadership Commitments to Improve Value in Health Care: Finding Common Ground. The sector statements and subsequent workshop discussion are summarized in this volume.

Embedded in these pages are insights gleaned from across the spectrum of healthcare stakeholders. Although each sector brought a unique set of challenges, skills, and expertise to its work, many common concerns, issues, and opportunities emerged, including the pressing needs to build more trust and transparency into the system, to identify national priorities and build the necessary capacity, to foster a shared commitment to evidence-driven care, and to build learning into the culture of health care by accelerating advances in medical informatics and engaging the frontline providers in change. Among the opportunities identified, the most essential was that these activities be taken up as a shared endeavor. No one sector, acting alone, can bring about the scope and scale of transformative change necessary to develop a system that can consistently and efficiently deliver the safe, effective, and quality care of value that should be our nation's standard. Stakeholder leadership from the Roundtable and beyond will be vital to success.

I would like to offer my personal thanks to Roundtable members for the leadership that they bring to these important issues, to the Roundtable staff for their skill and dedication in coordinating and facilitating the activities, and importantly, to the sponsors who make this work possible: the Agency for Healthcare Research and Quality, America's Health Insurance Plans, AstraZeneca, Blue Shield of California Foundation, Burroughs Wellcome Fund, California Health Care Foundation, Centers for Medicare and Medicaid Services, Charina Endowment Fund, Food and Drug Administration, Johnson & Johnson, sanofi-aventis, Stryker, and U.S. Department of Veterans Affairs.

Harvey V. Fineberg, M.D., Ph.D.
President, Institute of Medicine

Preface

The essence of this publication, *Leadership Commitments to Improve Value in Health Care: Finding Common Ground*, reflects the motivations and driving forces behind the Roundtable on Evidence-Based Medicine. That is, that no one sector can effect the transformation needed in health care and that collaborative work and action are vital to developing the learning healthcare system that provides care of the best possible value to all of our citizens. By value, we mean the full value equation—the best outcomes, safety, and service for the best price. The Institute of Medicine (IOM) Roundtable is made up of stakeholders with often different perspectives and incentives, but we are all stakeholders committed to obtaining better results and better value from the health care that we deliver and we receive. Outlined in this volume are exciting and important opportunities to collectively move toward our vision and goal.

This publication represents just one component of the Roundtable's work to help transform how evidence is both generated and used to improve health and health care. Our charter statement articulates a collective vision for a healthcare system that "draws upon the best evidence to provide the care most appropriate to each patient, emphasizes prevention and health promotion, delivers the most value, adds to learning throughout the delivery of care, and leads to improvements in the nation's health." Our goal is that by 2020, 90 percent of clinical decisions will be supported by accurate, timely, and up-to-date clinical information and will reflect the best available evidence. Although it is ambitious, this goal presents a tangible focus for progress and should be achievable given our nation's substantial investment in health care.

The guiding framework for the Roundtable's work is its focus on fostering the development of a learning healthcare system. Because our current system is so fragmented, achieving this aim will require the extraordinary creativity and energy discussed at the workshop and in this publication. Our initial workshop and resulting publication, *The Learning Healthcare System*, characterized the system that we seek, one that is designed to generate the best evidence and to apply that evidence to the healthcare choices that each patient and provider make in collaboration; to drive the process of discovery as a natural outgrowth of patient care; and to ensure innovation, quality, safety, and value in health care. The key characteristics of a learning healthcare system include adaptation to the pace of change; strong systemwide synergy and synchrony; a culture of shared responsibility; a practical clinical research paradigm in play; evidence standards that are consistent and tailored; clinical decision support systems that are fully applied; universal electronic health records; the establishment of clinical data as a public good; databases that are linked, mined in real time, and used; incentives that are aligned for practice-based evidence; patients who are engaged as evidence proponents; and a trusted scientific broker of needed guidance.

The Learning Healthcare System workshop series is designed to explore in greater detail these component issues. None is more important in this respect than the mutual commitment of the stakeholders discussed here. To identify the greatest opportunities and to begin the process of inter-sectoral collaboration, on July 24-25, 2007, the Roundtable convened a 2-day workshop titled Leadership Commitments to Improve Value in Health Care: Finding Common Ground. The third in the Learning Healthcare System series, this workshop convened representatives from a variety of sectors—patients, healthcare professionals, healthcare delivery organizations, healthcare product developers, clinical investigators-evaluators, regulators, insurers, employers-employees, and information technology professionals—to discuss the ways that each sector, individually and collaboratively, can contribute to the transformative change necessary to achieve the Roundtable's goal.

Workshop presentations resulted from several months of work by Roundtable members to develop, in cooperation with other participants recruited from their respective arenas, statements that laid out the issues and opportunities from the perspectives of each of the sectors. These statements detailed the important characteristics and activities of each sector with respect to evidence development and application and advanced some key opportunities and specific initiatives for individual and cross-sectoral work to bring about transformative change. These statements were presented over the course of the 2-day workshop and set the stage for rich discussion and debate. This publication includes the sectoral statements, a summary of the workshop proceedings, and identification of the common themes.

Among the participants, several important foundation stones were considered vital to progress. Common ground could be forged by building trust between the many stakeholders and fostering a shared commitment to evidence-driven care. Also needed are efforts to consistently build learning into the culture of health care and the establishment of a common focal point or trusted source to coordinate the development and dissemination of evidence. The greatest transformational opportunities identified include the clarification of core concepts, beginning with a sharper focus on the value proposition and the establishment of transparent principles and processes for evidence interpretation and use; identifying a set of national priorities around unused evidence and unavailable evidence and strengthening the national capacity for evidence development and guidance; reorienting the healthcare system to produce the evidence for today's decisions, with tomorrow in view; encouraging rapid progress in medical informatics; and engaging healthcare providers in establishing interdisciplinary evidence-driven team care as standard care. Above all, stakeholder leadership will be essential to encourage and promote the needed change.

We would like to acknowledge the many individuals and organizations that donated their valuable time to the development of this workshop summary. In particular, we acknowledge the contributors to this volume for their presence at the workshop and their efforts to further develop their presentations into the chapters contained within this summary. We would also like to acknowledge those who provided counsel during the planning stages of this workshop, including Patrick Anderson (Stryker), Helen Darling (National Business Group on Health), Michael Johns (Emory University), and Carmen Hooker Odom (Milbank Memorial Fund).[1] A number of IOM staff were instrumental in the preparation and conduct of the 2-day workshop in July 2007, including Rachel Passman, Kristina Shulkin, and Jamie Skipper. Roundtable staff, including Katharine Bothner, Alex Goolsby, LeighAnne Olsen, and Daniel O'Neill, helped to translate the workshop proceedings and discussion into this workshop summary. Stephen Pelletier also contributed substantially to publication development. We would also like to thank Michele de la Menardiere, Bronwyn Schrecker, Vilija Teel, and Jackie Turner for helping to coordinate the various aspects of review, production, and publication.

As illustrated in this publication, a shared commitment to evidence-driven care offers a means to define common goals, set priorities, and

---

[1]IOM planning committees are solely responsible for organizing the workshop, identifying topics, and choosing speakers. The responsibility for the published workshop summary rests with the workshop rapporteur and the institution.

identify practical ways to initiate action. However, collaboration is more than just a tool. Given the transformative change needed in health care, it is an imperative. The Roundtable looks forward to expanding the sphere of sector involvement, collaboration, and action in the field to build upon the substantial opportunities identified in this publication.

Denis A. Cortese, M.D.
Chair, Roundtable on Evidence-Based Medicine

J. Michael McGinnis, M.D., M.P.P.
Executive Director, Roundtable on Evidence-Based Medicine

Contents

APPENDIXES

Summary

This volume reports on discussions among multiple stakeholders about ways they might help transform health care in the United States. The U.S. healthcare system consists of a complex network of decentralized and loosely associated organizations, services, relationships, and participants. Each of the healthcare system's component sectors—patients, healthcare professionals, healthcare delivery organizations, healthcare product developers, clinical investigators and evaluators, regulators, insurers, employers and employees, and individuals involved in information technology—conducts activities that support a common goal: to improve patient health and well-being. Implicit in this goal is the commitment of each stakeholder group to contribute to the evidence base for health care, that is, to assist with the development and application of information about the efficacy, safety, effectiveness, value, and appropriateness of the health care delivered.

Because the nation falls far short of the possible in this respect, the Institute of Medicine (IOM) Roundtable on Evidence-Based Medicine was established in 2006 as a unique and neutral venue where the key stakeholders could work cooperatively to help transform the way in which evidence on clinical effectiveness is generated and used to improve health and health care and to drive improvements in the effectiveness and efficiency of medical care in the United States (Fisher, 2005; IOM, 2007; McGlynn et al., 2003; Wennberg et al., 2002).

The planning committee's role was limited to planning the workshop, and the workshop summary has been prepared by the workshop rapporteur and Roundtable staff as a factual summary of workshop discussions

Central to the Roundtable's work are the notions that, collectively, the healthcare sectors possess the knowledge, expertise, and leadership necessary to transform the healthcare system and that what is most acutely needed is a shared commitment to improving the development and use of information about the efficacy, safety, effectiveness, value, and appropriateness of the health care delivered. Roundtable members have developed a vision for a learning healthcare system needed to achieve their goal: by the year 2020, 90 percent of clinical decisions will be supported by accurate, timely, and up-to-date clinical information and will reflect the best available evidence.

Fostering the collaborative work necessary to achieve this goal is the aim of the IOM Roundtable's sectoral strategies process, which took place through the activities of nine sector-specific groups over several months in 2007 and culminated on July 23 and 24, 2007, in the third workshop in the Learning Healthcare System series, titled Leadership Commitments to Improve Value in Health Care: Finding Common Ground. The ideas presented and discussed at the workshop are summarized here. The three goals of the workshop were (1) to consider stakeholder capacity for stronger progress toward a learning healthcare system; (2) to explore transformational opportunities; and (3) to identify possibilities for collective initiatives that might be considered by Roundtable sectors.

In the months before the workshop, Roundtable members were asked to reach out to colleagues in their sectors to describe perspectives on the key challenges and opportunities for healthcare improvement, as well as how each sector might contribute to advancing progress toward the Roundtable's goal. Background papers summarizing these discussions were prepared and presented at the July workshop to provide context for cross-sector discussions. The elements of this process are presented in Appendix A and summarized as follows

- January: the initial formation of nine Roundtable sectoral discussion groups
- February and March: reaching out to other sectoral participants in preparing background material
- April: completion and circulation of strategy background paper to sector participants
- May: circulation of sector review draft to Roundtable members in each sector group
- June: consolidation of draft sectoral strategy background papers and dissemination to all Roundtable members
- July: presentation of authored background papers for public discussion at an IOM workshop on sectoral strategies

The workshop presentations of these sector-oriented perspectives were designed by presenters to highlight their views of the key advances, transformational opportunities, and cross-sector collaborations needed to achieve the stated goal.

The nine sectoral discussion groups were not Academy-appointed committees, and there was no attempt to ensure group consensus. The background papers reflect the views of the individuals who participated in the discussions prior to and during the workshop, as interpreted by the group coordinators and staff.

The purpose of this summary is to present lessons from experience; outline the range of key issues, stakeholder concerns, barriers, and challenges; and offer some potential responses as described by workshop participants. This chapter briefly summarizes workshop presentations, discussions, and relevant background materials and their relation to the workshop goals and to the overall Learning Healthcare System series of meetings. It has been prepared in consultation with the authors of sectoral background papers and reviewed independently by a committee appointed by the National Research Council to ensure that it is accurate and faithful to the meeting's purpose and content. It does not, however, represent an Academy consensus document, nor does it contain recommendations. Later chapters describe the presentations in more depth.

The greater part of workshop discussions focused on finding areas of common ground in which participants might join together on activities most important to the improvements necessary to fulfill the Roundtable's goal. Part One of this publication, Finding Value in Common Ground, presents a synthesis of the workshop discussions in the context of the Roundtable's focus and the workshop goals: the perspective guiding the sectoral strategies process (Chapter 1), important conceptual foundation stones needed for progress (Chapter 2), transformational opportunities recognized by participants as priority areas for focus and immediate work (Chapter 3), and areas for enhanced cross-sector collaboration (Chapter 4).

Drafts of the authored background papers were revised to incorporate the workshop discussions, and final versions are included in their entirety in Part Two of this publication, Leadership Commitments to Improve Health Care (Chapters 5 to 13). Appendix B provides the workshop agenda, Appendix C presents biographical sketches of the speakers, and Appendix D lists the workshop participants.

COMMON CONCERNS AND THEMES

The spirit of the workshop discussion was one of open exchange, and over the course of the 2-day meeting, participants underscored many pressing concerns common to all sectors, the following in particular:

- *Rising costs and limited resources.* Whether they are borne by those receiving or providing care or accrued during research on or the development of treatments and therapies, participants cited costs as limiting factors for access to and innovation in health care.
- *System inefficiencies.* The quality of health care in the United States is uneven and delivered by a system characterized by inefficiency and waste. The existing evidence is poorly applied, and the delivery of care for similar conditions varies widely throughout the country. Standards for care, healthcare system components, and even research are often inconsistent.
- *Increasing complexity.* Whether it is because of the increased importance of genetic variation, the rapidly evolving landscape of medical technologies, or the growing prevalence of chronic disease, medicine is becoming increasingly complex.
- *Expanding evidence gap.* Across the practice of health care, information is lacking for many key personal health or policy decisions. The "inference gap" between the evidence available and that needed to treat real-world populations will only widen as new interventions are introduced into the marketplace and health care moves further in the direction of personalized treatments.
- *Limited system capacity and flexibility.* The number of questions that need to be addressed to ensure appropriate care continues to expand exponentially, rendering impractical the current approach to the development of evidence. Although randomized controlled trials are important in certain circumstances, they cannot provide all the information necessary. The availability of technologies lags the demand. Whether through habit or other circumstances, evidence is neither getting translated to the extent that it needs to be nor distributed as widely as it should be.
- *Entrenched cultures.* Health care has various customs and practices often not conducive to reform. Caregiving and caregivers are often "siloed," with inadequate communications among the various functional areas of the healthcare system. Information is not shared as widely as it should be within specific healthcare systems, let alone between systems, contributing to inefficiency and distrust in the system. In general, providers, patients, and other sectors do not yet believe that the development of evidence is an activity relevant to their experience in the routine delivery of care.

Several general themes were recurrent over the course of the meeting as issues important across stakeholder categories (Box S-1).

BOX S-1
Common General Themes

- Build trust and collaboration
- Foster agreement on "value" in health care
- Improve public understanding of evidence
- Characterize the impact of shortfalls in the evidence
- Identify the priorities for evidence development
- Improve the level, quality, and efficiency of the research
- Clarify and promote transparency
- Establish principles for the interpretation and use of evidence
- Improve engagement in the full life cycle of interventions
- Focus on frontline providers
- Foster a trusted intermediary for evidence
- Build the capacity to meet the demand
- Create incentives for change
- Accelerate advances in health information technology

- *Build trust and collaboration.* How can the distrust that has emerged in health care—for example, distrust between and among patients and providers, providers and insurers, insurers and manufacturers, and manufacturers and regulators—be reduced? Health care depends for its effectiveness on the close cooperation of all parties involved. Building trust and facilitating transformative change will require broader-based collaboration and cooperative stakeholder engagement.
- *Foster agreement on "value" in health care.* What constitutes value in health care: reduced death or disease, better function, less pain, a better sense of well-being, fewer hospital days, or lower costs? Although all participants agreed on the centrality and importance of the value achieved from health care, different groups think of value in different ways. A multistakeholder effort might drive clarity and consensus on the principles and elements of value common to all stakeholders.
- *Improve public understanding of evidence.* What can be done to improve public understanding, acceptance, and demand for evidence-based care? Too often, people perceive that certain common terms such as "evidence based," "research," "medical necessity," and "risk" suggest a restrictive or experimental element to their care. It will take a systematic and coordinated communi-

cation strategy to better convey the central concepts that medical evidence is dynamic, that evidence-based medicine is the provision of care that the evidence suggests is best for any given patient at any given time, and that health care is a joint patient-provider endeavor.

- *Characterize the impact of shortfalls in the evidence.* What might be the tangible impact of broad improvements in the availability and application of appropriate evidence for healthcare decisions on patients, on providers, and on society? Documenting the consequences of provision of care on the basis of too little evidence or the potential benefits of providing care on the basis of the right evidence is a prerequisite to obtaining an improved understanding of and demand for evidence-based care and stakeholder activation.

- *Identify the priorities for evidence development.* Which medical care dilemmas represent the most challenging and pressing needs for better comparative information and guidance on choices among the available and the emerging diagnostic and treatment options? The first step toward a systematic and coordinated effort to conduct the most important assessments is identification of priorities as a sort of consensus national problem list and research agenda for the most pressing issues for medical care decisions.

- *Improve the level, quality, and efficiency of research.* How can the healthcare system take better advantage of emerging clinical record resources to gain insights into the evidence? Policies that facilitate the ability to use clinical data to monitor the effectiveness of interventions are needed. Novel approaches to the conduct of clinical trials are also needed. A more structured lexicon for "best practices" in undertaking observational studies may be necessary.

- *Clarify and promote transparency.* What principles define openness in health care, clinical research, the interpretation of evidence, coverage decisions, regulatory policy, marketing practices, oversight, and the governance of use of clinical data? Consensus is needed to establish common principles of transparency and standards for how they should be applied in each sector. One starting point might be with principles for evidence interpretation.

- *Establish principles for the interpretation and use of evidence.* What guiding principles related to application of the available evidence might be used to help decision makers determine when they should apply a proposed diagnostic or treatment intervention? Decisions about market approval, insurance coverage, provider use, and patient acceptance are all informed by some interpretation of the evidence. Clarity of the guiding principles is important.

- *Improve engagement in the full life cycle of interventions.* How should assessments and decisions on proposed healthcare services be tailored to ensure that each stage of the development and application process for a given intervention builds efficiently to the next? Many factors are at play for each intervention—for example, similarity to previously tested interventions, the safety and effectiveness of an intervention for some populations but not others, the availability of biomarkers predictive of efficacy, and costs that vary by scale and stage of application or by the need for later services. Facilitating innovation, access, and effective information gathering while emphasizing patient safety, appropriate application, improved outcomes, and efficiency will require a set of life cycle-oriented decision-making rules that are more carefully considered than they are at present.

- *Focus on frontline providers.* What key levers might help ensure that both primary care and specialty providers are taking full and appropriate advantage of the best available evidence in the care they provide? Accelerating the translation of clinical research into practice involves addressing matters of professional education, credentialing, licensure, practice support, economic incentives, patient acceptance, and the culture of care. It will require the central and coordinated involvement of the organizations that represent those providers.

- *Foster a trusted intermediary for evidence.* How can patients, providers, healthcare organizations, employers, insurers, and others know when they have the best evidence on which to base the healthcare decisions they make? In this information age, health-related information is presented constantly through news reports, marketing, professional organizations, journals, and the Internet; but it is often confusing and even contradictory. A trusted information source—one that is independent but that engages all stakeholders—is needed to identify gaps; set priorities; establish standards; and guide the development, interpretation, and dissemination of evidence on clinical effectiveness.

- *Build the capacity to meet the demand.* What mechanism is necessary to close the current and emerging gaps in evidence on the relative effectiveness of various interventions, to ensure the quality and integrity of the studies used to establish the evidence, and to provide a sustained capacity to meet the need? Currently, the combined resources of the various public and private organizations involved in studying comparative clinical effectiveness meet but a small and scattered fraction of the demand. The centrality of this problem to the quality and efficiency—the viability, according to some—of the nation's healthcare system may require the creation of a new independent entity devoted to the work.

- *Create incentives for change.* What practice-based economic and policy incentives might help enhance the next generation of new evidence and transform the ability and commitment of providers to use the best available evidence and more fully engage patients in the clinical decision-making process? Approaches include the alignment of purchasing incentives when value is determined; use of the reimbursement power of insurers and other financial incentives to generate new insights from medical care (e.g., coverage with evidence development); and the linkage of purchaser and payer decisions to performance incentives for best practices, outcomes, and the better secondary use of routinely collected data.

- *Accelerate advances in health information technology.* What can stakeholders do to accelerate the nation's progress toward the goal of the universal application of interoperable—or functionally accessible—personal and organizational electronic health records, as well as toward the goal of providing real-time electronic access to the best information available? Health information technology can facilitate the development of learning networks and accelerate the generation of evidence, enable data aggregation and utilization, deliver evidence to the point of care, and expand research capacities. Coordinated stakeholder action—and financial incentives—should be able to speed the progress necessary on both the basic interoperability issues (e.g., standards and vocabulary) and, possibly, the development of more radical data search innovations.

Several opportunities for collaborative activities by Roundtable members and participating sectors were identified by participants in the discussions:

- *Development of a priority assessment inventory.* Termed a "national problem list" by meeting participants, this is a multisector collaborative effort to develop criteria and a list of the diagnostic and treatment interventions that might be viewed as particularly important for the development of comparative effectiveness studies. The list will serve as a means of illustrating and prompting discussion on the key evidence gaps and on the design, support, and execution of the studies needed.

- *Pursue agreement on the value proposition.* Identify key concepts and elements to be considered in assessing and characterizing value from health care, setting the stage for discussions on approaches to assessing those elements and applying to add perspective and inform decision making. An IOM workshop, *Value in Healthcare:*

Accounting for Cost, Quality, Safety, Outcomes, and Innovation, was convened in November 2008, with publication of the workshop summary expected in 2009.

- *Identify common principles for evidence interpretation and use.* Identify the core principles underpinning activities in interpretation and use of evidence, as background for discussion of the implications and of the ways the principles might be applied in the development of a framework adaptive to different circumstances related either to the evidence base or the condition of interest.

- *Foster cooperative data sharing.* Several issues are important in this regard: platform compatibilities, standards, economic incentives and disincentives, the regulatory and privacy environment. Health Insurance Portability and Accountability Act issues are being addressed by an IOM Committee expected to issue its report and recommendations in 2009, including those related to the use of clinical data for knowledge development. The Roundtable's February 2008 meeting, *Clinical Data as the Basic Staple of Healthcare Learning: Creating and Protecting a Public Good,* addressed a number of the other issues related to sound data stewardship. And collaborative work has been sponsored by the Roundtable on mining electronic health records for postmarket surveillance and clinical safety and effectiveness insights.

- *Pursue a public communication initiative on evidence-based medicine.* Use the Roundtable membership's collective communication expertise to explore improving terminology and advancing public awareness on the nature and importance of evidence in medical care, the key needs, and the centrality of patient and provider communication around the state of the evolving evidence for individual treatment choices. The Roundtable's Evidence Communication Collaborative has a working group actively working on a communication initiative proposal.

- *Support progress on a trusted intermediary for evidence promotion.* The Roundtable's Sustainable Capacity working group oversaw the development of a comprehensive Issue Brief, framing the issues and options under discussion related to enhancement of the national capacity to develop, evaluate, organize, validate, and disseminate information on the comparative effectiveness of health interventions. Technical assistance and related information is provided on an ongoing basis to the various policy discussions of the issue.

- *Identify the potential from best practices in the use of evidence.* It is important to assess and underscore the best practices in evidence development and application, including consideration of ongoing methods of identifying and disseminating those best practices. A working group is underway to characterize the potential returns from implementing certain established best practices.

- *Enlist front-line healthcare providers more effectively.* Charge the sectoral working group on providers with proposing approaches to convening a coalition of provider groups, perhaps under Roundtable auspices, to consider sustained, coordinated work on health professions education, testing, credentialing, and practice setting tools and structure to improve focus, accessibility, use, and generation by providers of the best evidence. A Roundtable collaborative of providers is being formed to engage this issue.

PART ONE: FINDING VALUE IN COMMON GROUND

The Learning Healthcare System series of workshops sponsored by the IOM Roundtable on Evidence-Based Medicine is designed to both identify and discuss the most important advances needed to transform health care, with sector leadership and collaboration in this work. This workshop was aimed at considering how various sectors could make a difference. The sectoral strategies perspective development process engaged participants in the development of authored background papers to be presented during the workshop, as a first step toward the national conversation needed on how to facilitate a better alignment and better collaboration among the various sectors of the healthcare system. Part One provides a synthesis of the workshop discussion among participants from different sectors. The material presents the individual views of the participants of the workshop and does not represent the consensus of the discussion groups, the workshop participants, the Roundtable, or the IOM.

Guiding Perspective: The Learning Healthcare System

The Roundtable's goal for 2020 specifies what ought to be expected from a healthcare system that "draws upon the best evidence to provide care that is the most appropriate for each patient, emphasizes prevention and health promotion, delivers the most value, adds to learning throughout the delivery of care, and leads to improvements in the nation's health." Central to this vision is the development of a healthcare system that learns by generating and applying evidence as a natural component of the process of providing health care (IOM Roundtable on Evidence-Based Medicine, 2006).

The Learning Healthcare System

The guiding perspective for the Roundtable's vision and for the development of background papers from each sector is that of a learning healthcare system. Its key characteristics were discussed at the Roundtable's inaugural workshop and summarized in the annual report of the Roundtable, *Learning Healthcare System Concepts v. 2008* (Institute of Medicine, 2008):

- *Continuous improvement in the value delivered.* A learning healthcare system is one that maintains a constant focus on the health and economic value returned by care delivered and continuously improves in its performance.
- *Learning in health care as a partnership enterprise.* Broad culture change is needed to enable the evolution of the learning environment as a common partnership of patients, providers, and researchers alike.
- *Developing the point of care as the knowledge engine.* Given the rate at which new interventions are developed, along with new insights about individual variation in response to interventions, the point of care must be the central focus for the continuous learning process.
- *Full application of information technology.* The rate of learning—both the application and the development of evidence—will depend on the full and strategic application of information technology, including electronic health records central to long-term change.
- *Database linkage and use.* The emergence of large, electronically based datasets offers important new sources for quality improvement and evidence development. Progress requires fostering interoperable platforms, linking analyses, establishing networks, and developing new approaches for ongoing searching of those databases for patterns and clinical insights.
- *Advancing clinical data as a public utility.* Meeting the potential for using new datasets as central sources of evidence on the effectiveness and efficiency of medical care will require recognition of their qualities as a public good, including assessing issues related to ownership, availability, and use for real-time clinical insights.
- *Building innovative clinical effectiveness research into practice.* Improving the speed and reliability of evidence development requires fostering development of a new clinical research paradigm—one that deploys careful criteria for trial conduct, draws clinical research more closely to the experience of clinical practice, advances new study methodologies adapted to the practice environment, and engages cultural incentives to foster more rapid learning.

- *Patient engagement in the evidence process.* Accelerating the potential for better development and application of evidence requires improved communication between patients and healthcare professionals about the nature of the evidence base and the need for partnership in its development and use.
- *Development of a trusted scientific intermediary.* Greater synchrony, consistency, and coordination in the priority setting, development, interpretation, and application of clinical evidence require a trusted scientific intermediary to broker the perspectives of different parties.
- *Leadership that stems from every quarter.* Strong, visible, and multifaceted leadership from all involved sectors is necessary to marshal the vision, nurture the strategy, and motivate the actions necessary to create the learning healthcare system we need.

Patients, Providers, and Evidence Stewardship

In addition to these background features of the learning healthcare system, perspectives to inform the workshop discussions were provided by presentations on the issues of importance to patients, healthcare providers, and the evidence base for medical decisions. To frame these key perspectives, three authorities were asked to envision what an ideal experience for patients and providers and ideal stewardship of the evidence within a learning healthcare system might look like and, by contrasting the ideal situation in these areas with the current situation, to identify some priority areas for improvement. Margaret C. Kirk, chief executive officer of the Y-ME National Breast Cancer Organization and chairperson-elect of the National Health Council, commented from the patient's perspective. Terry McGeeney, a family physician and chief executive officer of a physician practice redesign initiative, commented from the provider perspective. Sean Tunis, founder and director of the Center for Medical Technology Policy, offered his thoughts on stewardship of the evidence. The full texts of their observations can be found in Chapter 1 of this document. Brief summaries follow here.

Patients   Drawing upon her experience working as a patient advocate, Margaret Kirk advised that because the ideal patient experience varies according to the patient's circumstance, maintaining the perspective of the patient as an individual is particularly important. Balancing the understanding that patients can react differently to treatments with the nation's urgent need to ensure quality care and use healthcare resources wisely will be a key challenge. Evidence-based medicine can be a powerful tool to ensure the best possible medical outcome; help close the quality chasm across geographic regions, treatment settings, and socioeconomic levels; and channel resources to their most effective use. However, to be applied successfully, evidence-based medicine must be structured to reflect the reality that what works for most patients may not be appropriate for others and that many other factors, such as patient life-stage and circumstances, should be considered alongside the evidence in determining any course of treatment. To achieve this vision of patient-centered care, the evidence base must be strengthened considerably; focus on outcomes important to patients, including quality of life; and account for variations among individuals. Better comparative, patient-directed risk-benefit information is needed, and the patient—as well as his or her family—must be considered an active and respected member of the healthcare delivery team from the outset of treatment decisions.

Fundamentally, patients who understand the evidence will make better decisions regarding their health care. However, studies have demonstrated that quality or a lack of adherence to evidence-based guidelines is not the primary concern of patients, emphasizing the importance of better communication with the general public about the importance of evidence to improve their health care, health, and well-being. Patients must also be encouraged to take an active part in healthcare decision making through a process in which both patients and providers engage in a thorough discussion of treatment options and consideration of patient preferences. The development of effective communication techniques and tools will rely on an improved understanding of patient needs and adherence to high standards of clear health communication to avoid patient misunderstanding and mistrust.

Providers   Terry McGeeney offered a perspective garnered from his years in practice as well as from his broader work dedicated to revitalizing family medicine. He began by noting that although all healthcare professionals strive to provide the best care to their patients, many practical realities present barriers to the consistent delivery of efficient, high-quality care. The medical home model was discussed as a possible approach to care that could help providers contend with these types of barriers and deliver care guided by the principles of patient centeredness, orientation toward the whole person, and a continuous relationship between provider and patient. Important supporting elements of the medical home include ensuring patient access both to care and to information, provision of information systems such as electronic health records with point-of-service reminders to support best practices, redesigned offices to increase practice efficiency, increased focus on quality and safety, efficient practice management, point-of-care services, and a team approach to providing care.[1] At the time of the

---

[1]The TransforMED Medical Home Model can be found at http://www.transformed.com.

workshop, four primary care organizations representing 365,000 physicians had signed on to this model, including the American Academy of Pediatrics, the American College of Family Physicians, the American College of Physicians, and the American Osteopathic Association.

Current practice experience falls short of this ideal in part because of inefficient workflows and support systems—which result in long delays for straightforward tasks such as patient follow-up or appointment scheduling—and because of the lack of adequate training and information systems needed to support the practice of evidence-based medicine. Overall, the fragmentation of information, expertise, and care delivery processes greatly compounds the complex task that healthcare professionals face when they try to deliver the right care at the right time.

McGeeney also viewed misaligned financial incentives and the poor adoption of technologies that support clinical practice as important barriers; however, he identified the need to change the culture of medicine as the most difficult challenge. Current practice is dominated by the notion of the physician as "captain of the ship," but it is characterized by weak coordination of care and limited information sharing. High-quality point-of-care services, including wellness promotion, disease prevention, and acute and chronic disease management, will increasingly depend upon the adoption of a team approach to care. Physicians and practices will have to work to coordinate their care with other providers, including colleagues in mental health centers, community health centers, social workers, pharmacists, physical therapists, nurse practitioners, and physician assistants. Communication and information sharing among healthcare professionals and with patients will be paramount, and clinical practices must gain a better understanding of how they should communicate with patients to encourage their participation in the decision-making process. Leadership by healthcare providers will be fundamental to progress but must be backed by broad changes to the healthcare system, including the development and availability of actionable comparative effectiveness information and electronic health records that meet the needs of patients and providers.

Stewardship of the evidence   To create the ideal experience for patients and providers, the development of evidence that is timely, reliable, and relevant is essential. Sean Tunis' work at the Centers for Medicare and Medicaid Services (CMS) and, more recently, the Center for Medical Technology Policy has informed his view that evidence stewardship should be characterized by the use of efficient and reliable methods for the development, dissemination, and application of evidence. Looking specifically at evidence development, Tunis noted that the ideal method for developing the necessary evidence is not yet known, and a willingness to support and try various approaches and strategies is of acute importance to improving stewardship of the evidence.

Several innovative approaches that are being used or are under development to improve and accelerate evidence generation were discussed.

Decision making—whether clinical or policy related—is based on the development of evidence through systematic reviews of the literature, decision modeling on the basis of the findings from literature reviews, retrospective analyses of administrative claims data or electronic health record data, and experimental or observational prospective studies. Confidence in the quality of the evidence derived by these methods ranges from low to high, but for decision makers, there is often no clear point at which evidence can be considered adequate to demonstrate improved net health outcomes. In the context of policy decisions this challenge is compounded by the evolving nature of the evidence, with important information about a technology or treatment not always available at the time that Food and Drug Administration (FDA) approval or coverage decisions are made. Because the necessary data are often accumulated only after the introduction of an intervention into clinical practice, some coverage policies have begun to provide options that allow decision making to be linked more precisely to evolving evidence. Examples of conditional approval policies include coverage with evidence development, value-based insurance design, and risk-sharing price models. These approaches allow postponement of further decision making until sufficient evidence is generated, allowing the reimbursement process to promote rather than create a barrier to the generation of additional evidence. Initial lessons learned include the need to ensure that the data collected are useful and informative and that appropriate mechanisms are in place to ensure support for projects carried out to obtain evidence. Other challenges include achieving stakeholder consensus on issues such as the adequacy of the evidence, determination of the additional evidence needed, and appropriate methodologies for the gathering of evidence.

The most pressing need is for work on study design and execution to better characterize the limits and appropriate uses of the various methodologies. The limits of randomized controlled trials (RCTs) and the promise of data from electronic health records have been widely touted, fueling an increased interest in pragmatic studies in real-world settings and observational methods using claims and electronic health record data. However, improvements in all study designs are needed to help develop a better understanding of what works under which circumstances. Prospective clinical trials will continue to be an important source of information, and exploration of the range of methodologies is needed to facilitate more efficient RCTs and, as appropriate, the increased use of pragmatic clinical trials and observational methods. In these efforts to improve methodologies, stakeholders must be engaged meaningfully, and patients and clinicians must be maintained as an organizing focus.

Finally, a recent proposal for the creation of a central enterprise for comparative effectiveness studies was discussed as a possible opportunity to improve stewardship of the evidence by improving the capacity for study execution and coordination of the dissemination of results. However, Tunis reminded workshop participants that some capacity for comparative effectiveness research exists and could be expanded without the creation of a new entity. Since previous efforts to conduct similar activities have largely failed, careful consideration is needed to determine whether and how these proposals will allow true progress.

Foundation Stones in the Common Ground

The first goal of the workshop was to consider elements of the stakeholder capacity to foster progress toward a learning healthcare system. As component players in health care, individuals from various sectors came to the workshop committed to exploring areas of common interest. The majority of the discussion was focused on achieving broader stakeholder cooperation and leadership. In 2 days of dialogue, frequent mention was made of certain basic characteristics of a more efficient and effective healthcare system (see Chapter 2).

Building Trust: Transparency and Value

The effectiveness of health care depends on the close cooperation of all parties involved, yet to some extent, certain levels of distrust pervade the healthcare system. Constructive steps are needed to build higher levels of trust into the fabric of the system. Workshop participants discussed the need for increased process transparency and establishing a shared sense of value in health care. Increased transparency was noted as a prerequisite for trust, meaning work to transform health care into a system whose processes, decisions, policies, and practices are developed in a manner that is more open to scrutiny and have appropriate levels of accountability. As a first priority, principles for the interpretation and use of evidence were mentioned several times as key. The push for greater transparency was also reflected in a discussion focused on clarifying various stakeholders' perspectives on value. In health care, value hinges on the ability to foster the best outcomes, ensure the best safety, and deliver the best service at the most affordable or the lowest cost; however, although stakeholders agree on the centrality and importance of the value achieved from health care, different groups conceptualize value in different ways. Clarification of the common elements of a value proposition for health care was viewed as essential to establishing a greater degree of trust among stakeholders.

Shared Commitment to Evidence-Driven Care

The presentations from various sectors included an array of opportunities and activities that could be used to better support evidence-driven care, ranging from the technical advances needed in information technology systems to the structuring of incentives to support an evidence-driven system that consistently applies evidence and captures the results for improvement. Importantly, a visible and shared commitment to evidence-driven care was constantly underscored as necessary to expand these activities across the healthcare system as a whole and to discover untapped resources and new opportunities for collaboration.

Building Learning into the Culture of Health Care

Making learning an explicit component of the experience and culture of heath care will require work on many important, interrelated dimensions. Participants noted the importance not only of developing the tools necessary for clinical experience to capture and apply new knowledge, but also of the culture change to ensure the priority given it by physicians. The value of evidence-based practice needs to be better incorporated into medical school curricula and made an integral part of continuing education for physicians. It was also noted that physician graduates often find a wide gap between discussions of evidence in medical school and applications of evidence in actual practice. Strategies are needed to embed the collection and use of evidence in individual medical practices, particularly for physicians in small private practices. Concomitant with cultural changes, mechanisms must be created to enable, support, and reward education and related practice support for evidence-based medicine. From more robust databases to improved methodologies for clinical trials and studies and the development of innovative tools by the use of information technology, systems need to consciously link research with practice in the development of knowledge. Frequent comments were made about the need for incentives to be structured so that they clearly support and reward practices that link evidence with learning. Education is needed, too, to help patients understand how the collection of evidence and the learning derived from that evidence can affect the quality of individual health care.

Common Focal Point and a Trusted Source

The need for coordination in the development and dissemination of information on clinical effectiveness was a prominent issue in workshop discussions. Most stakeholder presenters spoke in favor of the establishment of some version of a national entity, that is, a trusted source that is independent but engages all stakeholders; that has a certain degree of authority; and that could serve to identify gaps, set priorities for research, establish standards for interpretation and use of evidence, or otherwise guide the development, interpretation, and dissemination of evidence on clinical effectiveness. Such an entity might perform a number of important functions, including establishing a national research agenda on the basis of priority interventions for which the development of evidence about the relative risks and benefits of competing therapies is needed, ensuring the generation of valid and reliable evidence, and developing and interpreting research results. It could disseminate research-based knowledge to all stakeholders, including the public; discern where gaps in research now exist and marshal the resources, including the research expertise, infrastructure, and funding, needed to fill such gaps; or serve as a clearinghouse to ensure the ongoing and widespread sharing of evidence. Others felt that even if a new entity was not created, stronger coordination was needed to improve the consistency and effectiveness of the evidence development process. Some cautioned that care must be taken to ensure the ongoing encouragement of innovation.

Stakeholder Leadership for Change

Participants commented that illustrating the importance of evidence in improving health and guiding healthcare decisions should be a high priority for all sectors and that leadership is needed above all to promote the systemwide adoption of evidence-driven care. Although presenters for each sector commented on the clear potential of information about what works in health care and more rigorous application of clinical evidence to drive significant improvements in the outcomes derived from the healthcare system, this perspective was often not shared or articulated broadly within each sector. Fostering intrasectoral outreach and communication efforts could offer a substantial opportunity for stakeholders to demonstrate a shared commitment to evidence-driven care. In addition, sectors could develop a systematic, coordinated communication strategy to better inform the general public and other key audiences, such as opinion shapers and policy makers, about the central principles of evidence-based medicine. Together, these efforts would advance an important dimension of improving the generation and uptake of evidence by creating a demand for it. In this area, an important opportunity for collaboration among the sectors might be exploration of a follow-on approach to the sectoral strategies statements that would help expand the sphere of sectoral engagement, cooperative consideration, and action on crosscutting issues.

Transformational Opportunities

The second goal of the workshop was to explore potentially transformational opportunities for the sectors to help improve value from health care. Change on a significant scale is predicated to create the evolution of a learning healthcare system that returns the value needed, and the workshop discussions were therefore broad and ambitious in scope. Nonetheless, participants emphasized certain areas or activities as particularly key to progress. Areas of focus and some practical next steps are noted below and discussed in Chapter 3.

Focus on the Value Proposition

Already noted as essential to establishing a greater degree of trust between stakeholders, agreement on the value proposition in health care is clearly central to framing priorities, setting standards, and developing incentives that can produce the desired outcomes for the system as a whole. Cross-sectoral conversations about value were considered particularly pressing, given the number of reform efforts that focus on measuring and rewarding value. The perspectives of various stakeholders on the value proposition were discussed throughout the workshop, and as a priority item, participants suggested that a multisectoral effort is needed to explore how these perspectives might be brought into closer alignment. Roundtable members offered to provide input on the key elements that need to be considered in assessing and characterizing value from health care, as well as the ways in which those elements might be applied. Stakeholder input could be summarized and distributed for comment and discussion by the Roundtable and at a possible future workshop.

Transparent Principles and Processes for Evidence Interpretation and Use

Increased transparency was also suggested as being essential for greater stakeholder trust and collaboration. The principles and processes for evidence interpretation relate to questions of value, and ensuring transparency in these processes was viewed as a natural prerequisite to clarification of the value proposition. Discussants noted that work is needed to define the principles that guide the application of evidence when decisions between various diagnostic or treatment interventions have to be made, as well as the interpretation of evidence in processes such as market approval, insurance coverage, provider use, and patient acceptance. Some participants suggested that the Roundtable might seek input from stakeholders on the key elements to be considered in identifying principles that could govern the way evidence is interpreted and used and that should ensure the needed transparency. Input could be summarized and synthesized into a common set and then advanced for public and Roundtable discussion.

National Priorities: Challenges of Unused and Unavailable Evidence

Defining a set of national priorities for evidence production and application was viewed by participants as possibly enabling greater stakeholder focus and collaboration in more effective deployment of resources and improvement of the healthcare system. Participants suggested that a collaborative effort that engages all sectors is necessary to develop a set of priorities representing the key needs for evidence development and improved application of best clinical practices. The term commonly used was a "national problem list." Specifically, what are the most compelling needs for information about the relative benefits and risks of competing therapies, and what are the key opportunities to better apply interventions that are proven but unused? Exploring priorities could serve as the starting point for collaborative work on the support, design, and implementation of the studies needed. It was also noted that of equal importance is the utility of identifying criteria for determining priorities and learning more about the process challenges.

Producing the Evidence for Today's Decision with Tomorrow in View

Throughout a product's life cycle, from development and approval to introduction into clinical practice and use with broader populations, evidence continually evolves. However, healthcare decisions must be made at specific junctures, often in the absence of sufficient information. Any system designed to improve the way evidence is both applied and generated for healthcare decisions needs to consider how evidence relevant to today's decisions should be produced while providing the means to develop and integrate additional evidence throughout a product's life cycle. The ability to enable access and innovation while maintaining a constant focus on assessing the risks and benefits of treatments in practice will require a sophisticated capacity to capture and analyze data, particularly in the postmarketing environment, as well as a more carefully considered set of life cycle-oriented decision rules. Other needs that many participants identified included developing incentives to support the generation of new evidence, improving access to and use of secondary data to assess care delivered in the practice setting, building capacity for research by addressing infrastructural and methodological needs, and establishing a trusted source to serve as an evidence intermediary.

Medical Informatics: The Nerve Center of the Learning Healthcare System

The central value of medical informatics—which is where information sciences, technology, and health care intersect—is the capability to track and link the many processes and actors in the healthcare system. Because of this capability, informatics is an important driver of progress, and the participants viewed informatics as a key means of driving systemwide transformation in health care. Opportunities made available by health information technology include enhancing the development of evidence through learning networks, linked databases, registries, and electronic medical and personal health records and its application at the point of care and developing other types of clinical decision support systems to aid complex decision making. Stakeholder engagement via increased access for patients, providers, and the public to the best available evidence, along with systemwide tracking and improvement, is expected to benefit from advances in medical informatics. Fundamental to progress are broader access and system interoperability and standards that would enable information technology to serve as a conduit for the distribution and collection of knowledge throughout the healthcare system. Information technology tools could help provide a wider entrée, for example, to repositories of medical knowledge, evidence-based guidelines, and decision support systems in all care settings.

Interdisciplinary Evidence-Driven Team Care as Standard Care

Workshop discussions were largely predicated on a central belief that evidence-based care should be delivered by interdisciplinary teams, an approach that requires a significant shift in the culture of health care, including embracing the patient as part of the team. To make team-driven care the norm, attention is needed on retooling practices in the areas of clinical education, ongoing training, testing, and credentialing for frontline healthcare providers. The development of decision tools and prompts for use in the practice setting and the establishment of infrastructures to improve the focus, accessibility, use, and generation of the best evidence by providers would also help make evidence-based, team-driven care the norm. Similarly, practices could be designed and implemented to ensure that existing data from patient care loops back to inform the generation of new evidence. Other levers noted to promote broader uptake of the use of evidence in clinical practice include education, payments, measurement and assessment, enhanced patient engagement, and reporting requirements.

Moving Forward

As part of their preparation for this workshop, participants were asked to discuss specific areas in which cross-sector collaboration could inform the wider adoption of evidence-based practice in solving some of healthcare's most pressing problems. More than just a tool, broad stakeholder collaboration in health care is viewed as imperative for accomplishing what no single sector can accomplish on its own. Fundamentally, cooperative work among sectors offers an important way to define common goals, set priorities for the application of evidence to improve health care, and identify practical ways to move to action. Moreover, joint work among the sectors could facilitate the articulation, clarification, and definition of values, principles, and a vision for the reform of health care; help ensure better coordination of reform initiatives; and advance the identification of good practices and accelerate their wider dissemination as models.

The benefits of collaboration mentioned include possible advances in several critical areas, including the establishment of standards and common terminology; the development of new tools, products, and methodologies, particularly those driven by information technology; further development of an improved information technology infrastructure; improved thinking and practice in healthcare finance; the education of important audiences, from policy makers to the public, about the value of evidence-informed health care; and the support of additional evidence-based research.

PART TWO: LEADERSHIP COMMITMENTS TO IMPROVE HEALTH CARE

The core preparatory activity for the workshop discussion was the work of those from the nine sectors—patients, healthcare professionals, healthcare delivery organizations, healthcare product developers, clinical investigators and evaluators, regulators, insurers, employees and employers, and individuals involved with information technology—to develop authored background papers on sector perspectives. These papers were summarized in presentations at the workshop and provided an opportunity for participants to present an overview of sector activities relevant to improving the generation and application of evidence and to articulate some promising, potentially transformational opportunities for individual and collaborative work. The authored sector papers are included in their entirety in Part Two (Chapters 5 to 13) of this publication. Each chapter contains an overview of the sector, key activities, leadership commitments, and initiatives. Final content was left to the discretion of sector authors, and similar elements may be presented in slightly different formats. The sector background papers are included in this publication to inform the discussions of the Roundtable and do not represent recommendations of the Roundtable or the IOM. During the workshop, the sector authors highlighted the key components of their papers and identified their priorities for work to advance the Roundtable's goal. Their comments are summarized below; each section begins with a description of the sector profile.

Patients and Consumers

Patients and other "consumers" in health care do not represent a monolithic profile, and neither do the organizations that represent them. Just as demographic characteristics, education, and socioeconomic factors distinguish individuals, organizations representing consumers and patients differ by size, purpose, organizational structure, governance, and source of funding. Consumer organizations representing the patient's point of view include condition-specific advocacy groups, public education organizations, labor unions, population-specific organizations, targeted-purpose organizations, and crosscutting, consensus-building groups. Although each organization is dedicated to improving patient health and health care, collectively they come to the table with various levels of decision-making skills, patient engagement, health literacy, access to information, and knowledge about the use of evidence in medicine. Their core focus is engaging the public, enhancing public understanding of issues in health care, and ensuring meaningful consumer participation in health care. Their primary activities include advocacy, education, training, and the development and distribution of information. Generally, patient organizations participate as stakeholders in policy development and research design to ensure that such work is transparent, is clinically important, and reflects consumers' interests and preferences.

The goal of consumers is to generate more and better evidence to support a patient-centric approach to healthcare delivery that reflects evidence-informed clinical and patient decision making and leads to improved healthcare outcomes and an improved quality of life for patients. Integral to achieving this goal will be ensuring that patient decisions are informed by evidence, that greater patient activation is realized, that self-management and physician-patient communication are enhanced, and that care is patient focused and coordinated across healthcare settings.

The patient sector presentation emphasized the importance of establishing an independent, public–private entity tasked with coordinating comparative effectiveness research. Noting that the better use of health information technology will facilitate patient access to and dissemination of valuable information, it underscored that health information technology has the potential to help patients become more active partners in their health care, improve patient-physician communication, and revamp medical education curricula to help providers recognize the need to engage their patients' decision-making skills and preferences. A related goal would be medical education designed to help physicians and other healthcare professionals acquire motivational communications skills to increase consumer and patient engagement in their own health care. Finally, the sector material encouraged transformation to a healthcare system that is patient focused, better integrated, and better coordinated and that embeds more rational incentives around desired outcomes in the provider payment system. Any large-scale change will require patient participation as partners in decision making on every dimension.

Healthcare Professionals

The presentation focused on the healthcare professionals who ultimately determine and deliver care, noting that by the fundamental nature and scope of their work, they are cornerstones in any effort to reform health care. With more than 600,000 physicians, 3 million nurses, and 200,000 pharmacists currently practicing in the United States, these groups represent the frontline of health care. Engaging this sector, the primary interface for patients, is essential to making progress in the wider application of evidence in health care.

Although efforts are under way to ensure the standard application of best evidence in many sector activities—through education, accreditation, and leadership—a refocusing of these efforts to better support the training in and adoption of evidence-based methods, lifelong learning, and interdisciplinary team-based care is important to improve current practices. Specific suggestions include the development and implementation of innovative cross-disciplinary curricula that train integrated teams of faculty and students for a stronger focus on the evolution of evidence at all stages of a practitioner's career and for credentialing criteria that align with core competencies in evidence-based medicine. To increase the generation of medical evidence, the sector paper discusses the enhanced education of healthcare professionals about how existing information from patient care can be used as clinical research data. To expose healthcare professionals to the generation of the science base from which evidence-based recommendations are developed, increased opportunities are needed for them to participate in practice-based research.

Related changes in practice setting systems are also discussed, as government agencies, insurers, and hospitals invest in the acquisition of electronic health records. Full use depends on the development and implementation of a common vocabulary and interoperable technology.

A more robust information technology infrastructure will enable more universal access to electronic medical records; allow inquiry of databases containing patient data for quality assessment; and enable broader access to repositories containing medical knowledge, evidence-based guidelines, and decision support systems in all care settings.

Healthcare Delivery Organizations

Although 89 percent of the physicians in the United States work in solo practices or small-group practices (less than 10 physicians), larger healthcare delivery organizations—including integrated delivery systems, large physician or multispecialty groups, hospitals, and hospital systems—care for a significant number of patients and account for a significant proportion of healthcare expenditures. For example, the nearly 5,800 hospitals in the United States account for about 30 percent of all healthcare expenditures. Because of their size and integrated capacities, these organizations play a critical role in the provision of health care overall by virtue of their ability to drive practice trends, set standards, and influence smaller practices by sharing information, resources, and guidelines. Because of the substantial investment that many of these organizations have made in implementing an information technology infrastructure as well as developing a substantial research capacity, they lead the field in the generation and use of evidence in clinical decision making. Several case studies illustrate the potential for systems that can identify relevant evidence and embed it in the practice setting by providing decision support that makes the relevant knowledge available to clinicians and patients at the point of care and enables the tracking and continual improvement of performance. Informed by these experiences, discussions in this sector emphasized the fundamental importance of enabling significant data aggregation as well as establishing a culture that uses everyday healthcare delivery as a learning tool and a means of generating evidence.

Expanding the evidence base and improving practice guidelines depend on access to data from large patient populations. Information technology is essential in this respect not only for supporting increased data aggregation and use across care settings and time but also for establishing research networks. Information technology is central to improving the application of evidence by providing decision support at the point of care and enabling systematic quality measurement and reporting to monitor, improve, and support evidence-based practices. In addition, a culture and leadership that support transformative change are needed—particularly given the need for interoperable healthcare information technology systems that bring greater coherence to the multiple—and often conflicting—reporting requirements for different payers. The existing adversarial relationships between hospitals and physicians reduce hospitals' leverage to effect the needed changes in practice behavior and culture and have to be ameliorated.

As entities at the interface of patients, providers, and payers, healthcare delivery organizations have a unique opportunity to identify and implement the needed change. The background paper from this sector emphasized the interest in creating a national entity to develop and disseminate needed evidence, increasing the demand for evidence-based care through communication efforts, and increasing the support for evidence-based care through improved linkage of evidence with performance standards and incentives. Finally, large healthcare delivery organizations can lead the way in the adoption of electronic health records as well as encouraging their broader adoption by smaller physician groups through the provision of technical assistance and expertise and the provision of assistance with the establishment of learning networks of organizations that have implemented electronic health records to disseminate knowledge to all providers—both organized and nonorganized.

Healthcare Product Developers

More than 20,000 companies worldwide produce more than 80,000 brands and models of medical devices and diagnostics for the U.S. market. The biopharmaceutical portion of the market includes more than 2,000 companies worldwide that collectively introduce 25 to 30 new innovative products each year and that currently have some 2,000 products in development. In bringing pharmaceuticals to the market, developers often invest an average of 15 years and more than $800 million. By conducting high-quality clinical research to meet regulatory requirements, to adhere to coverage and coding policies, and for clinical decisions, product developers play a pivotal role in the development of evidence. Likewise, participants from the health product sector discussed their work to interpret evidence to meet formulary access and coverage requirements and to encourage the application of evidence through the dissemination and communication of information on specific clinical issues to providers, patients, and payers. Because the tasks of developing and translating evidence into practice are core capabilities of the industry, members of this sector underscored their potential to add far more value to healthcare delivery and the appropriate use of medications and devices than has yet been realized.

Several key questions were presented as pivotal in developing a system that better generates and uses evidence in healthcare decision making: who will decide the priorities for more evidence, who is responsible for generating evidence, who is responsible for synthesizing evidence, who pays for the generation and synthesis of evidence, and who is responsible for ensuring that evidence is translated into practice? Thus, three key transformational opportunities were identified by participants for this sector's work: (1) establishing principles for interpretation of the evidence, (2) developing new methods for the generation of evidence, and (3) accelerating the application of evidence by identifying behavioral approaches that speed the translation of clinical research into practice, thereby driving the learning healthcare system.

The extensive experience of this sector across the spectrum of activities related to the development and application of evidence creates numerous opportunities for collaboration. As critical stakeholders, product developers believe that they can contribute extensively to discussions related to the interpretation and use of evidence. Their understanding of evidence development and the potential methodological or data limitations, for example, could be used to inform the development of standards of evidence for product approval, healthcare policy decision making, and patient care decisions. Other relevant conversations might focus on the development of principles governing how evidence is integrated into coverage decisions; the development of best-practice standards for interpretation of the evidence; and education about the uncertainties of decision making from studies conducted with nonrepresentative populations. The sector's methodological expertise was also noted as potentially useful to discussions about how to develop evidence that better addresses individual patient needs.

In the area of application of the evidence, the sector paper emphasized the needed development of a process for setting coverage and payment policies that are open, transparent, and trustworthy; that consider a wide range of relevant evidence; and that can help foster a better understanding of real-world data requirements for the developers of clinical practice guidelines. Additionally, communications expertise developed through investments in sophisticated advertising offers possible utility in the development of refined methods of communicating evidence to consumers to assist with (1) consumer-based decision making and (2) the development and implementation of a research agenda focused on systems changes and behavioral approaches important to improving the translation of evidence-based guidelines into clinical practice and adherence to therapeutic regimens. To achieve all of these goals, discussions of healthcare product developer opportunities recognized the need to partner with many stakeholders, particularly the patient sector, healthcare delivery organizations, clinical investigators and evaluators, insurers, and regulators.

Clinical Investigators and Evaluators

The work of clinical investigators and evaluators includes quantitative and qualitative evaluations of specific healthcare interventions, projects that improve population health, cost-benefit analyses, and organizational studies. The principal activities of the sector include those involved in evidence development: design and implementation of clinical trials and registries, database development, study reviews, standards development, evaluation of the application of evidence in clinical practice, methodology development, and modeling and simulation studies.

Sector discussants identified several important and overarching challenges. Resources for research and development are limited both in terms of participation in research activities by healthcare providers and the public and in financial terms. Investigators must also contend with what is characterized as the inefficient use of existing data—including, for example, the inefficient secondary use of data. Systemic constraints inherent in the way healthcare organizations deliver care or use information are barriers to the creation of new evidence. Needs for new and improved research methodologies permeate the sector's work.

Sector presenters suggested several major transformational initiatives if clinical investigators are to promote a learning healthcare system: improved and sustained investment in applied research and development; reengineering of healthcare delivery to facilitate structured learning about best practices; use of information developed during the routine delivery of health care to assess outcomes; clarifying the ways in which outcomes assessment can be performed in compliance with HIPAA regulations; better standardization of institutional review board practices; greater interaction between regulators, payers, and investigators in the generation of evidence; and the development of new policies and approaches concerning advanced coverage for new therapies. Of central importance is expanding the use of a broad range of clinical research designs to compare approved treatments. Examples of these designs include not only conventional RCTs but also large pragmatic trials and cluster randomized trials. To allow this expansion, creating an environment in which both providers and patients see participation in such trials as an expected, desirable activity was considered especially important. To improve data quality, use, and access, presenters emphasized the development of improved database architectures, policies, and governance procedures. Finally, participants felt that increased activity is needed to expand the workforce of trained investigators and evaluators and to develop innovative methodologies that will improve research quality and accelerate the translation of evidence into practice.

Regulators

Federal agencies, including FDA and CMS, regulate different aspects of the healthcare system: the former regulates the introduction and use of medical products, whereas the latter regulates the quality of care through its reimbursement decisions for healthcare products and services under Medicare and Medicaid. With expenditures of approximately $650 billion in 2006 and serving more than 90 million beneficiaries, CMS naturally plays a key role in the overall direction of the healthcare system, particularly through management of coverage decisions, payment structures, and accountability measures under Medicare. With Medicaid, although CMS sets global policy, each state has substantial flexibility to determine the final form of the program as carried out in its jurisdiction. Moreover, the states directly regulate the practice of medicine, the healthcare workforce, and the commercial (including nonprofit) health insurance that is purchased from health insurance companies or commercial managed care health plans.

Participants noted that regulators share a critical mandate and interest in the safety and effectiveness of the pharmaceuticals, devices, and services used in medical care. Because regulators are responsible for assessing medical products at various points in their life cycles, they collect and analyze substantial amounts of data to evaluate whether a product is safe and effective for its indicated use. As the nation moves toward personalizing treatment, those developing the background paper for the regulatory sector underscored the centrality of a better evidence base to their work. FDA's contribution to this effort resides primarily in its ability to improve the quality and type of evidence generated during the early phases of a medical product's life cycle, as well as to improve the development, communication, and use of risk information throughout a product's life cycle. CMS's key contribution—at the state and federal levels—lies in its ability to leverage the broad healthcare system through the implementation of initiatives and incentives that advance evidence-based medicine, as well as the potential value of coverage requirements to generate new evidence

Unique challenges in regulation lie in the tension between innovation and access to new therapies and the need for greater evidence about performance. For example, the FDA Critical Path Initiative includes programs aimed at reengineering and streamlining clinical trials, facilitating better understanding of product performance, hastening the implementation of personalized medicine, increasing the quality and quantity of information that can be derived from clinical trials and other data analyses, and easing administrative and other burdens associated with the conduct of complex, multisite studies. In addition, work is under way to modernize management of the nation's medical product safety information by developing a national electronic standard for a medical product adverse event report, called the individual case safety report, as well as laying the foundation for a sentinel system, a national postmarketing surveillance system. CMS uses coverage with evidence development policies to accelerate the development of evidence and has several other programs aimed at modernizing and supporting the use of information technology capabilities. Projects under development include Lifecycle Evidence Development, which embodies a substantial culture change by way of continuous data acquisition, evaluation, and response to findings, and the Chronic Condition Data Warehouse, a new research resource. CMS is also working to build pay-for-performance incentives into its payment systems.

Certain initiatives emphasized by participants focused on the state level. With Medicaid coverage decisions made locally, for example, it is anticipated that states will continue to work with each other and with not-for-profit organizations, federal partners, and others—as they are doing now—to expand the use and availability of evidence in clinical and administrative decision making. Increasingly, deliberations among state insurance policy makers are shaped by the inclusion of research evidence, as is work to articulate state standards of effective medical practices. State regulators are playing a catalytic role in moving toward a more consistent, relevant, and accessible approach to measuring and communicating information about a physician's competence throughout his or her career.

The regulatory sector presentation focused on two key possibly transformational initiatives. First, a national think tank or large national collaborative effort is considered important to identify evidence needs, agree on priorities, and assign projects to fill gaps in the evidence knowledge base. Second, a national problem list or national research agenda is needed both to illustrate the pressing need for more evidence development and to identify areas and projects of priority for research on the basis of the most significant evidence gaps in health care today.

Insurers

In 2005, private health insurance plans and other private spending, including consumers' out-of-pocket costs, accounted for almost 55 percent of total U.S. healthcare expenditures (approximately $1.09 trillion of $2 trillion). Public spending, including spending by Medicare, Medicaid, the State Children's Health Insurance Program, the U.S. Department of Defense, and the U.S. Department of Veterans Affairs health benefits program, accounted for the remaining 45 percent of total healthcare expenditures. The insurance industry operates in a variable and volatile marketplace. After a period of relatively low cost increases in the mid-1990s, healthcare costs again began to rise, resulting in the growth of health insurance premiums that peaked at 13.9 percent in 2003. The number of uninsured Americans grew during the same period, rising from 14 percent in 2000 to 15.3 percent in 2005. Although the growth in premiums slowed during from 2003 to 2006, healthcare costs continue to outpace inflation and place significant pressure on the cost of insurance coverage, as evidenced by the approximately 46 million Americans who remain uninsured and the recent increase in the numbers of uninsured or inadequately insured.

Presentation and discussion noted that, in addition to the general challenges related to rising costs, waste, and the provision of ineffective care that characterize the healthcare system, insurers face issues related to new treatments and higher-priced technologies; the increased bargaining power of providers; increased consumer demand; an aging population; and chronic conditions associated with obesity, smoking, and substance abuse. Accompanying pressures on the insurance industry are wide regional variations in treatment, the significant underuse and misuse of recommended best practices, and an undue reliance on treatments of little or no value. In some cases, legislative mandates and regulatory processes have contributed to the challenge of basing decisions on evidence.

The payer sector has been deeply engaged in the promotion of medical policy based on evidence. For example, committees of physicians, pharmacists, and other healthcare professionals research the scientific evidence on drugs, depending in part on comparative effectiveness data, to determine which drugs to place on formularies. New technologies are assessed before insurers pay for them. Patients and providers are offered customized tools to modify their behavior, encourage the use of preventive care, monitor potential medication interactions, and improve health. Both public and private health insurers have begun to offer performance-based incentives measured by selected evidence-based standards and performance measures.

The insurer sector discussion suggests four major transformational activities: (1) a comparative effectiveness board, to help coordinate reform and set priorities; (2) a national research strategy focused on gaps in the evidence that, if filled, have the potential to significantly improve patient outcomes; (3) the transparency of actionable information that is used to make healthcare decisions; and (4) increased investment in the healthcare infrastructure, including improved workforce training. In addition, insurers called for focused, coordinated research efforts to address the gaps in evidence that have been identified and factors that drive physician decision making. One model might come from health insurance plans that are collaborating to implement a national strategy to aggregate data from multiple plans and other sources to produce and report on an increasingly sophisticated set of quality and cost measures throughout the country. Sector participants also supported policies that would both reinforce the FDA's capacity to assess the long-term safety and effectiveness of new drugs and strengthen the FDA's review of certain devices and its capacity to track device safety. Also emphasized were investments in several key areas of infrastructure, including improved systems for aggregating administrative data and electronic health record information reliably.

With respect to cross-sector collaboration, sector participants underscored, in addition to a national comparative effectiveness board, the development of a more transparent and consistent approach to judging evidence with broad-based involvement of plans, product developers, evaluators, patients, employers, and government; collaboration among providers, payers, and developers to balance evidence with the effects of demographics, genomics, patient preferences, family history, and other factors; and aligning benefit language with the language of innovations in evidence-based medicine to ensure that the public understands that the goals of evidence-based medicine and comparative effectiveness are not a reduction in access, but an improvement of health care.

Employers and Employees

Employers and employees shoulder a large share of healthcare expenditures in the United States. In return, they depend on the healthcare system to ensure the well-being and productivity of the workforce. Rising costs over the last decade have led to an erosion of employer-sponsored healthcare coverage, and healthcare benefits are an increasingly major factor in labor negotiations between employers and potential employees. Currently, only two-thirds of employees under 65 years of age have employer-sponsored coverage, and 40 percent of the employer market is self-insured. Employer expenditures rose 140 percent over the last decade, and healthcare spending is projected to continue to rise at a rate of 7 percent annually over the next decade, twice the rate of inflation. In 2006, employee premiums and out-of-pocket spending averaged $3,136, up 12 percent from 2005. Costs, however, are only part of the challenge. In the face of wasteful spending and poor outcomes because of the overuse, underuse, and misuse of healthcare services, employers have increasingly supported efforts to improve healthcare quality, safety, and efficiency, including the use of combined purchasing power to strengthen the system by improving quality and managing costs.

The primary opportunities for employers and employees to encourage evidence-based medicine include provider contracting, benefit plan design, employee decision support, and public policy advocacy. As provider contracts are set, vendors can be selected and rewarded as they incorporate standards of medical evidence. Through benefit design, differential coverage encourages effective care—as, for example, when coverage tiers are based on the strength of the evidence of effectiveness; network selection is based on performance; employee cost sharing encourages the use of high performers; and physicians, hospitals, and networks recognized for excellence receive higher payments. By developing and using decision support tools and resources, employers and employees can promote decision making informed by the evidence as well as risk-benefit profiles; and in a broader sense, employers and employees can shape public policy and advocate for patient safety, healthcare information technology, and comparative effectiveness research.

Participants from the employer and employee sector identified several opportunities for immediate progress. First, the expansion of the evidence base through comparative effectiveness research and the improved capture and use of information generated as part of clinical experience could, in part, be assisted by policy advocacy and the provision of support for the adoption and implementation of health information technologies. Second, the evidence could be appropriately incorporated into coverage and payment policies by targeting purchasers and payers, building on existing performance measurement and payment programs, and establishing cross-sector agreement on transparent methods and standards. Last, creating a demand for evidence-based medicine through a collective communications campaign is fundamental to the success of the other initiatives. Such a campaign should build on existing efforts and bring to bear the research and marketing expertise of stakeholders to promote the development of a learning environment and sustained change toward an evidence-based healthcare system.

Healthcare Information Technology

As key players in the healthcare arena, those in information technology have evolved from a focus on the delivery of stand-alone "smart" medical equipment (echocardiography systems, radiology systems, etc.) to the development and delivery of increasingly integrated clinical systems, full-function electronic health records, and related complex and evolving systems for healthcare professionals. Key players in healthcare information technology include clinical source system providers that create systems for use in specific functional areas (e.g., laboratories, radiology departments, and surgeries); electronic health record companies, which provide consolidated and integrated clinical systems that support inpatient and outpatient practices; administration and chain data management companies, which develop administrative systems in support of clinical care and research; World Wide Web–based patient and consumer information companies; personal health record companies; and niche companies, such as those that provide education tools, data warehousing, enterprise information management, and data analysis. Fundamentally, the work of this sector focuses on improving consumer access to reliable health and disease management information, enhancing patient-provider communication and interaction, developing operational effectiveness and efficiency, improving the ability to manage and analyze large quantities of data, and improving research on clinical effectiveness and quality of care.

The background paper from the information technology sector identified seven priority areas or challenges on which current work aims to improve the sector's ability to support the transformative change implied in the Roundtable's goal. Perhaps the single most transformational step toward achieving the goal of a learning healthcare system lies in the development and implementation of information technology industry standards. In conjunction with these standards, healthcare information technology sector participants underscored the need for collaboration with other sectors to develop a common vocabulary to facilitate the interoperability of clinical systems and the interpretation of clinical data across multiple sites. In the area of workflow, the dual goals of seamless movement of data between various patient care environments and just-in-time delivery of the right information are important to ensure that the best decisions can be made in partnership with patients. In part, this requires streamlining the complex tools that enable the collection, aggregation, synthesis, delivery, and interpretation of and access to data as part of provider clinical decision support systems. It also requires developing new ways to view clinical data, and their relationship to other data, to help users interpret the significance of relationships and make appropriate and informed patient care decisions. Other sector themes included addressing questions in the area of connectivity to ensure that healthcare networks connecting various stakeholders provide the seamless transfer of relevant and appropriate information, minimizing the sources and number of data inputs while increasing data integrity and reliability.

The paper from the information technology sector translated these challenges into three transformational initiatives. The first involves building and promoting the foundational technologies needed to enable healthcare information technology-assisted evidence-based medicine. Achieving the goal of a learning healthcare system would be enhanced by the development and implementation of information technology industry standards and common vocabularies in health care. This would support healthcare information technology at every level and provide building blocks for bringing computational intelligence to aid human cognition in evidence-based medicine.

The second initiative involves the establishment of a government-industry collaborative ecosystem for the ongoing evolution and development of clinical information technology standards. A virtuous cycle, or the continual feeding of outputs back into the cycle as inputs—as illustrated by eBay, Flickr, and YouTube—would result in more users of the standards and therefore more feedback. In the term "ecosystem," it is assumed that both community and technology are included, as they are in blogs and wikis. Participants suggested that an evaluation of technical barriers to the adoption of existing publicly supported, open-standard vocabularies and tools by healthcare information technology providers would be useful. Initiatives could be provided to remedy technical barriers, and success could be measured by determination of the rates of adoption and utilization of the technologies. Because information in the healthcare system is partitioned into silos without connectivity, a clinical data and analytic infrastructure must be created to enable evidence-based medicine, especially given the fact that doctors spend 60 percent of their time seeking data. To achieve this, convening or supporting initiatives would be useful, perhaps by the IOM, to identify metrics around accessibility of core clinical data and core analytic tools (e.g., reporting specifications and data visualization).

To speed these initiatives and realize the goals of the information technology sector, the third initiative discussed would involve the provision of an incentive for dramatic innovation similar to the robot race of the Defense Advanced Research Projects Agency in which researchers competed with each other to create a driverless car. The collective investment of resources by competitors and the innovative research that resulted far exceeded what could have been achieved by direct investment of the $1 million prize. This contest might act as a model for healthcare information technology because a diverse population should be engaged in the radical technological innovation needed in evidence-based medicine. Such innovation could guide clinical decisions based on individual data, along with relevant clinical evidence and experiential information gathered from the mining of data on previous patients with similar conditions, all with just-in-time evidence delivery, alerts, and flexible data views. One option might be a challenge sponsored by the IOM as an Advanced Technical Strategies Innovations Initiative.

REFERENCES

Fisher, E. S. 2005. More care is not better care: Regional differences show that spending more does not improve—and may hurt—patients. More accountability can help. *Expert voices* (7). Washington, DC: National Institute for Health Care Management Foundation.

Institute of Medicine. 2007. *The learning healthcare system.* Washington, DC: The National Academies Press.

———. 2008. *Learning healthcare system concepts, v. 2008.* Washington, DC: The National Academies Press.

IOM Roundtable on Evidence-Based Medicine. 2006. *Charter and vision statement: Roundtable on evidence-based medicine.* Washington, DC.

McGlynn, E., S. Asch, J. Adams, J. Keesey, J. Hicks, A. DeCristofaro, and E. Kerr. 2003. The quality of health care delivered to adults in the United States. *New England Journal of Medicine* 348(26):2635-2645.

Wennberg, J., E. Fisher, and J. Skinner. 2002. Geography and the debate over Medicare reform. *Health Affairs* Suppl. Web Exclusives:W96-W114.

PART ONE

Finding Value in Common Ground

1

Guiding Perspective:
The Learning Healthcare System

OVERVIEW

This volume reports on discussions among multiple stakeholders about ways they might help to transform health care in the United States. The U.S. healthcare system is large, multifaceted, unorganized, and influenced by so many commercial forces, interest groups, and myriad decision points that it is sometimes described as a "nonsystem." This character translates also to the challenges of evidence development and application, with fragmentation and silos of expertise, services, and knowledge, as well as gaps in quality and shortfalls in the ability to translate biomedical research into clinical treatments and improved health outcomes (Institute of Medicine, 2000, 2001, 2007). The various sectors involved in the U.S. healthcare system share an interest in delivering better value for our healthcare investments, and many are working to achieve change. Some efforts have resulted in important movements in specific areas, such as quality improvement and assessment of the clinical evidence, but stronger efforts are needed to coordinate these reforms across the many component sectors of the U.S. healthcare system. In particular, stakeholders in the healthcare system need the opportunity to discuss and collaborate on issues of common concern and to identify areas in which they may work collectively.

The Roundtable on Evidence-Based Medicine was convened as a forum to facilitate collaborative assessments and actions needed to help improve the way evidence is generated and applied to improve health care. The participants define evidence-based medicine as the notion that "to the greatest extent possible, the decisions that shape the health and health care of

Americans—by patients, providers, payers, and policy makers alike—will be grounded on a reliable evidence base, will account appropriately for individual variation in patient needs, and will support the generation of new insights on clinical effectiveness" (IOM Roundtable on Evidence-Based Medicine, 2006). As a tangible focus and as a means of charting progress, Roundtable members specified a goal that by 2020, 90 percent of all clinical decisions will be supported by accurate, timely, and up-to-date clinical information and will reflect the best available evidence. In preparation for a workshop to consider the possibilities for collaboration within and between sectors on behalf of better evidence in health care, the Roundtable initiated a sector-by-sector strategy assessment process.

This effort, described below, engaged dozens of participants from multiple sectors in coordinated work to identify opportunities within and among sectors to improve value in health care by making the evidence needed more widely available and used. The content of these discussions was captured in papers authored by participants and presented at the workshop. This publication summarizes the elements of their discussions and presentations at the July 2007 workshop on sectoral strategies, entitled Leadership Commitments to Improve Value in Health Care.

THE LEARNING HEALTHCARE SYSTEM

The context for the work is set by the Roundtable's commitment to work toward building a learning healthcare system. Rapid advances in scientific understanding of the basis of disease and the quickening pace of technological change present challenges to improving the development and application of evidence common to all healthcare sectors. Although evidence-based medicine sets a basic standard of care that patients should expect, it must be delivered by a system that learns, in which evidence development and application are built into the routine processes of care and results are fed back into the system to improve the entire healthcare system.

To characterize the learning healthcare system and explore the key advances needed, the Roundtable initiated the Learning Healthcare System series of workshops to build on the findings and recommendations of earlier Institute of Medicine (IOM) reports on the need for system reform (Institute of Medicine, 2000, 2001). The inaugural workshop in the series discussed key elements of a learning healthcare system, as summarized in the Annual Report of the Roundtable, *Learning Healthcare System Concepts v. 2008* (Institute of Medicine, 2008).

- *Continuous improvement in the value delivered.* A learning health-care system is one that maintains a constant focus on the health and economic value returned by care delivered and continuously improves in its performance.

- *Learning in health care as a partnership enterprise.* Broad culture change is needed to enable the evolution of the learning environment as a common partnership of patients, providers, and researchers alike.

- *Developing the point of care as the knowledge engine.* Given the rate at which new interventions are developed, along with new insights about individual variation in response to interventions, the point of care must be the central focus for the continuous learning process.

- *Full application of information technology.* The rate of learning— both the application and the development of evidence—will depend on the full and strategic application of information technology, including electronic health records central to long-term change.

- *Database linkage and use.* The emergence of large, electronically based datasets offers important new sources for quality improvement and evidence development. Progress requires fostering interoperable platforms, linking analyses, establishing networks, and developing new approaches for ongoing searching of the databases for patterns and clinical insights.

- *Advancing clinical data as a public utility.* Meeting the potential for using new datasets as central sources of evidence on the effectiveness and efficiency of medical care will require recognition of their qualities as a public good, including assessing issues related to their ownership, availability, and use for real-time clinical insights.

- *Building innovative clinical effectiveness research into practice.* Improving the speed and reliability of evidence development requires fostering development of a new clinical research paradigm—one that deploys careful criteria for trial conduct, draws clinical research more closely to the experience of clinical practice, advances new study methodologies adapted to the practice environment, and engages cultural incentives to foster more rapid learning.

- *Patient engagement in the evidence process.* Accelerating the potential for better development and application of evidence requires improved communication between patients and healthcare professionals about the nature of the evidence base, and the need for partnership in its development and use.

- *Development of a trusted scientific intermediary.* Greater synchrony, consistency, and coordination in the priority setting, development, interpretation, and application of clinical evidence requires a trusted scientific intermediary to broker the perspectives of different parties.

- *Leadership that stems from every quarter.* Strong, visible, multi-faceted leadership from all involved sectors is necessary to marshal the vision, nurture the strategy, and motivate the actions necessary to create the learning healthcare system we need.

These basic elements of healthcare innovation and progress were revisited throughout the workshop and served as the common point of reference for sectoral perspectives.

THE SECTORAL STRATEGIES PROCESS

The IOM Roundtable on Evidence-Based Medicine initiated the sectoral strategies process (see Appendix A) in January 2007. Key participants were from sectors represented on the Roundtable: patients, healthcare professionals, healthcare delivery organizations, healthcare product developers, clinical investigators and evaluators, regulators, insurers, employees and employers, and information technology developers. Coordinators were identified by Roundtable members for each sector and were asked to reach out to their sectoral colleagues to help describe that sector's perspectives on relevant key issues and opportunities, as well as a collaborative program of activities that could be used to address them. The final content and structure of these statements were left to the discretion of each group, but the process was guided by a shared vision for healthcare improvement, a perspective informed by the key characteristics of a learning healthcare system and a focus on three central system elements: patients, providers, and the stewardship of evidence.

The sectoral strategies process was conducted over several months in 2007 and included the following activities:

- January: the initial formation of nine Roundtable sectoral discussion groups
- February and March: reaching out to other sectoral participants in preparing background material
- April: completion of circulation of strategy background paper to sector participants
- May: circulation of sector review draft to Roundtable members in each sector group
- June: consolidation of draft sectoral background papers and dissemination to all Roundtable members
- July: presentation of authored background papers for discussion at an IOM workshop on sectoral strategies

The process culminated in the July 2007 workshop Leadership Commitments to Improve Value in Health Care: Finding Common Ground, which aimed to

- consider ways in which major healthcare sectors can contribute to transformative progress toward the development of a learning healthcare system and achievement of the Roundtable's goal for improvements in evidence-driven health care;
- explore, from the perspective of these major sectors, some immediate opportunities for action both within and among sectors, and discuss approaches to taking those steps; and
- through focused discussion around specific crosscutting issues, develop suggestions for collective efforts—through the Roundtable and beyond—to support the highest-priority transformational initiatives.

PATIENTS, PROVIDERS, AND STEWARDSHIP OF THE EVIDENCE

The workshop began with presentations from perspectives that are central foci of concern and attention regardless of the sector: patients, providers, and issues in stewardship of the evidence. Primary among these are the patients and providers, whose needs each sector endeavors to support. Also vital to health care is the stewardship of clinical evidence, a responsibility that all stakeholders share. Perspectives on these three components of the healthcare system were presented at the workshop to emphasize their fundamental importance and to orient the discussion toward opportunities for collaborative work. Three individuals were asked to present the ideal healthcare system experience from the perspective of patients, providers, and the stewardship of the clinical evidence. These perspectives, described below, provide a rich set of observations illustrating the myriad issues that must be considered to draw on the best evidence and provide the care most appropriate to each patient.

Patients

Margaret C. Kirk[1]

To provide a simple illustration of one of the challenges of moving the current patient experience to the ideal, consider the following situation: a

---

[1]The patient perspective summarized here was presented by Margaret Kirk, chief executive officer of Y-ME National Breast Cancer Organization and chairperson-elect of the National Health Council. The opinions are hers.

woman has just received a diagnosis that her breast cancer has returned and has metastasized to her spine. She had previously had a mastectomy and 2 years earlier had completed her second course of chemotherapy, which was, of course, intended to be her last. She thought that she was through battling the disease, but, in fact, her cancer has returned and her life is once again thrown into confusion. She has so many questions: "Why did this happen?" "Can I really make it through chemotherapy again?"

In one scenario, imagine that this patient is 38 years old with three children living at home. In another, she is a 65-year-old retiree with a husband of 40 years; both are looking forward to spending more time visiting their two grown children and grandchildren. In yet another scenario, she is an 80-year-old widow with three middle-aged children and eight grandchildren. On the surface, at least, each of these patients has the same medical diagnosis. However, when their backgrounds are considered, it becomes clear that these three patients cannot be thought of in monolithic terms when potential treatment plans are evaluated.

One important challenge in health care is to develop an evidence base that acknowledges that even with identical diagnoses, patients' life stages, underlying health, social support networks, attitudes about health and illness, faiths, cultures, and many other factors are important considerations in determining the course of treatment appropriate for each patient. The ideal patient experience would have to include the patient and his or her family as respected members of the healthcare delivery team from the outset of treatment decisions, which is equivalent to the National Health Council's definition of "patient-centered care." Although various stakeholders have emphasized the central role of patients and the importance of evidence-based medicine, the perspectives of these patients—the group that all other stakeholders in the healthcare system serve—must still be heard. Although it is assumed that all stakeholders work in the patient's best interest, the competing interests at play create an urgency, from the patient's perspective, to better understand what it will take to build an evidence base in which his or her unique needs remain at the forefront.

Evidence-based medicine is a powerful tool that can be used to ensure the best possible medical outcome, and when it is used in the context of a strong patient-provider relationship, it is a necessary component of an ideal patient experience. It can help close the quality chasm across geographic regions, treatment settings, and socioeconomic levels. It also channels resources to their most effective use. The challenge, however, is to balance the nation's urgent need to ensure quality care and to use resources wisely with the understanding that patients react differently to different treatments and have different priorities and personal values with respect to different treatment options. In some cases, patients have reported the use of evidence or a lack of evidence to deny Medicaid coverage for various treatments for asthma, epilepsy, and depression. Although this shortsighted view may save money for the payer in the near future, it could also result in costly emergency room visits and hospitalizations as well as physical and emotional suffering for the patient, all of which might have been averted if care had been delivered in a timely and an appropriate manner.

For evidence-based medicine to be applied systematically, it must be structured to support the reality that what works for most patients may actually cause harm or be inappropriate for others. In other words, as an epidemiological view is embraced and public health decision-making models are used, providers should also remember and embrace the promise of personalized medicine. In the patient-centered world of personalized medicine, individual patient data in the hands of an individual healthcare professional are given equal standing with aggregated public health data. The pressure to use evidence-based medicine thus sometimes seems counter to the goals of personalized medicine, because it tends to measure outcomes in a population rather than a personal level. Decisions based on evidence that also account appropriately for individual variation in patient needs are, of course, the ideal and the goal of both evidence-based medicine and personalized medicine.

The focus should not be which medicines work the best, the fastest, or the cheapest but, rather, which treatment options are available under different circumstances and how they are best communicated to individual patients. Most of the data currently available tend to be cost based instead of informing best practices or even relative costs. The healthcare system needs to move beyond "one size fits all" to which treatment will work best for the individual patient. Breast cancer is one of the few areas that is building a body of research to allow more individualized treatment plans, but this kind of information has begun to be developed for few other chronic diseases. In research carried out in the future to expand the evidence base, improved transparency of research at the bedside will help patients make better-informed choices.

To facilitate patient-centered care, increased attention around better understanding of patient needs is also warranted. Although many stakeholders in the healthcare system have come together to improve the effectiveness, safety, efficiency, and affordability of health care, these efforts seldom acknowledge that engaging patients more fully in their own care can positively affect medical outcomes. To make progress, communication is key. It is crucial to utilize the higher standards of clear health communication in which the components of the healthcare industry and healthcare professionals engage in useful dialogues with patients. An emphasis on and the utilization of clear health communication principles is essential to avoid patients' misunderstanding and mistrust of the information they receive.

The National Health Council has done extensive research on communicating with patients on a variety of health topics. The council's findings consistently show that language, tone, content, and context should not be taken for granted. As a successful example, the Y-ME National Breast Cancer Hotline empowers those touched by breast cancer with ways to communicate with their healthcare providers, encouraging callers to "become the lead player on their healthcare team." There is also the Partnership for Clear Health Communications and its Ask Me 3 program, which encourages patients to ask and keep asking three critical questions until they get satisfactory answers (National Patient Safety Foundation, 2008): (1) What is my main problem? (2) What do I need to do? (3) Why is it important for me to do this? In addition, the National Breast Cancer Coalition has been successful in creating models for survivors to be more fully informed about their future treatment options and engaged in choosing from among those options, specifically through education, advocacy, and participation in the U.S. Department of Defense Breast Cancer Research Program; but there is still a need for a more systemic effort to address communications.

If providers truly wish for patients to comply with medical advice or, rather, to mutually agree to share responsibility, then every communication must be carefully planned, tested, and refined to effectively influence the audience. In addition, there should be a clear distinction between health communications and health literacy. Although the onus is largely on providers to communicate health information more clearly, health literacy involves reaching a much larger audience and perhaps a complete overhaul of educational and cultural systems. There have been several proposals for improving the ability of healthcare professionals to communicate more effectively with patients, including financial incentives and additional classes as part of the educational process.

Finally, patients must perceive the problem before they seek a solution. Studies have shown that to patients, quality or a lack of adherence to evidence-based guidelines is not their primary concern. In fact, most patients are unaware that the care they receive may not be the best and, therefore, have little perspective from which to judge the evidence. Demonstrating to patients the current lack of evidence and its impact on improving the health care that they receive will help them better understand the importance of evidence. All stakeholders must be willing to explain the value of evidence to patients and demonstrate how it can be used to improve their health care, health, and well-being. There must also be built into the system a mechanism that informs and educates patients about all options based on good evidence, including securing second opinions, but that allows patients and their caregivers to ultimately decide what is the right treatment for their unique personal circumstances. In this area also, additional research must be done on the best ways to meaningfully involve patients in these difficult decisions. Such true engagement of the patient and clear and honest communication about evidence-based medicine will help to raise awareness and address the misperception that "the system" is simply using evidence to limit access to care. It only makes sense that the patient who has an understanding of the evidence will make better decisions regarding his or her health care

In short, the key is protecting, honoring, and establishing the patient-provider relationship such that the parties are on equal footing and the relationship carries the same weight as public health and epidemiological evidence when providers and patients make clinical decisions. To do this, communication is essential. It is crucial for all stakeholders to begin the difficult work to achieve this goal. To quote my mother: "If it was easy, everybody would be doing it." The task is not easy, but we simply must make it happen.

Providers

Terry McGeeney[2]

Several years ago, the seven family medicine organizations realized the need for a fundamental change in the specialty within the U.S. healthcare system. In response, the Future of Family Medicine Project emerged in 2001 to assess the healthcare and technology needs of patients and providers and to identify the fundamental changes necessary to address these issues and transform family medicine. The final report highlighted existing issues in the practice of family medicine and identified a new model of practice that employs a patient-centered team approach, eliminates barriers to access, advances the use of information systems and electronic health records, operationally redesigns offices to function more efficiently, focuses on quality and outcomes, and improves overall practice finance and cost savings (Martin et al., 2004; Spann, 2004).

The report also called for the creation of a financially self-sustaining national resource to provide practices with ongoing support during the transition to a new model of family medicine, thus inspiring the genesis of TransforMED, a practice redesign initiative affiliated with the American Academy of Family Physicians, which seeks to lead and empower family medicine practices and transform the specialty of family medicine and which is the reference point for the issues discussed here. Several lessons have emerged from the current work that can inform the development of

---

[2]The providers' perspective summarized here was presented by Terry McGeeney, M.D., M.B.A., a family physician for 30 years and head of an American Academy of Family Medicine-initiated project to revitalize family medicine.

a learning healthcare system and identify the steps needed to achieve the Roundtable's goal.

The model of care emphasized in this work is that of the "personal medical home." The medical home model represents the transformation of the family medicine practice experience in which the principles of patient centeredness, a whole-person orientation, and a continuous relationship between the provider and the patient guide patient care. As of the date of the workshop, four primary care organizations representing 365,000 physicians had signed on to this model, including the American Academy of Pediatrics, the American College of Family Physicians, the American College of Physicians, and the American Osteopathic Association. Key supporting elements of this model include patient access to care, patient access to information, information systems such as electronic health records with point-of-service reminders of best practices, redesigned offices to increase practice efficiency, an increased focus on quality and safety, efficient practice management, the provision of point-of-care services, and a team approach to providing care within the practice (TransforMED, 2007).

Two components are of particular importance. First, information systems, including those that provide information for patients such as online portals with laboratory results, online appointment scheduling, and electronic (or virtual) visits, hold great promise for improving care. However, emphasis is needed not only on the implementation of such systems but also on ensuring that patients have access to the necessary technology (e.g., computers) to connect with these information technology resources. Second, high-quality point-of-care services, including wellness promotion, disease prevention, and acute and chronic disease management services, depend on the adoption of a team approach to care. To make this work, practices will have to accept greater responsibility for their patients' care as a whole and work to coordinate their care with other providers. This is not the sole responsibility of the provider. The development and utilization of a multidisciplinary team approach that includes those inside and outside the practice—colleagues in mental health and community health centers, social workers, pharmacists, and physical therapists, as well as nurse practitioners and physician assistants—will be particularly important in the face of emerging healthcare workforce shortfalls to ensure the provision of appropriate and timely care. In addition, the provider is not the sole decision maker but provides information and support to allow the patient to participate in decisions affecting his or her own care and wellness.

To demonstrate the value of this model of care, a 2-year national demonstration project is under way and is funded in part by the American Academy of Family Physicians and in part by the Commonwealth Fund. The purpose of the national demonstration project is to demonstrate that the new medical home model of care enables providers to deliver higher-quality, patient-centered care that results in improved patient satisfaction and improved practice staff satisfaction while providing a successful business model for the practice. The national demonstration project has been deemed a learning laboratory that has evaluated initiatives addressing various points along the continuum of providing medical homes for patients. For example, the residency-based demonstration project, referred to as Preparing the Personal Physician for Practice, seeks to train family physicians for practice in the twenty-first century with a prominent focus on evidence-based medicine and technology. Since existing residency training methods have not significantly evolved since the 1970s, this project examines new techniques for improving the training of primary care physicians.

Some initial results from previous national demonstration projects mark the potential of this approach. For example, some studies have indicated that at present, most providers either completely lack the ability to use information systems or underuse them. By one estimate, only 10 percent of practices use their information systems to their fullest capacity. Within family medicine practices, 40 percent use electronic health records, which is up from 30 percent just since 2006. However, a national study that focused on improving the use of electronic health records and information systems indicated that that proportion has already risen to as high as 42 percent (Center for Health Information Technology, 2007).

In addition to physician training and the utilization of electronic health records, the current practice experience falls short of the ideal in many areas. Evidence-based medicine is poorly defined and poorly understood; queries for evidence to inform clinical decisions are inefficient and often produce information that is outdated or not useful for decision making. For example, outcomes are typically measured only in the context of payment, with little value placed on outcomes important to patients (patient feedback and information on patient satisfaction are not actively sought). Also, because many practices do not look for opportunities to improve efficiency, acute care is often not available because of scheduling constraints, chronic care is episodic and fragmented, and prevention and wellness services are viewed as afterthoughts and often are not reimbursed.

A key contributing factor endemic to current medical practice is the perception that the doctor is the "captain of the ship," a view that does not allow coordination in the provision of health care or the use of multidisciplinary team approaches to care. Regular, productive staff meetings are nearly nonexistent and contribute to low staff morale and increased office inefficiencies. Compounded by the lack of an efficient workflow and support systems, these issues result in long delays in patient follow-up, difficulty with information gathering, and problems with appointment scheduling.

To overcome these current problematic patterns, the most difficult challenge may be to change the culture of medicine itself. Most people outside of medicine do not know or understand that the culture of medicine needs to change, let alone that physicians and practices are not equipped to make the challenging and difficult transition. To illustrate the resistance to change in the medical community, consider a description of the stethoscope from a nineteenth-century *London Times* editorial that now is obviously quite shortsighted:

> That it will ever come into general use, notwithstanding its value, is extremely doubtful because its beneficial application requires much time and gives a good bit of trouble, both to the patient and to the practitioner, because its hue and character are foreign and opposed to our habits and associations.

In addition to a culture of medicine that strongly resists change, other barriers to achieving the ideal exist. Misaligned incentives are present at all levels, greatly adding to the inefficiencies and costs of care. For example, because payments for procedures are often higher, healthcare professionals could be encouraged to perform more procedures than necessary instead of providing other effective services, such as cognitive services. Likewise, healthcare professionals employed by hospitals are usually not paid unless an oftentimes unnecessary patient visit is involved—again, prompting avoidable and costly patient care. Finally, there is a lack of incentives for the next generation of healthcare professionals to practice family medicine, where a great deal of care is delivered. In the United States, specialists are paid 300 percent more than primary care doctors. In comparison, in most countries outside the United States, specialty practitioners are paid 30 percent more than primary care doctors (Gajilan, 2007; Snyder, 2007).

Barriers also exist on a basic practice level. For example, a lack of leadership within a practice can stymie progress before it even gets started. Poor communication, poor understanding of the team concept of care, misaligned financial incentives, the silo mentality of care with its lack of coordination and information sharing, and the proprietary nature and lack of interoperability of electronic health record systems with other systems used in healthcare practices—all can combine into an insurmountable hurdle that needs to be overcome.

Providers must be encouraged to overcome these barriers to provide improved care for their patients, such as using evidence at the point of care to determine the proper course of treatment. When it is used at the payer level, the designation "not medically necessary" often prompts procedural, diagnostic, and pharmaceutical coverage denials that waste time and money, creating a tremendous financial drain and barrier to practice efficiency, not to mention creating tremendous tension among all parties—payers, providers, and patients. In addition, improved communication is needed at the practice level, for physicians as well as patients, on the importance of evidence in improving health and the health care provided. One notable issue is that many of the current evidence-based guidelines serve specialty care well in the context of a narrow focus on limited organ systems. Physicians should be better engaged in the development of evidence by becoming involved in practice-based, primary care-focused research. The key for primary care is evidence-based decision support (not guidelines) that addresses the complexity of the patient in accordance with a whole-person orientation of care.

Care is often inappropriate or delivered without consideration of the available alternatives, as a result of patient pressure or because of narrow information provided by pharmaceutical company representatives. A better understanding of the importance of evidence and the use of evidence-based guidelines by patients and providers alike would help to reduce requests for unnecessary therapies as well as the perception of some physicians that it is more time-efficient to carry out patient wishes than to follow evidence-based guidelines. Physician-patient communication will also be improved by the increased availability of comparative effectiveness information, which will provide physicians with the evidence they need to appropriately tailor a patient's course of treatment. Furthermore, improved provider and staff satisfaction can lead to a lower level of staff turnover, greater office efficiency, and improved team communication. These improvements lend a greater opportunity to provide patients with a continuity of care—a practice that studies have shown to be important. Patients who have access to comprehensive primary care experience both better health outcomes and lower medical costs (Schoen et al., 2007).

These barriers to progress also have effects on the healthcare system as a whole. All of the barriers listed above, in addition to misaligned and disproportionate financial incentives, result in a continued decrease in interest among medical students to pursue a primary care specialty, contributing to a significant shortage of primary care physicians in the foreseeable future. One of the motivating issues of the demonstration project described above is that transforming medical practices to meet the needs of today's patients and healthcare system, while improving the chance of financial viability of primary care practices, will also increase interest in the specialty.

All parties in the healthcare system—physicians, patients, payers, vendors, and suppliers—are part of the solution in moving clinical practice to the ideal. Cross-sector meetings and collaboration are needed to align incentives and determine how best to provide physicians with the information and flexibility they need for evidence-based decision making. Some opportunities for achieving this transformation include making practices more patient centered by working to communicate better with patients and facilitate shared decision making, rewarding processes and practices that are based on evidence, and increasing the focus on developing actionable information (for example, diagnostics should provide results that physicians can act on to better treat their patients).

Development of the electronic health data infrastructure will be necessary to bring about the needed transformation, although that action alone is not sufficient to bring about the transformation. Some advances of particular help to providers will be the development of electronic health records that meet the needs of both the provider and the patient. These records should be interoperable with other systems used in healthcare practices so that patient data can be accessed from all sites at which a patient receives care; they should contain evidence-based guidelines that can be accessed easily at the time of care; and they should be linked to population-based registries. These aims could be supported by the development of a national health data repository and the capacity to self-populate electronic health records with patient data. A narrowing of the number of vendors (currently, more than 220 vendors maintain and sell proprietary electronic health record data) might allow the market shift needed to allow greater electronic health record flexibility and data entry. Patient portals should also be supported, particularly if they are based out of the patient's medical home, to ensure physician access and use to support the continuity of care.

From a coverage and reimbursement standpoint, instead of labeling procedures as not medically necessary, which creates office inefficiency, perhaps the designation "not supported by the evidence" should be used. As opposed to physicians relying on representatives from healthcare product manufacturers to accurately represent their drugs and devices, comparative effectiveness studies must be undertaken regularly. Finally, the medical legal system must be reworked to better support evidence-based medicine: specialists often advise the use of additional tests and local standards of care that take precedence over what is based on evidence.

To make progress toward the Roundtable's goal, stakeholders must collectively discuss current barriers and take collaborative action to resolve these key issues. The new reality that healthcare providers and all stakeholders should collectively seek is an evidence-based, patient-centered, personal medical home for all. Milestones should be developed to provide practice steps that gauge progress toward a learning healthcare system, including the establishment of a national data repository on quality outcomes, self-populating population-based registries that provide recommendations, and proactive evidence-based patient management. Primary care practices must be encouraged to participate in office-based research that allows the development of meaningful evidence-based decision support at the point of care. This research should also incorporate a proactive means of managing populations of patients with open sharing and adoption of results to maintain a focus on the totality of the patient, not simply a disease or an organ system.

Stewardship of the Evidence

Sean Tunis[3]

The ideal in health care might be characterized by the utilization of efficient and reliable methods for the development, dissemination, and application of evidence. In focusing on improving the development of evidence and, in particular, on how to move from theory to practice, examples from the Centers for Medicare and Medicaid Services and the Center for Medical Technology Policy (CMTP) illustrate some of the challenges of implementation and offer some lessons and recommendations for future work.

Evidence-based medicine is commonly defined as an approach that "de-emphasizes intuition, unsystematic clinical experience, and pathophysiologic rationale as sufficient grounds for clinical decision-making and stresses the examination of evidence from clinical research" (Evidence-Based Medicine Working Group, 1992). In this definition, evidence-based medicine has a function in clinical decision making rather than policy decision making. However, the same definition currently has been adopted for policy making. Therefore, in today's context, the term "clinical research" might be expanded to encompass broader notions such as "comparative effectiveness research" or "knowledge about what works."

Evidence is derived through four main methods: (1) systematic reviews of the literature, (2) decision modeling on the basis of literature reviews, (3) retrospective analyses of administrative claims data or electronic health record data, and (4) experimental or observational prospective studies. These four methods vary in terms of the level of confidence in the knowledge generated, as generally reflected in the hierarchy of evidence. For decision making, the evidence gathered by these methods is weighted according to the levels of confidence in and the reliability and rigorousness of the methods.

The issue that emerges, however, is determining when the evidence is adequate to demonstrate that an item or service can improve net health outcomes or can be labeled by Medicare's standards as medically necessary. The quality of evidence is continuous, with confidence in the evidence ranging from low to high, and a clear inflection point at which the evidence changes from insufficient to sufficient is lacking. Adequacy is a judgment about the evidence rather than a characteristic of the evidence itself.

As an example of this dilemma, consider the natural history of a hypothetical imaging technology from the initial development phases through Food and Drug Administration (FDA) approval and entry into the marketplace (Figure 1-1). For a diagnostic method, FDA approval might be granted

---

[3]The perspective on stewardship of the evidence summarized here was presented by Sean Tunis, M.D., M.Sc., former chief medical officer at the Centers for Medicare and Medicaid Services and now head of the Center for Medical Technology Policy.

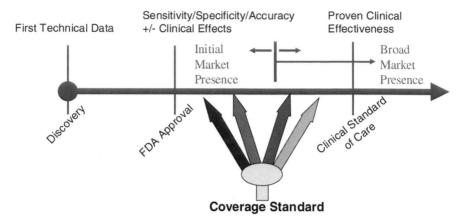

FIGURE 1-1 The natural history of imaging technology.

on the basis of initial studies of sensitivity and specificity, and FDA would allow an initial, limited presence in the marketplace. Somewhere between the time of FDA approval and the time of generation of incontrovertible evidence of clinical effectiveness, there is, at least for many payers, a point at which evidence becomes adequate for coverage. However, considerations related to cost, a willingness to support innovation, or the importance of personal choice vary significantly between individual payers. These variations define a range rather than a precise point at which an intervention can be deemed as having adequate evidence to support its use. In terms of evidence-based medicine, it is important to keep in mind that it is not a binary question of whether evidence exists or not but, rather, a question of how a clinical or policy decision is superimposed on the available evidence.

Because many critical healthcare decisions are dichotomous, one approach to coverage policy is to provide some options that meter decision making more precisely to the quality of the evidence. Medicare's coverage with evidence development policy, for example, provides additional coverage options that are linked to requirements such as patient participation in registries or clinical trials. Instead of a "yes" or a "no" decision, the coverage with evidence development policy allows decisions to be made conditionally on the basis of further data collection and evidence development. Coverage decisions are then revisited when a larger body of evidence is available.

A second example, value-based insurance design (VBID), varies the amount of copayment that patients provide on the basis of the level of evidence or cost-effectiveness of an intervention. VBID is the alignment of clinical and financial incentives to encourage the use of high-value interventions and services that are based on a more solid foundation of evidence. Thus, the more clinically beneficial the evidence suggests that a therapy is, the more out-of-pocket cost savings will a specified patient population receive for using that intervention.

A third approach is the risk sharing on price model, which allows payers to pay a certain price for a newer drug, contingent upon demonstration of long-term benefits and effectiveness. For example, Johnson & Johnson recently reached a deal with the United Kingdom's National Institute for Clinical Excellence regarding use of the company's drug for multiple myeloma, bortezomib (Velcade). The drug is made available in the United Kingdom and is paid for by the National Health Service (NHS) based on the expectation that it effectively shrinks a patient's tumors. Johnson & Johnson has agreed to reimburse the NHS for the full cost of the treatment ($48,000 per patient) if these results are not demonstrated.

The coverage with evidence development, VBID, and risk-sharing price model approaches acknowledge that all of the information needed about a technology or a treatment is not always available at the time of FDA approval. They provide ways to make decisions and postpone further decision making until sufficient evidence is generated, essentially allowing the reimbursement process to move forward and promoting the generation of additional evidence rather than creating a barrier to its generation.

These approaches have not always yielded the desired results, and some useful examples illustrate the many challenges that have emerged upon policy implementation. After years of disputes with the positron emission tomography (PET) scanning community over coverage issues, Medicare adopted a coverage with evidence development approach, paying for the use of this technology only in the context of a prospective registry. Additionally, Medicare agreed to cover PET scans for suspected dementia only in the context of a pragmatic clinical trial. However, although the trial for suspected dementia was designed, it was never funded, and as a result, no coverage for PET scans exists for patients with suspected dementia. In May 2006, the National Oncologic PET registry was initiated under the coverage with evidence development approach and requires self-reporting of changes in patient management by physicians in response to PET scan results. The lack of data on diagnostic utility makes this registry of questionable immediate value. However, 80 percent of PET imaging sites now participate in the registry, making it arguably the largest practice-based research network in the world. By using this approach, an infrastructure for the collection of data from PET imaging sites has been created and could be used for real-world simple trials of diagnostic utility, if funding for such studies were made available.

Encouraged by the potential of these approaches, CMTP has been active in encouraging similar types of work in the private sector. Recent work by CMTP on a study related to coronary computed tomography (CT) angiography illustrates many of the challenges and issues that an ideal evidence-based healthcare system will have to confront. In April 2006, the Medicare Coverage Advisory Committee reviewed a Duke University evidence-based practice report on CT angiography that found that only 10 studies had been performed at single centers, all with sample sizes of less than 100 subjects, and requested that more research on this intervention be conducted. In the meantime, Medicare coverage for CT angiography will be provided at the local level by use of consensus-based American College of Cardiology appropriateness guidelines rather than research-based guidelines.

To address these issues, a workgroup was convened at CMTP that included all the major vendors of CT angiographs (Siemans, Phillips, General Electric, and Toshiba), key payers (Aetna, Kaiser Permanente, United Healthcare, and BlueCross/BlueShield Association), healthcare professional groups (the American College of Cardiology and the American College of Radiology), and the patient perspective (the American Heart Association). Initially, the group agreed that a potential future use of CT angiography would be for asymptomatic, intermediate-risk patients, and it considered conducting a registry study. However, it was decided that a prospective controlled study was needed, and as discussion progressed, the various perspectives at the table became evident. For example, although the vendors sought to include asymptomatic intermediate-risk patients and intermediate outcomes, the payers thought that such patients should be excluded and sought clinical end points such as cardiac death and myocardial infarction instead. Other questions emerged around the type of coverage policy to be used, specifically whether coverage with evidence development should be applied, because this would effectively constrain use of the technology to those in the trial until initial results became available in 4 to 5 years. The discussion is ongoing and illustrates the point that because perspectives on when the evidence is adequate for decision making differ among stakeholders, arriving at a clear consensus on the additional evidence needed and the methods to be used to obtain that evidence will be a continuous challenge.

In terms of the methodologies used to generate evidence, there is much discussion and certainly some promise in the improved utilization of alternatives to randomized controlled trials as well as the potential data from improved electronic health records. Along with these discussions, the notion has emerged that when the electronic health record is perfected, there will be a substantially reduced need for prospective controlled studies. This belief is bolstered by common negative views of randomized controlled trials: that they are expensive, are slow, and need to enroll very large numbers of subjects; that they often raise more questions than answers and cannot evaluate effects on typical patients treated by average clinicians; and that they encounter great difficulty both in securing physician participation and in recruiting and retaining subjects. These drawbacks have fueled increased interest in observational methods, claims data, electronic health records, and pragmatic studies or controlled studies in real-world settings and with real patient populations. However, prospective clinical trials will continue to be an important source of information because there are many questions for which it is difficult to control for the baseline differences in patient selection. Therefore, work is needed to better understand the appropriate use of all research activities available. Work should aim to facilitate more pragmatic clinical trials, promote the use of observational methods, and improve the data from electronic health records. The advances needed for these various methods are very different and will entail confronting distinct challenges. Therefore, a real effort should be made to promote all these types of research activities in concert.

Finally, the creation of a central agency for comparative effectiveness studies or a substantial increase in funding for this type of research has recently been proposed as a way to develop the comparative effectiveness information needed. However, a large capacity to support comparative effectiveness research in the form of systematic reviews, clinical trials, and cost-effectiveness modeling already exists, and numerous organizations have undertaken similar activities but have not been successful. Therefore, it is important to consider how these proposals differ and what will allow true progress to be made. Perhaps there will be more funding, greater political insulation through the use of an independent board, greater participation from all stakeholders in the healthcare system, more access to health information technology, more transparency and credibility in the process, increased interest in developing cost-effectiveness or comparative value information, or a larger support base formed on the basis of a greater consensus of the need for comparative effectiveness research. The case has not yet been made clear as to which, if any, of these elements are key to developing the needed information or leading to the improvements in health care that are sought. The worst outcome would be to add millions or billions of dollars to work that has already been done without clarifying why those past efforts have not met the perceived need.

The ideal approach for comparative effectiveness research or evidence generation is not known; however, the important technologies and the priority issues that have to be tackled are well recognized. Rather than priority setting, what is now needed is the willingness to support and try various approaches, including reviewing claims data and using data from electronic health records. All methods and strategies should be advanced and used so that through trial and error, the healthcare system can begin to learn what works. It will be critical to engage stakeholders meaningfully in this process and maintain patients and clinicians as an organizing focus. Ultimately, all stakeholders seek simply to provide information that helps clinicians and patients make decisions. Therefore, as the creation of an evidence-based healthcare system proceeds, the notion that evidence-based medicine is itself a subjective notion must be remembered.

REFERENCES

Center for Health Information Technology. 2007. *EHR adoption.* http://www.centerforhit. org/ (accessed May 19, 2008).

Evidence-Based Medicine Working Group. 1992. Evidence-based medicine. A new approach to teaching the practice of medicine. *JAMA* 268(17):2420-2425.

Gajilan, A. C. 2007. Analysis: "Sicko" numbers mostly accurate; more context needed. *CNN Medical News.* http://www.cnn.com/2007/HEALTH/06/28/sicko.fact.check/index.html (accessed June 30, 2007).

Institute of Medicine. 2000. *To err is human: Building a safer health system.* Washington, DC: National Academy Press.

———. 2001. *Crossing the quality chasm: A new health system for the 21st century.* Washington, DC: National Academy Press.

———. 2007. *The learning healthcare system.* Washington, DC: The National Academies Press.

———. 2008. *Learning healthcare system concepts, v. 2008.* Washington, DC: The National Academies Press.

IOM Roundtable on Evidence-Based Medicine. 2006. *Charter and vision statement: Roundtable on evidence-based medicine.* Washington, DC.

Martin, J. C., R. F. Avant, M. A. Bowman, J. R. Bucholtz, J. R. Dickinson, K. L. Evans, L. A. Green, D. E. Henley, W. A. Jones, S. C. Matheny, J. E. Nevin, S. L. Panther, J. C. Puffer, R. G. Roberts, D. V. Rodgers, R. A. Sherwood, K. C. Stange, and C. W. Weber. 2004. The future of family medicine: A collaborative project of the family medicine community. *Annals of Family Medicine* 2(Suppl 1):S3-S32.

National Patient Safety Foundation. 2008. *AskMe3 Patient Brochure.* www.npsf.org/askme3/ PCHC/download.php (accessed November 2007).

Schoen, C., R. Osborn, M. M. Doty, M. Bishop, J. Peugh, and N. Murukutla. 2007. Toward higher-performance health systems: Adults' health care experiences in seven countries, 2007. *Health Affairs* 26(6):w717-w734.

Snyder, D. 2007. Vanishing breed: What happened to the family doctor? *Fox News online.* http://www.foxnews.com/story/0,2933,306439,00.html (accessed October 30, 2007).

Spann, S. J. 2004. Report on financing the new model of family medicine. *Annals of Family Medicine* 2(Suppl 3):S1-S21.

TransforMED. 2007. *The new model.* http://www.transformed.com/newModel.cfm (accessed May 19, 2008).

2

Foundation Stones in the Common Ground

The first goal of the workshop was to consider elements of the stakeholder capacity to foster progress toward a learning healthcare system. Discussing these elements was key to progress, because health care in the United States is composed of diverse, sometimes competing, interests that imperfectly relate to each other under the assumption that they will collaborate around common interests to achieve common goals. Indeed, any system's long-term viability is predicated on the ability of its disparate stakeholders to find ways to work together productively. Stakeholder cooperation was a driving force behind the workshop, Leadership Commitments to Improve Value in Health Care, and an imperative for the development of a learning healthcare system.

As an initial step toward broader understanding of stakeholder capacities, individuals identified from each Roundtable sector—patients, healthcare professionals, healthcare delivery organizations, clinical investigators, healthcare product developers, regulators, insurers, employers and employees, and information technology experts—were asked to develop an authored background paper that outlined the nature of each sector's activities relevant to evidence generation and application, as well as the primary opportunities for individual and collective work to drive progress toward the Roundtable's goal of ensuring that by 2020, 90 percent of clinical decisions are supported by accurate, timely, and up-to-date clinical information.

These papers were made available in advance of the workshop, and key elements were presented at the workshop as a way to share the rich perspectives of each sector, as well as to develop a sense of the intersecting interests and potential alignments among the sectors. Indeed, stakeholders present at the workshop came to the discussion committed to exploring opportunities to work together, and the resulting exchange of ideas was both frank and constructive. In the 2 days of dialogue, participants acknowledged areas of contention as well as those around which they had substantive agreement. Throughout the workshop, participants noted the unique nature of these discussions, and their importance was underscored by the emergence of opportunities for sectors to work together not only in areas in which they have a common purpose but also in those in which uncertainty exists or more discussion was needed to broker a greater level of agreement among them.

True to the spirit of the meeting, the greater part of the discussion focused on finding areas in which participants might work to effect the improvements necessary to accelerate progress. This chapter summarizes portions of the workshop discussions focused on elements essential for concrete and sustained system change. Over the course of the discussions, participants emphasized certain elements: trust, commitment to evidence-driven care, embedding learning into the culture of health care, development of a common focal point and a trusted source of evidence, and stakeholder leadership. A consistent understanding and commitment to these "foundation stones" among the various sectors of the healthcare system would constitute an important starting point for progress.

BUILDING TRUST: TRANSPARENCY AND VALUE

As noted throughout the workshop and this publication, participants felt there are ample opportunities for increased collaboration, ranging from the development of national research priorities to streamlining policies and procedures that affect the whole healthcare system (e.g., financial incentives and reimbursement). Discussions also revealed the tensions and even mistrust that pervade the healthcare system—between patients and providers, providers and insurers, insurers and manufacturers, manufacturers and regulators, and so forth—and have historically impeded progress. In these instances, trust—or a belief in the reliability, truth, or ability of other stakeholders—has been compromised by doubts about motivations or perceived conflicts of interest. This context poses a significant barrier to the emerging vision for health care as a system that is guided by evidence, is broadly interactive, and is continuously evolving and improving. Opportunities to work together constructively are possible only if a higher level of trust among stakeholders is established, and without evidence, trust is at risk. The presumption of this workshop, and of the Roundtable, is that increased opportunities for cross-sector conversations will help break down misperceptions and encourage a new degree of honesty and candor within and among sectors. Priorities in this respect include increasing system transparency and defining a shared value proposition for health care.

Transparency

As a prerequisite for progress, participants emphasized the need to embrace an ethos whereby processes, decisions, policies, and practices are established and carried out more in public than in private, with greater openness and accountability. Achieving the vision of the Roundtable will require stakeholders to make concessions. The risks and benefits of possible approaches must be articulated clearly so that each sector can weigh the merits and the relative trade-offs.

A starting point suggested for the creation of greater transparency was the establishment of principles for the interpretation and use of clinical evidence. Individuals in a number of different sectors make these judgments to provide actionable information to decision makers at all levels: patients, physicians, providers, employers, and policy makers. However, despite the broad impact of coverage decisions or guideline development, there is often little transparency in how information is gathered, synthesized, or weighted in making decisions; as a result, there is little accountability. Participants felt that the increased transparency of these processes not only would provide a needed context for decision makers but also would help clarify what types of information are most helpful for decision making, essentially, what constitutes consistent, accurate, usable, and meaningful evidence.

Transparency is particularly needed in areas in which stakeholder responsibilities and obligations overlap. In addition to the interpretation and use of evidence, these areas include regulatory decision making, marketing practices, and data collection and governance. Also important are instances in which financial transactions occur, including general funding structures and payment practices. Establishing, clarifying, and publicizing principles, or rules of the road, will be vitally important, and collaboration among stakeholders is needed to determine the principles and areas of focus that will bring greater openness to health care.

Value

Increased transparency ensures a shared understanding of important processes, and perhaps no element has greater need for shared perspective than the notion of value in health care. Although commenters pointed to the centrality and importance of realizing value from health care, different stakeholders evaluated this value in different ways. Depending on the perspective and circumstances, value might mean reduced death or disease, better function, less pain, a better sense of well-being, fewer hospital days, or lower costs. As a result, the healthcare system is often structured to deliver value as defined by different sectors, and these definitions are potentially at cross-purposes. It will be increasingly important to design a common approach to the delivery of value-driven healthcare services. To provide a better sense of common purpose and goals, workshop participants suggested that a multistakeholder effort is needed to drive clarity and consensus on common principles and elements of value in health care.

SHARED COMMITMENT TO EVIDENCE-DRIVEN CARE

The sectoral background papers cataloged a growing number of efforts within each sector to improve the development and application of evidence and identified a large set of overlapping priorities among stakeholders, providing an important and encouraging basis for discussion. There was an overarching interest in embedding evidence throughout the healthcare system, and participants discussed the importance of a shared commitment among all stakeholders to evidence-driven care to facilitate the identification and use of untapped resources in various sectors that could promote dramatic systemwide improvements.

For example, as one of its fundamental functions—and belying the many gaps in evidence available to support current care—the U.S. healthcare system captures important knowledge that could be used to provide insights into healthcare practices. Healthcare clinics, laboratories, offices, and organizations across the country collect important information on a daily basis. Both a commitment to sharing information developed during the routine delivery of health care to improve the understanding of what works and for whom and a commitment to developing new capabilities to generate evidence that cannot be acquired from routinely collected data are needed. Similar examples were cited for application and dissemination of the evidence, reinforcing the notion that each sector has much to contribute to the transformation of health care. The collective expertise, resources, and experiences in health care are needed to broaden access to clinical decision support systems and electronic health records, bring clinical research closer to clinical practice, improve the quality and accessibility of healthcare data, and create decision support systems that produce actionable information with the end user in mind. Likewise, each sector can help structure the healthcare environment to offer incentives for and reward activities that support a system that consistently applies evidence and captures the results for improvement. In each of these areas, participants believed that the collective commitment of all sectors to evidence-driven health care holds the potential to create transformative innovation and progress.

BUILDING LEARNING INTO THE CULTURE OF HEALTH CARE

Throughout the workshop, it was emphasized that to manage complexity, organizations must emphasize a culture of teamwork, adaptability, synchrony, and tracking and measurement oriented toward continual learning and improvement. Health care has become increasingly complex, resulting in hyperspecialization, the fragmentation of knowledge and care, unnecessary variations in practice patterns, and the slow diffusion of best practices. Despite the increasing sophistication of decision support technology and its ability to provide knowledge when needed and despite the availability of tools that help orchestrate team-based approaches to health care, little priority has been placed on integrating these technologies and tools into the process of providing health care. Enhancing the focus of health professions training on the dynamic nature of evidence, how to track and apply it, and how to contribute to its development will require both a different approach by schools of health professionals and a shift to a culture that values and emphasizes the importance of ongoing training or lifelong learning.

Concomitant with educational efforts should be the acceleration of advances in health information technology and the incorporation of those advances into the healthcare setting. Technology can be an important tool that supports a culture of learning—for example, creating learning networks to improve the way in which evidence is shared. Other opportunities for the use of technology include enabling data aggregation and utilization, delivering evidence to the point of care, and expanding research capacities.

In these efforts, a focus on frontline providers is necessary to ensure that healthcare professionals take full and appropriate advantage of the best available evidence when they provide care. Accelerating the translation of clinical research into practice will require the organizations that represent providers to address matters of professional education, credentialing, and licensure. However, other sectors that develop evidence and support its use will also have to make the needs of healthcare professionals more central to their work. For example, clinicians may require tools that help them understand how to best access and use evidence in their decision-making processes or why they should spend their time on what might appear to be mostly an operational or administrative function. For physicians and patients to truly engage in a learning healthcare system, they need to understand how they might benefit from it. Accordingly, patients need to become more involved in their own care, including their involvement in both the development and the use of evidence.

COMMON FOCAL POINT AND TRUSTED SOURCE

The fragmented nature of evidence development compromises its accuracy and efficiency and can result in guidance that is conflicting, of limited relevance, or out of date. Too much information of varying quality is now available. Some workshop participants believed that coordinated efforts in evidence development might be much more productive and that some process or repository might be needed to coordinate data collection and access to those data. In particular, most participants and working groups who addressed this issue supported the establishment of a national entity—a trusted, independent source that engages all stakeholders—that could serve to identify gaps; set priorities; establish standards; and otherwise guide the development, interpretation, and dissemination of evidence on clinical effectiveness. To most stakeholders, the lack of clinical effectiveness information represents a "missing link" in the healthcare system, and various ways to create the needed capacity were proposed. The funding, organization, and governance suggested by participants for the proposed coordinating capacity varied, and several basic functions were proposed for the entity: agenda-setting for the generation of evidence; coordination of the development and interpretation of comparative effectiveness research; and dissemination of knowledge to all stakeholders and beyond, including the public. This entity could foster cross-sector collaboration in the development and distribution of evidence and could help both standardize and synthesize evidence-based knowledge at the national level. Other participants suggested that the entity could serve as a clearinghouse to ensure the ongoing and widespread sharing of evidence generated in the field. It could spark and support collaboration among stakeholders. Importantly, it could also serve to communicate advances in the development of evidence.

STAKEHOLDER LEADERSHIP FOR CHANGE

It was generally acknowledged that the ultimate driver of widespread support for evidence-driven care will be strong leadership within and among the various healthcare sectors that can articulate the tangible impact of broad improvements in healthcare decisions on patients, providers, and society. Although the representatives of various sectors recognized the potential of evidence-based practice to drive dramatic improvements in patient health and to guide the necessary transformation of the nation's healthcare system, they indicated a strong need to make a better case. Some individuals still see evidence-based medicine either as "cookbook medicine" that restricts the use of provider judgment or as a way to ration or limit patient access to care. In creating a case to strengthen intrasectoral support for change, efforts can also be made to improve the demand for evidence more broadly, particularly by purchasers, consumers, hospital and other industry boards, and regulators. It was felt that the public deserves to know how improvements in the generation and application of evidence-based medicine might translate to their own care. Ways to better illustrate the impact of evidence-driven care are important to improved communications. Participants asked for collaboration in documenting the consequences of care based on too little evidence and the potential benefits of having the right evidence in hand for real-world decision making. Participants provided a collection of compelling examples viewed as means of improving the understanding of and demand for evidence-based care and stakeholder activation. They also suggested that efforts are needed to more effectively convey the central concepts that medical evidence is dynamic, that evidence-based medicine is knowing what the evidence suggests is best for any given patient at any given time, and that health care is a joint patient-provider partnership.

3

Transformational Opportunities

The second goal of the workshop was to identify and discuss potentially transformational opportunities for the sectors to help improve value from health care. The Roundtable on Evidence-Based Medicine's vision for health care is *a system that draws upon the best available evidence to provide the care most appropriate to each patient, emphasizes prevention and health promotion, delivers the most value, and adds to learning throughout the healthcare delivery system.* Workshop participants felt that achieving this vision will require transformational change—from incentives aligned for the application and generation of the best evidence and a greater emphasis on wellness and disease prevention to the adoption of interoperable personal and electronic health record systems that support both individual patient care and improvement of the evidence base. Progress toward this long-term vision is possible only if reform efforts focus on broad, crosscutting initiatives that seek to catalyze transformative, systemwide change. For example, information gleaned as part of routine practice might be made more central to discovery, innovation, and research; the culture of health care might define new stakeholder roles and responsibilities to better support value in health care; and increased investment might produce comparative effectiveness information to better inform decision making by patients and healthcare professionals about the risks and benefits of a particular treatment and the role of patient preference in determining courses of treatment.

As part of the discussion of sectoral strategies, workshop participants were asked to specifically consider what initiatives and opportunities represented the most promising approaches to bringing about transformative change within health care. During the 2-day workshop, individuals from each sector presented for discussion the highest-priority transformational opportunities identified by members of that sector. This chapter summarizes those opportunities and relevant workshop discussions not only to illustrate where leadership is needed but also to offer some possible priority items for immediate action.

Briefly, these items highlight the need for a set of principles and priorities and the need to address issues related to stakeholder engagement and capacity development. Each sector coordinator addressed the need to clarify certain core concepts, such as the value proposition in health care and principles for evidence stewardship. The establishment of a set of national priorities for evidence development and application was viewed by most as a means of coordinating stakeholder action. Similarly, participants from different sectors called for better streamlining and coordination of the research enterprise to produce more timely and relevant information. Finally, advancing healthcare informatics and shifting the culture of health care to support evidence-driven team care were often mentioned as essential for systemwide transformation. This chapter explores some of those opportunities in more detail.

FOCUS ON THE VALUE PROPOSITION

Workshop participants viewed an effort to drive clarity and consensus around the principles and elements of the value proposition common among all stakeholders as a first priority for multistakeholder collaboration. Because participants cited increased value as a desired outcome of sector activities, a focus on value offers an opportunity to align stakeholder interests around a common goal, a step considered potentially transformative in building a greater sense of trust and a willingness of the sectors to collaborate. Initial discussions revealed substantial disagreement on what constitutes value in health care. It might best be expressed as improvements in physical and mental health and a sense of well-being. This means getting the right care at the right time to the right patient for the right price. However, what is "right" about care, time, and price depends on perspective and circumstances. What weight is given to clinical outcomes, increased productivity, improved safety, better service, innovation, or cost savings? The perceived importance of these outcomes varies according to one's point of view as a patient, caregiver, family member, employer, healthcare manager, healthcare product developer, or regulator. Moreover, the determination of value is often complicated by the fact that a benefit received is the result of a cost shared or borne elsewhere. Although most participants believed that determination of the value proposition for a specific intervention must begin with an understanding of its relative safety and effectiveness across populations, others believed that innovations in healthcare delivery, advances in understanding genetic variations, and accounting for patient preferences are opportunities to create value at entirely new levels.

Although a product developer's definition of value might differ considerably from an insurer's, a patient's, or a practitioner's, a focus on defining value in health care is important to help frame priorities, set standards, and develop incentives that can produce the desired outcomes for the system as a whole. Cross-sector conversations about value were viewed as particularly important, given the number of reform efforts that focus on measuring and rewarding value. As noted above, defining core concepts in health care was viewed as essential to establishing a common ground. Defining value, in particular, was viewed as having a strong potential to improve stakeholder trust and advance the collaboration and cooperation needed for progress.

TRANSPARENT PRINCIPLES AND PROCESSES FOR EVIDENCE INTERPRETATION AND USE

As noted in Chapter 2, increased transparency in the processes and decision-making rules used in health care will also promote trust and cooperation among stakeholders. The interpretation and use of evidence are particularly important, because the effectiveness and efficiency of health care depend on the quality and reliability of the underlying evidence base. Because the care, integrity, and timeliness with which medical evidence is produced, interpreted, and applied are fundamental to identifying, confirming, and improving on best practices for different circumstances, evidence stewardship is the shared responsibility of all stakeholders.

Guiding principles on the application of available evidence are needed not only to help decision makers determine when they should apply a proposed diagnostic or treatment intervention, but also to guide other processes informed by some interpretation of the evidence, such as market approval, insurance coverage, provider use, and patient acceptance. Such clarity is needed because without mutual understanding among all parties involved of the bases on which the evidence will be interpreted and applied, the generation of new evidence may result in little or no benefit to patient care. Without a mutual understanding, payers may lack consistency in their coverage decisions, regulators may request more studies, manufacturers may demur on product development because of what they see as ambiguous requirements and decision-making criteria, caregivers may be uncertain about the appropriate intervention, and patients may feel confused about what is best for them. All of these dynamics impede innovation, progress, efficiency, and the dissemination of results that should be expected from the healthcare delivery system.

The workshop discussion emphasized the importance of the need for guiding principles; participants noted that the term "evidence based" is increasingly used as a driver or benchmark for proposed reforms in guideline development, coverage decisions, and incentives in the healthcare system. For example, the potential impact of stronger linkages between evidence and incentives was the basis for a number of different efforts, including aligning existing policies to pay for care on the basis of the evidence, structuring reimbursement decisions to encourage widespread sharing of best practices and notable outcomes, designing benefits that link coverage to the determination of effectiveness and the strength of the evidence or that reward positive consumer behaviors supported by evidence-based medicine, and assigning preferential status to hospitals or physicians who meet evidence-based quality and safety standards.

In these discussions, some participants voiced concern over the potential implications for patient care, depending on how the evidence is interpreted and used. For example, disease-specific evidence or determinations of efficacy in a broad population cannot be generalized to all settings and all patients but nevertheless are often used to develop practice guidelines. If such evidence is linked too tightly with rewards and incentives, the care provided might not be appropriate for individual patients. Some participants believed that the interpretation and use of evidence should be structured so that individual care needs are not superseded by population-level evidence.

When coupled with the discussion of the myriad ways in which evidence might be used to transform health care, the uncertainty around what constitutes appropriate evidence underscores the need to establish principles and transparent processes to guide its interpretation and use. This was viewed as a precondition not only for coordination and synchronization of reform efforts but also for the effectiveness of such efforts in bringing about transformative change. Achieving a learning healthcare system requires not only a robust capacity to generate and apply new insights but also clear principles to guide the use of evidence. Using the neutral forum provided by the Roundtable, stakeholders could be queried on the key elements to be used in establishing a common set of principles for evidence interpretation and use.

NATIONAL PRIORITIES: CHALLENGES OF UNUSED AND UNAVAILABLE EVIDENCE

Many issues confound the delivery of appropriate care to patients, but perhaps the most fundamental issue is the absence of information that could be used to guide treatment decisions. In most instances, the available information is insufficient or not appropriately organized to guide the selection of choices from among competing treatment options. Often, when guiding evidence exists, it remains unused. The identification of national priorities for evidence development and improved application of that evidence constitute a simple but potentially powerful step toward better use of the healthcare system's collective resources. For example, which medical care dilemmas have the most pressing needs for better evidence to guide the selection of choices from among available and emerging diagnostic and treatment options? What proven best practices are not adequately applied, and what approaches are needed to accelerate the adoption and diffusion of best practices into care?

To tackle these challenges effectively, many participants supported the development of national priorities that would identify both specific interventions in need of research and current best practices that are underused in practice. Ideally, each list would be limited in length to keep its focus crisp and would be sufficiently flexible so that new items could be added as existing treatment options are addressed. The specific areas in need of exploration and prioritization are discussed in more detail below.

Many participants spoke in favor of a list of priority assessments—to identify specific research areas in which the need for clinical effectiveness information, that could be used to inform decision making, is the most acute. Such a list would form the basis of a cohesive plan and action agenda for an improved healthcare system. The process of developing inclusion criteria presents the opportunity to gather expertise from relevant sectors for collective identification of the most important answerable scientific questions. The resulting inventory would provide a common reference point for identifying key evidentiary uncertainties and gaps, as well as serve as a basis for identifying how stakeholders might initiate the needed studies. The latter is particularly important, given the current emphasis on understanding the comparative clinical effectiveness of new interventions but the limited resources available to support head-to-head assessments. Greater consensus provided by what several participants called a "national problem list" might allow the nation to focus limited resources on those interventions that are of the highest priority.

Taking advantage of existing resources will require not only a prioritization of areas in need of evidence development but also efforts to address the limited adoption and diffusion of many practice interventions of demonstrated benefit. Recent analyses have demonstrated not only that care varies significantly for reasons unrelated to appropriateness, but that even when the available evidence strongly supports a regimen of care—or best practice—such care is received, on average, only half of the time. To move toward a system that generates insights on what works best for whom and under what circumstances, work must focus on ensuring the ability of the healthcare system to select and use established best practices for care. The identification of a set of best clinical practices that are underapplied in practice would be an important first step in highlighting systems that effectively apply existing knowledge as well as the improvements needed by the healthcare system.

A set of national priorities not only would illuminate the most pressing common concerns, but also would provide a framework for illustrating the importance of a healthcare system oriented toward the application and generation of clinical evidence. Collaboration between sectors to help develop national priorities would serve to engage stakeholders in a common agenda and inform strategic decisions about who is responsible for generating evidence, synthesizing it, paying for its collection and interpretation, and ultimately ensuring that the evidence is translated into practice. In a world of limited resources for research and development, participants emphasized that priority setting would help stakeholders best apply the existing resources.

PRODUCING EVIDENCE FOR TODAY'S DECISIONS WITH TOMORROW IN VIEW

Evidence continually evolves over the life cycle of any one product or intervention. Beginning during the research and development phase for a product or intervention, investigators create evidence with which regulators may evaluate the safety and efficacy of the product or intervention for regulatory approval. Once approved for use, studies on effectiveness investigate the associated outcomes in clinical practice. In clinical environments, the effects of treatment with the product or intervention might vary because of differences within delivery systems or patient characteristics, such as genetic variation or multiple comorbidities, or for other reasons, such as level of adherence to the treatment or protocol. Some participants noted that studies conducted to assess various end points are often lengthy, resulting in a significant lag between when evidence is needed and when it is available, as well as significant additional expense. Moreover, with the rapid pace of technological changes in diagnostic and treatment patterns, incremental improvements present an additional challenge to the creation of evidence that is both timely and relevant.

Patients and providers are compelled to make healthcare decisions at specific junctures throughout the course of care, and because of the ever-evolving nature of evidence, most participants acknowledged that they often make decisions in the absence of sufficient information. As a result, many felt that any system designed to improve the way evidence is applied and generated for healthcare decision making needs to consider both how evidence should be produced for today's decisions and how additional evidence should be developed and integrated throughout a product's life cycle.

Engaging the Life Cycle of Interventions

Throughout the life cycle of an intervention, critical assessments and decisions occur at specific points in the care process (e.g., approval, coverage, and application). Facilitating innovation, access, and effective information gathering, while emphasizing patient safety, appropriate application, improved outcomes, and efficiency, will require a set of life cycle-oriented decision-making rules that have been more carefully considered than they are at present. In part, economic and policy incentives are needed to enhance the generation of new evidence. Approaches suggested included aligning purchasing incentives to value, using the reimbursement power of insurers and other financial incentives to generate new insights from medical care (e.g., coverage with evidence development), linking purchaser and payer decisions to performance incentives to support best practices and outcomes, and designing practical and immediately implementable solutions to support the generation of evidence.

Also emphasized were incentives for the better secondary use of the data that have been collected. Health data are collected routinely for financial and administrative purposes and are increasingly collected during the course of care through electronic health records and other mechanisms. However, the available data are not systematically used to assess the results of treatments employed in routine practice. In addition, regulatory change may be needed to obtain greater access to healthcare data. Although patient privacy should be adequately protected, a school of thought suggests that healthcare data represent a public good and therefore need to be made transparent and accessible to clinical researchers, albeit with stringent oversight. Proactive steps would have to be taken to ensure that access to patient healthcare data becomes more open. Suggestions for stakeholder action included a comprehensive review of privacy issues in the context of the practice of evidence-based medicine and the development of principles and standards for the proprietary treatment of data. Practical approaches are needed to improve the quality of data and the transparency of their stewardship. A February 2008 Learning Healthcare System workshop, *Creating a Public Good: Clinical Data as a Basic Staple of Healthcare Improvement*, explored the notion of clinical data as a public good and evaluated a variety of perspectives on the issue. Publication of the workshop summary is expected in 2009.

Another opportunity noted to make better secondary use of data might be the creation of a distributed healthcare data researcher network. Existing healthcare service delivery settings could make better use of the data already in their databases. Existing data obtained from real-world patient care could be used more widely as feedback for continuous improvement in clinical practice and for the generation of evidence. In addition, a more robust information technology infrastructure could likely lead to new ways of using the data that do exist and to wholly new ways of mining the data collected in the future. Keys to success in these endeavors might include stakeholder participation in developing data oversight principles and data governance procedures and the specification of a technical design that accommodates existing data systems, along with careful coordination of current federal and private data collection initiatives.

Building Capacity

To take advantage of the new streams of healthcare data generated throughout a product's life cycle and to close the gaps in evidence of the relative effectiveness of various interventions, stakeholders also noted the importance of ensuring that a sustainable capacity for clinical effectiveness research is developed. Currently, the combined resources of the various public and private organizations involved in assessing clinical effectiveness meet a small fraction of the demand. The centrality of this problem to the quality and efficiency—the viability, according to some—of the nation's healthcare system suggests that more investment is needed. Specific capacity needs include innovation in the development of tools and methodologies that can be used to ensure the quality and integrity of clinical studies, development of the human capital needed to conduct complex studies and analyses, and expansion of the infrastructure for research.

Better tools and processes for collection and analysis of the data required to generate evidence are needed. One way to expand the evidence base would be to find ways to improve the capture of data relevant to comparative effectiveness research and to informing clinical experience, in part by drawing more comprehensively on the expertise of researchers, healthcare delivery systems, and healthcare professionals as well as by making more effective use of information technologies. More funding, a priorities list, and better clinical tools would all contribute to a goal of seeing that the generation of evidence throughout the life cycle of an intervention is more of a focus and a priority.

A central challenge to building capacity is the need for innovative approaches for generating evidence. For example, an in-depth evaluation of what constitutes best practices in using observational studies might be undertaken and guidelines developed. Key questions in this regard are how better insights can be obtained from the evidence available in clinical records, and what research innovations can improve their utility. Accordingly, participants emphasized the need for policies that address the broad interoperability of information technology across various clinical and research data systems and also ensure a modernized and updated approach to health information policies and management. Also needed is the development of a better understanding of when the use of different methods of evidence development, including observational and data-mining methods, is appropriate. A related challenge is the need to blend new ways of incorporating new types of knowledge into older research approaches. Today's evidence interpreters, for example, need to meld traditional ways of gathering and assessing evidence with such emerging approaches as genomics, pharmacogenetics, imaging, and proteomics. The factoring in of new technologies is also part of this mix.

Discussants referenced the need to enhance the nation's ability to conduct formal prospective comparisons of treatments in common use when observational studies alone are insufficient. Examples of methods that might be well suited to such comparisons include pragmatic clinical trials and cluster randomized trials, in addition to conventional randomized clinical trials. Investments in technology will also broaden the ability to generate evidence. For example, the Food and Drug Administration (FDA) is working to develop standards and processes that can be used to optimize the retrieval and analysis of information from electronic healthcare databases. FDA has also put forth the concept of establishing a sentinel network for safety surveillance, which relies on a sophisticated ability to mine electronic databases, and created the Critical Path Initiative, which was designed to modernize the scientific process that transforms a potential human drug, biological product, or medical device from a discovery into a medical product.

A Trusted Source

As the capacity to produce evidence—particularly the ability to engage the life cycle of products and interventions—expands, the information available to guide decision making may become overwhelming. Particularly in the era of the Internet, many patients and other decision makers readily access healthcare information, but a means must be developed to help navigate emerging information and guide decision makers. Participants spoke to the need for a trusted source of information that patients, providers, healthcare organizations, employers, insurers, and others can rely on to ensure that they have the best evidence available. An entity of this sort could also act as an evidence intermediary that is independent but engages all stakeholders in identifying gaps; setting priorities; establishing standards; and guiding the development, interpretation, and dissemination of evidence on clinical effectiveness. The utility of such an organization in unifying and coordinating the disparate voices and interests that currently speak for the status of clinical evidence was also noted. Some participants cautioned that care must be taken not to stifle innovation.

MEDICAL INFORMATICS: THE NERVE CENTER OF A LEARNING HEALTHCARE SYSTEM

Information technology is key to a learning healthcare system, in improving both the generation and the application of evidence to improve health care. The value of medical informatics—where the information sciences, technology, and health care intersect—is its ability to track and link the many processes and actors involved in the healthcare system. Because of this capability, most participants spoke to informatics as one of the most important drivers of progress. Throughout the workshop, participants mentioned ways in which medical informatics could enhance the development of evidence (through learning networks and the use of information gleaned from linked databases, registries, and electronic and personal health records); the application of evidence (through clinical decision support systems that encourage best practices at the point of care and assist with complex decision making); stakeholder engagement (by giving patients, providers, and the public access to the best available information); and systemwide tracking and improvement (via feedback mechanisms, performance measurement, and rewards and incentives).

Fundamentally, broader access, system interoperability, and standards are essential for progress in evidence-based medicine. On the issue of access, virtually all commenters spoke to the need to expand the adoption of technology so that it is used as universally as possible across the whole healthcare system. Such expansion would, ideally, include across-the-board access to repositories of medical knowledge, evidence-based guidelines, decision support systems in all healthcare settings, and the wider and more equitable distribution of medical technology. Having wide access to robust, fully functional electronic healthcare databases that can provide clinical decision support and link to research findings is seen as a critical goal. It was noted that stakeholder commitment is needed to provide the financial support to foster the wider application of evidence in clinical practice through the use of medical informatics.

The lack of compatibility in technology is a well-known impediment to progress. Frequent reference was made to the need to facilitate clinical information technology standards and a common information technology vocabulary, as well as to standardize data collection, metrics design, and the development and application of formulas. The development of these and other global standardizations will help create a common understanding of the data among all users.

Today, some organizations already have the ability to aggregate data across practice sites and times and to understand in real time what is working or not working for patients. They also have the potential to use information technology to deliver evidence at the point of care and to use data from their large patient healthcare information databases to add to the evidence base. These are all positive trends, but the sense at the workshop was that wider access to these capacities is needed urgently and that further development is necessary to improve the existing medical informatics technologies and develop new capabilities.

Beyond the challenge of interoperability, participants also pointed out that electronic medical record systems should be improved. They need to be made more sophisticated and universal in design and to provide more comprehensive information. They should be linked more effectively to essential data in ways that readily help researchers connect the pieces of evidence in their assessment of individual datum points. Electronic health records have to be redesigned to reduce the need for entry of redundant data, to provide recommended practices, and to accommodate a common language once such language standards have been developed. There is also the need to ensure wider, universal access to electronic health records by healthcare professionals; increased investment is needed to advance this goal.

Medical informatics can provide important infrastructure for evidence development and application. However, to have an impact on practice and health, several systems changes are also required. Specific needs include guidelines for the use of evidence-based medicine in healthcare settings, more investment by government and insurers in providing access to electronic health records and in utilizing medical informatics, enhanced guidelines to increase the use of evidence-based practice recommendations, strategies to motivate and support expertise in the use of these practices among healthcare professionals, and better practical training in such practices for students in the medical and healthcare professions, including practice competence for licensure and certification.

INTERDISCIPLINARY EVIDENCE-DRIVEN TEAM CARE AS STANDARD CARE

The need to coordinate the many different actors and expertise in a healthcare system reflects the complexity of delivering the appropriate care to individual patients that often spans disciplines, organizations, and various levels of intensity. Participants emphasized that to ensure the best health outcomes, not only must healthcare practice be evidence-driven but the culture of care itself must shift to reflect and embrace the complexity of patient care. Rather than the current hierarchical approach, the provision of patient-focused health care would be coordinated by a team of healthcare professionals. In this approach, leadership and expertise might vary based on specific needs. Although the use of interdisciplinary teams may be an effective method for the delivery of evidence-based care, institutionalization of this approach will require a significant shift in the culture of health care.

The fundamental nature of evidence is that it is constantly evolving, which creates a need for continuous learning to be built into the system. There is thus a need for reevaluation of the various roles and responsibilities of healthcare professionals and for stronger clinical education—both ongoing training for practitioners and better training for students.

The background paper for the healthcare professions sector in particular emphasized the importance of facilitating greater collaboration and discussion among the various professions. Collaborative work might focus on identifying opportunities in education, credentialing, and practice to encourage team approaches to the provision of evidence-based care. Greater healthcare provider engagement in these issues will be critical to embedding evidence into the structures and processes used to deliver health care. As a practical first step toward achieving this goal, participants proposed the convening of a coalition of healthcare provider groups to discuss the approaches, incentives, and supports needed.

Patient involvement in and engagement with providers' decision making have to be enhanced, and stakeholders should create and implement strategies that support this goal. The better availability of decision support tools for patients would also help encourage patient involvement. The goal of helping patients become more engaged in the management of their own care will require enhanced physician-patient communication and better exchange of information, including information about the best treatment options. In this context, patients need to be able to access their personal health information and evidence-based decision support programs more easily. To help ensure the centrality of the patient, sector participants suggested that providers develop skills that allow them to assess their patients' preferences and communicate better with them. Better communication will require providers to have tools, strategies, and even specific messages that will help improve provider-patient communications, particularly in ways that would keep those conversations focused on the evidence and inform physician and patient decisions with the available evidence.

4

Moving Forward

OVERVIEW

The third goal of the workshop was to consider suggestions and possibilities for cross-sector work. The process of developing background papers on the work and possibilities of each sector, as well as the workshop itself, brought together a wide variety of interests and voices. The papers of the sector groups—patients, healthcare professionals, healthcare delivery organizations, healthcare product developers, clinical investigators and evaluators, regulators, insurers, employers and employees, and individuals involved with information technology (IT)—provided important contextual information for workshop discussions. Key elements of those papers included an overview profile of each sector, a description of the key evidence-related activities within the purview of that sector, and a sample set of sectoral initiatives and priorities that could help transform health care. Finally, each sector was asked to suggest areas for possible collaboration and cooperation with other sectors. The key priorities identified by each sector were presented by sector representatives during the 2-day workshop.

In the course of the discussions at the workshop, sector participants identified pressing challenges in the development and application of evidence for use in health care from their unique perspectives. Substantial overlaps in priority activities emerged, as did specific areas in which the sectors were uncertain about how best to proceed. Importantly, however, participants agreed that the spirit of the sectoral strategies process as well as the nature of the workshop discussions was unique and refreshing. Few platforms for cross-sector discussion exist, and participants considered the opportunity to meet in the neutral venue provided by the Roundtable on Evidence-Based Medicine important to accelerating improvement in the healthcare system. This chapter summarizes workshop discussion that focused on and highlighted the potential impact of collaborative work. What follows is not intended to be an exhaustive exploration of the subject matter, but rather a synopsis of what participants stated during the workshop including suggested opportunities for Roundtable action.

BUILDING ON COMMON GROUND

Several important considerations drive the sector participants' interest in collaborative action. Clearly, collaboration is needed to accomplish what no single sector can achieve on its own. Furthermore, joining in common work offers the representatives of each sector a means to define common goals, set priorities for applying evidence to improve health care, and identify practical ways to move to action. Importantly, too, collaborative work holds the fundamental potential to expand basic knowledge and understanding of the use of evidence in medicine by collecting and distilling data from multiple practice settings and observational perspectives. Working jointly was also seen as a way for the sectors to help ensure that the limited resources available for evidence-based initiatives can be distributed equitably and cost-effectively. Moreover, in the spirit of the Roundtables, cross-sector cooperation can help ensure that all voices in health care are given a chance to contribute to and participate in transformational initiatives. Finally, working together was seen as a means to resolve the ill-founded misperceptions and stereotypes about other sectors. However, collaboration is more than just a tool. Indeed, for the scope of reforms that are needed across health care today, a mutual effort among sectors is nothing short of an imperative. Many reforms simply will not take place without input and buy-in from different stakeholder groups. A number of possible activities for multisectoral collaboration identified for Roundtable consideration during the workshop are discussed below.

PRIORITIES FOR COLLABORATION

Clarify Core Concepts

An initial set of potential cooperative Roundtable projects focus on the articulation and, whenever possible, the establishment of agreement on commonly held values and principles related to evidence-based medicine (EBM), including the related tasks of setting standards and establishing a common language and terminology for EBM. Workshop participants referenced agreement among the multiple sectors on fundamental assumptions and key elements of the value proposition in health care and on principles guiding the application and use of evidence as priorities for providing a foundation on which additional agreements can be built.

Because general agreement on the principles of EBM and common understanding of a basic language for EBM are essential for further reform, several workshop participants proposed additional discussions similar to those described here to foster a greater consensus on the standards to be used in EBM. Suggestions included collective work to design standards for the practice of EBM, product development and approval, patient care decisions, the collection and use of data, the implementation of studies, and the terminology used in the field of EBM and technology.

Cooperative work involving multiple sectors was noted as necessary for development of a common language through which various sectors can speak to each other productively about areas in which they have similar concerns. An example given was IT, in which there is a critical need for a common vocabulary and lexicon, including redundancy-reducing protocols for entering information into electronic health records and terms that can be widely recognized across platforms and applications.

Joint projects across sectors are also vital to improved thinking and practice about financial issues in evidence-based health care, particularly areas such as reimbursements and incentives. Collaborative dialogues will help establish principles governing how evidence is integrated into coverage decisions—for example, in cases that might include the denial of access to medicines or might promote the swift introduction of a new technology with evidence of superior benefit. Moreover, dialogues among the sectors will create a feedback loop that can better link evidence, performance, and results with reimbursement rates and the establishment of incentives. In turn, these conversations will drive appropriate cultural and procedural changes in the healthcare system. Cross-sector projects could foster agreement on processes for translating research into improved policies for coverage and provider payment.

Agreement on basic principles, standards, and language was noted by many as having a cumulative effect, fostering an environment of openness and transparency across the healthcare system. Collaboration among sectors could bring heightened transparency to the judging of evidence in the process of making medical policy decisions. Similarly, the collaborative process could bring welcome transparency and enhanced trust in considerations of coverage and payment policies. Cross-sector collaborations could result in greater access to databases, storehouses of medical knowledge, guidelines for evidence-based practice, information about decision support systems, comparative performance statistics, and other important data. Such open cooperation among sectors will facilitate the development of better quality and efficiency measurements, standards, and guidelines for EBM.

Identify Priorities and Develop Capacity

Initial Roundtable collaborative efforts could focus on developing, clarifying, and articulating a shared vision of how evidence can best be brought to bear to improve health care. As has been noted, many participants supported the development of a national problem list and an inventory of best practices as priority areas for action. Many also believed that a shared vision would be further defined and inculcated through the establishment of an independent body for consideration of comparative effectiveness that engages all stakeholders in the development of more transparent and consistent approaches to judging evidence, especially in the context of decision making regarding medical policy, and provision of a neutral venue in which controversial issues can be resolved.

In addition to a coordinating entity, the development of capacity related to data and research methods might also be an important focus. Joint work among the sectors could perhaps expand the sources of data from which evidence is derived to draw data more directly from practice settings and other sources of observational data. A research-focused collaboration might work to implement studies designed to investigate systems changes or behavioral approaches that can be used to improve the translation of evidence-based guidelines into clinical practice or to look at the effectiveness of understudied interventions.

Research is also needed on innovative approaches to encourage the broader use of evidence-supported healthcare decision making among physicians, perhaps with links to outcomes evaluations. Cross-sector projects fostered by Roundtable members might provide an opportunity for controversial or highly innovative research to be discussed and conducted safely. Similarly, it was felt that such collaborations might provide a means to focus attention on research-oriented questions that no one sector can address effectively on its own, such as the development of evidence-based guidelines for patients with complex medical challenges (e.g., multisystem diseases).

As a specific example, the representative from the regulatory sector spoke to an interest in working with other members of the healthcare community to enhance the ability to identify problems with medical products and disseminate information as quickly as possible. Agencies within the U.S. Departments of Health and Human Services, Defense, and Veterans Affairs, for example, have begun to explore the feasibility of creating a distributed, electronic, national medical product safety initiative. Such a sentinel network would help make information about the safe and effective use of medical products accessible to patients and healthcare professionals in a timely and efficient fashion. The network would be assembled through public–private collaborations and would connect to existing efforts rather than require the creation of a new system.

Accelerate Digital Progress

Broad collaboration among sectors is also vital for success in building a stronger IT infrastructure in health care and warrants more attention by the Roundtable in the view of many participants. Workshop participants emphasized stronger practice support systems for healthcare professionals and for the rapid design of an interoperable technology that enables providers to have ready access to the variety of information available across the healthcare system. Participants specifically noted the need for cross-sector support for broader access to electronic health records, particularly to help smaller healthcare practices adapt the systems and processes that larger practices now use.

Collaboration was noted as essential to the development of new tools, products, and methodologies driven by IT. The potential of IT to advance the goals of linking evidence more definitively and broadly with health care can hardly be overstated. Collaborative input from multiple sectors in work to build, improve, and share IT-based tools—including electronic health records, registries, and interoperable systems—will ensure that these tools can support the specific needs of all sectors. Contributions from many sectors, for example, might also result in the kind of innovation needed to develop a new format for technology appraisals that allows the integration of ratings of clinical and cost-effectiveness in ways that can support value-based insurance benefits and guide patient and clinician decision making toward higher value.

Productive new thinking about IT-based ways to share information expeditiously throughout the healthcare system, such as procedures for sharing alerts about medications, is also seen as critical to the development of IT-based tools to assess quality in health care. An IT-focused collaborative could serve as an effective channel for the distribution of models of good practices. In addition, cross-sector work in IT could improve the patient experience through the use of such applications as personal health records that promote patient safety, systems that give patients better access to their own records, processes that improve the security and privacy of patient records, and procedures that reduce duplicative efforts and result in cost savings. Cooperation among sectors is also critical to the development of the next generation of IT tools, whose capacities are not yet known.

Input from a wide variety of sectors mobilized by Roundtable members might help ensure that evidence-based tools and products for healthcare consumers are straightforward, are easy to use, and fully meet the needs of the end users. Such tools could help consumers weigh the risks and benefits of various treatment options and explain the evidence behind coverage decisions. Specific target groups could include retirees, frequent users of health care, and those with limited English proficiency or health literacy. Similarly, conversations among sectors could lead to the development of new methodologies—perhaps supporting large population studies that use electronic health records—and the collective exploration of their benefits.

Engage Healthcare Providers

The central importance of healthcare providers in driving the adoption of evidence-based practice was underscored by the range of opportunities identified for collaboration—within the healthcare provider sector and between that and other sectors—around issues important to all healthcare professions. Primary among these was possible convening by the Roundtable of professional organizations to discuss issues such as the transformation of healthcare professions education to one that emphasizes just-in-time and lifelong learning, as well as approaches to credentialing that better support evidence-based practice. Other areas mentioned for collaborative work included initiatives to improve the development of comparative effectiveness information, practice workflow efficiency, and decision support systems as well as initiatives to promote shared decision making.

A primary opportunity underscored by several participants to support and engage healthcare providers is through the development of better information to help guide clinical decision making. Research on the comparative risks and benefits of competing interventions would benefit from collective work among researchers, clinicians, and healthcare professionals to identify research questions, research priorities, and opportunities to draw research closer to the clinical practice environment. Also, there are opportunities to speed the development of information about clinical best practices as well as the clinical decision support systems needed to accelerate the adoption and use of such information.

Workshop participants viewed the patient-provider relationship as paramount in health care and suggested that improving and supporting productive communication at the point of care would provide opportunities to improve the delivery of appropriate care. Work is needed to improve understanding of how information is best communicated to patients and clinicians as well as how best to support their engagement in shared decision making.

Foster Stakeholder Collaboration Around Communications

Collaboration also sets the stage for sectors to work together to support a stronger national presence of EBM. Virtually all commenters believed that the sectoral strategies process provided an important starting point for progress and that participants should work within and between sectors to expand the sphere of cross-sector involvement and action on the opportunities identified.

Several participants discussed the possible impact of a multisector effort to design and implement a national strategy to educate important audiences, ranging from opinion leaders and policy makers to the general public, about what EBM is, what its goals are, and why it is important. Research might explore the need for better communication about EBM, perhaps by prioritizing the questions to be addressed or suggesting strategies that can be used to appropriately educate select audiences. Work already under way was described that engages multiple sectors in developing refined methods of communicating evidence to consumers both to educate them about health care informed by evidence and to assist them with decision making. Such efforts might focus on ways to better educate patients to manage their own care, such as the development of training programs to help them find accurate information about medications. Education programs could also be targeted to physicians and other healthcare providers to better educate them about the value of evidence-based decision making and to influence clinical behaviors so that providers consider the evidence more broadly. Another appropriate use of collaborative education would be public information and education strategies that pique the public's demand for evidence-supported health care.

Cross-sector collaboration is seen as an appropriate means of designing and implementing public information outreach programs and marketing campaigns. As part of such efforts, the sectors would work together to increase media understanding of EBM and their level of attention to the application of evidence in medicine. One sector cited an example of a current multistakeholder collaborative, the Alliance for Better Health Care, which promotes comparative effectiveness research and its dissemination through advocacy. Its goals include increased federal funding for comparative effectiveness research; the identification of knowledge gaps and the prioritization of areas for further research; and the broad dissemination of research findings to clinicians, patients, and others in formats that diverse audiences can understand.

If collaboration is an important tool in educating the public about the use of evidence in health care, it is also necessary for ensuring that individuals better engage the use of evidence in clinical care. In this regard, cross-sector partnerships will be necessary to balance evidence in health care with such factors as the effects of demographics, genomics, patient preferences, and family history. Such joint projects might advocate the concept of using observational patient data as evidence, encourage the development of patient materials to support consumer adoption of EBM concepts and practices, and support the development of robust methods that would allow the inclusion of patient values and preferences in complex decision making. A related dimension would focus on the generation of broad-based evidence of the safety and efficacy of procedures or products in controlled populations and the generation of evidence with a high degree of relevance to individual patients and specific patient subgroups. Another aspect would center on understanding the proper role of evidence in healthcare decisions in terms of patient care versus, for example, policy or reimbursements.

CONCLUDING COMMENTS AND NEXT STEPS

Overall, the spirit conveyed at the workshop was of a sense of opportunities for a variety of sectors to work together productively to link evidence and the practice of health care, and the important facilitative role that the Roundtable can play in this effort. Although participants recognized that collaboration implies a certain amount of give and take and that countless barriers might hinder such work, truly important innovations are within reach, and now is the time for sectors to join together to advance policies and practices to ensure that evidence is applied more broadly, more consistently, and more effectively to all decisions in health care.

Comments offered at the workshop's conclusion summarized and emphasized the pressing and well-established concerns common to all sectors, particularly the following:

- *Rising costs and limited resources.* Whether they are borne by those receiving or providing care or accrued during research on or the development of treatments and therapies, participants cited costs as limiting factors for access to and innovation in health care.
- *System inefficiencies.* The quality of health care in the United States is uneven and delivered by a system characterized by inefficiency and waste. The existing evidence is poorly applied, and the delivery of care for similar conditions varies widely throughout the country. Standards for care, healthcare system components, and even research are often inconsistent.
- *Increasing complexity.* Whether it is because of the increased importance of genetic variation, the rapidly evolving landscape of medical technologies, or the growing prevalence of chronic disease, medicine is becoming increasingly complex.
- *Expanding evidence gap.* Across the practice of health care, information is lacking for many key personal health or policy decisions. The "inference gap" between the evidence available and that needed to treat real-world populations will only widen as new

interventions are introduced into the marketplace and health care moves further in the direction of personalized treatments.

- *Limited system capacity and flexibility.* The number of questions that need to be addressed to ensure appropriate care continues to expand exponentially, rendering impractical the current approach to the development of evidence. Although randomized controlled trials are important in certain circumstances, they cannot provide all the necessary information. The availability of technologies lags the demand. Whether through habit or for other reasons, evidence is not getting translated to the extent that it needs to be or distributed as widely as it should be.
- *Entrenched cultures.* Health care has various customs and practices that often are not conducive to reform. Caregiving and caregivers are often "siloed," with inadequate communications among the various functional areas of the healthcare system. Information is not shared as widely as it should be within specific healthcare systems, let alone between systems, contributing to inefficiency and distrust in the system. In general, providers, patients, and other sectors do not yet believe that the development of evidence is an activity relevant to their experience in the routine delivery of care.

In addition, participants revisited a number of the common themes that recurred throughout discussions on key advances and issues, on which stakeholders could work together (Box 4-1).

- *Build trust and collaboration.* How can the distrust that has emerged in health care—for example, distrust between and among patients and providers, providers and insurers, insurers and manufacturers, and manufacturers and regulators—be reduced? Health care depends for its effectiveness on the close cooperation of all parties involved. Building trust and facilitating transformative change will require broader-based collaboration and cooperative stakeholder engagement.
- *Foster agreement on "value" in health care.* What constitutes value in health care: reduced death or disease, better function, less pain, a better sense of well-being, fewer hospital days, or lower costs? Although all participants agreed on the centrality and importance of the value achieved from health care, different groups think of value in different ways. A multistakeholder effort is needed to drive clarity and consensus on the principles and elements of value common to all stakeholders.
- *Improve public understanding of evidence.* What can be done to improve public understanding, acceptance, and demand for

---

BOX 4-1
Common General Themes

- Build trust and collaboration
- Foster agreement on "value" in health care
- Improve public understanding of evidence
- Characterize the impact of shortfalls in evidence
- Identify the priorities for evidence development
- Improve the level, quality, and efficiency of research
- Clarify and promote transparency
- Establish principles for the interpretation and use of evidence
- Improve engagement in the full life cycle of interventions
- Focus on frontline providers
- Foster a trusted intermediary for evidence
- Build the capacity to meet the demand
- Create incentives for change
- Accelerate advances in health information technology

---

evidence-based care? Too often, people perceive that certain common terms such as "evidence based," "research," "medical necessity," and "risk" suggest a restrictive or experimental element to their care. A systematic and coordinated communication strategy is needed to better convey the central concepts that medical evidence is dynamic, that evidence-based medicine is the provision of care that the evidence suggests is best for any given patient at any given point in time, and that health care is a joint patient-provider endeavor.

- *Characterize the impact of shortfalls in the evidence.* What might be the tangible impact of broad improvements in the availability and application of appropriate evidence for healthcare decisions for patients, for providers, and for society? Documenting the consequences of provision of care on the basis of too little evidence or the potential benefits of providing care on the basis of the right evidence is a prerequisite to obtaining an improved understanding of and demand for evidence-based care and stakeholder activation.

- *Identify the priorities for evidence development.* Which medical care dilemmas represent the most challenging and pressing needs for better comparative information and guidance for choices among the available and the emerging diagnostic and treatment options? The first step to a systematic and coordinated effort to conduct the most important assessments is identification of the priorities as a sort of consensus national problem list and research agenda of the most pressing issues for medical care decisions.

- *Improve the level, quality, and efficiency of research.* How can the healthcare system take better advantage of emerging clinical record resources to gain insights into the evidence? Policies that facilitate the ability to use clinical data to monitor the effectiveness of interventions are needed. Novel approaches to the conduct of clinical trials are also needed. A more structured lexicon for "best practices" in undertaking observational studies may be necessary.

- *Clarify and promote transparency.* What principles define openness in health care, clinical research, the interpretation of evidence, coverage decisions, regulatory policy, marketing practices, oversight, and the governance of use of clinical data? Consensus is needed to establish common principles of transparency and standards for how they should be applied in each sector. One starting point might be with principles for evidence interpretation.

- *Establish principles for the interpretation and use of evidence.* What guiding principles related to application of the available evidence might be used to help decision makers determine when they should apply a proposed diagnostic or treatment intervention? Decisions about market approval, insurance coverage, provider use, and patient acceptance are all informed by some interpretation of the evidence. Clarity on the guiding principles is important.

- *Improve engagement in the full life cycle of interventions.* How should assessments and decisions on proposed healthcare services be tailored to ensure that each stage of the development and application process for a given intervention builds efficiently to the next? Many factors are at play for each intervention—for example, similarity to previously tested interventions, the safety and effectiveness of an intervention for some populations but not others, the availability of biomarkers that are predictive of efficacy, and costs that vary by scale and stage of application or by the need for later services. Facilitating innovation, access, and effective information gathering while emphasizing patient safety, appropriate application, improved outcomes, and efficiency will require a set of life cycle-oriented decision-making rules that are more carefully considered than they are at present.

- *Focus on frontline providers.* What are the key levers that might help ensure that both primary care and specialty providers are taking full and appropriate advantage of the best available evidence in the care that they provide? Accelerating the translation of clinical research into practice involves addressing matters of professional education, credentialing, licensure, practice support, economic incentives, patient acceptance, and the culture of care. It will require the central and coordinated involvement of the organizations that represent those providers.

- *Foster a trusted intermediary for evidence.* How can patients, providers, healthcare organizations, employers, insurers, and others know when they have the best evidence on which to base the healthcare decisions they make? In this information age, health-related information is constantly presented through news reports, marketing, professional organizations, journals, and the Internet; but it is often confusing and even contradictory. A trusted information source—one that is independent but that engages all stakeholders—is needed to identify gaps; set priorities; establish standards; and guide the development, interpretation, and dissemination of evidence on clinical effectiveness.

- *Build the capacity to meet the demand.* What mechanism is necessary to close the current and emerging gaps in evidence on the relative effectiveness of various interventions, to ensure the quality and integrity of the studies used to establish the evidence, and to provide a sustained capacity to meet the need? Currently, the combined resources of the various public and private organizations involved in studying comparative clinical effectiveness meet but a small and scattered fraction of the demand. The centrality of the problem to the quality and efficiency—the viability, according to some—of the nation's healthcare system may require the creation of a new independent entity devoted to this work.

- *Create incentives for change.* What practice-based economic and policy incentives might help enhance the next generation of new evidence and transform the ability and commitment of providers to use the best available evidence and more fully engage patients in the clinical decision-making process? Approaches include alignment of purchasing incentives accordingly when value is determined; use of the reimbursement power of insurers and other financial incentives to generate new insights from medical care (e.g., coverage with evidence development); and the linkage of purchaser and payer decisions to performance incentives for best practices, outcomes, and the better secondary use of routinely collected data.

- *Accelerate advances in health information technology.* What can stakeholders do to accelerate the nation's progress toward the goal of the universal application of interoperable—or functionally accessible—personal and organizational electronic health records, as well as toward the goal of providing real-time electronic access to the best information available? Health information technology can facilitate the development of learning networks and accelerate the generation of evidence, enable data aggregation and utilization, deliver evidence to the point of care, and expand research capacities. Coordinated stakeholder action—and financial incentives— should be able to speed the progress necessary on both basic interoperability issues (e.g., standards and vocabulary) and, possibly, the development of more radical data search innovations.

Finally, in reflecting on priority next steps for Roundtable consideration, a number of opportunities were mentioned, including the following:

- *Development of a priority assessment inventory.* Termed a "national problem list" by meeting participants, this is a multisector collaborative effort to develop criteria and a list of the diagnostic and treatment interventions that might be viewed as particularly important for the development of comparative effectiveness studies. The list will serve as a means of illustrating and prompting discussion on the key evidence gaps and on the design, support, and execution of the studies needed.
- *Pursue agreement on the value proposition.* Identify key concepts and elements to be considered in assessing and characterizing value from health care, setting the stage for discussions on approaches to assessing those elements and applying to add perspective and inform decision making. An IOM workshop, *Value in Healthcare: Accounting for Cost, Quality, Safety, Outcomes and Innovation,* was convened in November 2008, with publication of the workshop summary expected in 2009.
- *Identify common principles for evidence interpretation and use.* Identify the core principles underpinning activities in interpretation and use of evidence, as background for discussion of the implications and of the ways the principles might be applied in the development of a framework adaptive to different circumstances related either to the evidence base or the condition of interest.
- *Foster cooperative data sharing.* Several issues are important in this regard: platform compatibilities, standards, economic incentives and disincentives, the regulatory and privacy environment. Health Insurance Portability and Accountability Act issues are being addressed by an IOM Committee expected to issue its report and recommendations in 2009, including those related to the use of clinical data for knowledge development. The Roundtable's February 2008 meeting, *Clinical Data as the Basic Staple of Healthcare*

Learning: Creating and Protecting a Public Good, addressed a number of the other issues related to sound data stewardship. And collaborative work has been sponsored by the Roundtable on mining electronic health records for postmarket surveillance and clinical safety and effectiveness insights.

- *Pursue a public communication initiative on evidence-based medicine.* Use the Roundtable membership's collective communication expertise to explore improving terminology and advancing public awareness on the nature and importance of evidence in medical care, the key needs, and the centrality of patient and provider communication around the state of the evolving evidence for individual treatment choices. The Roundtable's Evidence Communication Collaborative has a working group actively working on a communication initiative proposal.

- *Support progress on a trusted intermediary for evidence promotion.* The Roundtable's Sustainable Capacity working group oversaw the development of a comprehensive Issue Brief, framing the issues and options under discussion related to enhancement of the national capacity to develop, evaluate, organize, validate, and disseminate information on the comparative effectiveness of health interventions. Technical assistance and related information is provided on an ongoing basis to the various policy discussions of the issue.

- *Identify the potential from best practices in the use of evidence.* It is important to assess and underscore the best practices in evidence development and application, including consideration of ongoing methods of identifying and disseminating those best practices. A working group is underway to characterize the potential returns from implementing certain established best practices.

- *Enlist front-line healthcare providers more effectively.* Charge the sectoral working group on providers with proposing approaches to convening a coalition of provider groups, perhaps under Roundtable auspices, to consider sustained, coordinated work on health professions education, testing, credentialing, and practice setting tools and structure to improve focus, accessibility, use, and generation by providers of the best evidence. A Roundtable collaborative of providers is being formed to engage this issue.

The issues and questions heard throughout the workshop explicitly underscored the importance of the unique approach of the Roundtable's activities: convening disparate stakeholders and sectors to engage in issues about which they have common concerns but, as yet, little collective vision or will to drive the changes needed. Participants noted frequently the sense of the opportunity presented by the sectoral strategies process and were encouraged to expand the sphere of engagement of each of their sectors in the priority issues and initiatives. Real prospect exists for moving forward on common ground, but it will take diligence, commitment, and leadership.

PART TWO*

Leadership Commitments to Improve Health Care

---

*This section includes papers authored by the conveners for each sector in the sectoral strategy process and presented at the workshop. The papers report the perspectives identified in the course of the discussions and are not intended as consensus statements.

5

Patients

Coordinator

Joyce Dubow, AARP

Other Contributors

Jennifer Bright, Mental Health America; Maureen Corry, Childbirth Connection; Carolina Hinestrosa, National Breast Cancer Coalition; Ann Kempski, SEIU; Carol Sakala, Childbirth Connection; Gail Shearer, Consumers Union

SECTOR OVERVIEW

The U.S. healthcare system is in crisis. Healthcare quality is, at best, uneven, with wide variation based on geography and patient characteristics, such as age, gender, race, and ethnicity. Although the United States spends more of its gross domestic product on health care than any other nation, higher spending does not necessarily yield better outcomes.

Since 2000, health insurance costs have increased by 87 percent (Kaiser Family Foundation/Health Research and Educational Trust, 2006). As healthcare costs continue to escalate, employers and workers find it increasingly difficult to afford coverage. The percentage of those with employer-sponsored coverage dropped from 60.2 percent in 2005 to 59.7 percent in 2006 (U.S. Census Bureau, 2007). Although the decline between 2006 and 2005 was slight, the continuing trend is troubling. Moreover, 47 million were uninsured (U.S. Census Bureau, 2007). In the United States, 42 percent of people with chronic conditions report that they have skipped medications, not seen a doctor, or forgone recommended care because of costs (Schoen et al., 2007). A principal factor contributing to increasing long-term health expenditures is adoption of new technologies and innovations that have not undergone adequate scrutiny to determine comparative clinical or cost-effectiveness (Centers for Medicare and Medicaid Services, 2007; Davis et al., 2007; U.S. House Committee on Appropriations, Subcommittee on Military Construction, Veterans Affairs, and Related Agencies, 2007) as well as regional differences in the use of supply-sensitive services (Regenstreif, 2005).

In addition, as noted by the Institute of Medicine, patients are often frustrated with their inability to participate as full partners in their health care (Institute of Medicine, 2001). Inconvenient access to care, a lack of information to inform decision making, cultural and linguistic barriers, financial impediments to service, and, too often, the "tone" of the physician-patient relationship are just a few of the reasons for patient frustration and dissatisfaction.

Exacerbating the problems of escalating costs and quality gaps is the dearth of reliable evidence to inform clinician and patient decisions. A substantial portion of the medical care delivered in the United States is not based on or supported by evidence, although experts differ on the degree to which this is the case (Learning What Works Best, 2007). Despite the potential that the development, dissemination, and implementation of better evidence holds for patients, the infrastructure and financing required to pursue the necessary research are lacking. As a result, information on effectiveness is "almost never available" (Smith, 1991). Even when it is available (for example, for pregnancy and childbirth), it is not widely applied or may be used or interpreted inconsistently.

As the end users of health care, consumers and patients would realize great benefit from a reengineered healthcare system designed to achieve improved quality and safety as well as greater efficiency and cost reduction (Shortell et al., 2007). Thus, they have a vested interest in seeing that the scientific basis for care expands. Yet, in general, the public is not aware of the concept of evidence-based medicine (EBM), nor does the current terminology used to describe the concept resonate with consumers when it is presented to them (Shore and Carman, 2006).

The structure and process for generating evidence and evaluating comparative effectiveness must instill confidence among all stakeholders, including consumers-patients, that the research supporting the information is valid and fair. An independent, unbiased entity could potentially have the requisite credibility among all parties if it conducted investigations in accordance with acceptable scientific standards and operated in a fully transparent manner. Such a trusted intermediary for evidence could build and maintain public support by disseminating meaningful and reliable information.

For consumers and patients, trust in the process would be enhanced if research topics were significant and important to them. Full transparency and disclosure, as well as open and inclusive processes in the identification of research priorities, the formulation of research questions, and the development and application of evidence, are essential.

Consumers believe that they are justifiably suspicious of the motivation of entities offering healthcare guidance and advice if these organizations have conflicting interests. Instilling confidence in EBM is further complicated by the fact that choice—a cherished value among consumers and a proxy for quality—could be constrained by the application of evidence (e.g., the tiering of benefits and coverage determinations) (Office of New York State Attorney General Andrew M. Cuomo, 2007). Some consumer groups consider that the application of EBM may be a backdoor way to ration healthcare benefits or deny coverage. Therefore, steps must be taken to ensure that, in the guise of applying the "best evidence," individuals are not inappropriately denied the needed care. Education would help consumers better understand EBM as a means to improving quality and safety and ensuring appropriate care, not as a tool to unfairly or arbitrarily justify the denial of treatment. As a policy matter, it will be necessary to determine the proper balance between the need for standardizing care and addressing individual needs by allowing appeals and exception processes when the need for deviating from standard practices arises.

Consumers need to be supported to help them understand options, benefits, harms, probabilities, and scientific uncertainties (O'Connor et al., 2003). They also need assistance to clarify their personal values in relation to the benefits and the potential harms of particular interventions. The research literature finds that consumers have an "optimism bias" that causes them to consistently underestimate personal risk, particularly when they consider hazards that they perceive as having a low probability of occurring (Hibbard et al., 2003). Therefore, they may overestimate the benefits of a particular treatment option, whereas they may downplay potential harms (Brownlee, 2007). Decision aids or shared-decision-making programs can supplement the counseling that practitioners provide. Findings from studies assessing decision support programs suggest that patients who use these tools achieve increased knowledge, have more realistic expectations about the benefits and harms of the treatment options, and feel less uncertainty about feeling uninformed (O'Connor et al., 2003). For example, patients using decision aids were 21 to 44 percent less likely to choose a surgical procedure for back pain, excessive bleeding, and angina (O'Connor et al., 2003). Nevertheless, although many decision tools have been tested in randomized trials and can help patients formulate decisions, far too few tools have undergone such rigorous investigation, considering the breadth of decisions that consumers must make (O'Connor et al., 2003). Experts also advise that patients and physicians perceive the decision tools to be fair, accurate, and balanced (Kasper et al., 1992).

In addition, comparative reports using measures that are based on evidence-based guidelines could inform consumer decisions in selecting health plans and providers. Appropriate research methods, such as cognitive and usability testing, should be applied to ensure that the intended audience understands the materials developed for consumer use. The difficulties that consumers may have with information on healthcare quality are not necessarily because they are "confused" or because the information is too technical. Rather, the information that is currently available is not always interesting or relevant to consumers, particularly because it is not typically available at the level of analysis that is the most meaningful to patients (i.e., at the physician or practice level).

However, there are strategies that could mitigate some of these concerns. Efforts are under way on many fronts to guide the development and presentation of information used to inform consumer choices. To cite just two examples from multistakeholder consensus initiatives, a workgroup on cost/price transparency of the Quality Alliance Steering Committee (Health Care Quality Leaders Join Forces, 2006) has drafted principles for reporting cost and price information to consumers; and in April 2006 the AQA Alliance, a multistakeholder consensus group that focuses on physician-level measurement, endorsed principles for public reports that include specific guidance for consumer reports (AQA Alliance, 2006). In addition, the Aligning Forces for Quality program is doing extensive research, including focus groups and surveys, to determine how best to communicate with the public on health care quality.

Evidence-based content to help consumers understand healthcare quality needs to be supported by communication strategies that promote clear, understandable messages directed to target audiences through appropriate channels (Robert Wood Johnson Foundation-Aligning Forces for Quality, 2007). Strategies to advance EBM should include communication and educational approaches designed to engage consumer organizations as well as help individuals understand how EBM relates to their personal experience and its potential to improve quality and safety and to achieve savings. These messages need to recognize the uncertainty in medicine and the need for patients to make trade-offs as they weigh the available options with input from their clinicians (Fraenkel and McGraw, 2007). Communication strategies can be designed to improve understanding and allay confusion. Although health information is clearly more complex and laden with subjective factors, communication initiatives can be informed by other disciplines, such as the financial industry, that have found ways to communicate effectively with consumers about complex topics (Pronovost et al., 2007).

Sector Profile

Before the sector is described, it is important to address the fact that "consumer" organizations do not all refer to themselves using this term. For example, some prefer to call themselves "patient advocates." A recent survey of 2,809 people determined that of the possible labels—patient, individual, person, consumer, client, customer, or other—healthcare recipients preferred the terms *individual* and *patient* (32 and 31 percent, respectively). Only 7 percent of those surveyed preferred the term *consumer* (Robert Wood Johnson Foundation, 2007). In general, the most suitable term depends on the context in which it is used. Thus, when an individual is receiving healthcare services, she or he is appropriately described as a *patient*. When the individual is considering insurance options, the term *customer* or *consumer* may be more suitable. This statement attempts to take the context into account, but this is not necessarily a signal for a strong preference for any particular descriptor except to recognize that terminology is situational.

Consumers are not monolithic, nor are the organizations that represent them. Just as demographic characteristics, education, and socioeconomic factors distinguish individuals, organizations representing consumers and patients differ with respect to size, purpose, organizational structure, governance, and source of funding. Financial support may come from membership fees, dues, philanthropy, or other sources. It should be noted that the source of funding is often a contentious and divisive issue among consumer organizations. Finally, some consumer organizations emphasize local action and rely on grassroots support. Others have broad-based memberships and have both a local and a national orientation. Still other groups gain impact from targeted expertise, whereas many consumer organizations provide services for members and advocate for public policy change.

Table 5-1 offers a typology of the types of organizations that represent and reflect consumer perspectives; groups rarely belong in only a single category, and they typically engage in multiple activities and have multiple objectives and purposes.

Consumer organizations affect public policy in various ways. For example, Consumers Union emphasizes its objectivity and independence from vested interests. Labor unions, such as Service Employees International Union, affect the healthcare marketplace through their influence on employer-sponsored benefit design and their advocacy before state and federal policy makers. Others, such as AARP, bring the strength of numbers as well as a politically active cadre of volunteers to influence federal and state legislative and regulatory bodies. The National Breast Cancer Coalition establishes public policy and legislative priorities in research and access to health care and mobilizes its nationwide grass roots to enact its agenda and also trains and educates its members to promote systems change to achieve its mission of ending breast cancer.

In addition to individual organizational efforts, consumer groups work collaboratively among themselves as well as with other stakeholders or in ad hoc coalitions to improve quality, advance public accountability, promote health insurance coverage, and carry out other initiatives. For

TABLE 5-1 Typology of Organizations That Represent and Reflect Consumer Perspectives

Focus	Example
Condition specific	National Breast Cancer Coalition, Childbirth Connection, Mental Health America, Epilepsy Foundation, American Diabetes Association
Advocacy	AARP, Consumers Union, National Breast Cancer Coalition, Childbirth Connection, Mental Health America, Families USA, National Consumers League, National Health Council
Public education	Consumers Union, AARP, NBCC, Childbirth Connection, Mental Health America, Center for the Study of Services/ *CheckBook* magazine, National Health Council
Labor unions	Service Employees International Union, National Education Association, American Federation of Labor and Congress of Industrial Organizations
Population specific (e.g., by age, gender, or race/ethnicity/culture)	National Partnership for Women and Families, AARP, Children's Defense Fund
Targeted purpose (e.g., family support)	Family Voices, National Alliance on Mental Illness, Alzheimer's Association
Broad, crosscutting/ consensus building	Consumers United for Evidence-Based Healthcare, National Health Council

NOTE: Many organizations represent consumers from multiple perspectives.

example, the Alliance for Better Health Care, is a coalition of consumers, employers, unions, providers, health plans, pharmacists, and researchers who share the conviction that high-quality health care requires good evidence to support sound medical decision making (Alliance for Better Health Care, 2007). The National Working Group on Evidence-Based Healthcare is a mixed stakeholder coalition consisting of consumers, disease-specific groups, caregivers, practitioners, and caregivers that educates and advocates for issues about evidence.

ACTIVITY CATEGORIES

Policy advocacy and participation in national policy development to promote quality, safety, comparative effectiveness, and consumer protections.

A considerable amount of public policy advocacy is already under way among consumer organizations. Several advocate (independently or collaboratively with other organizations) in support of funding for comparative effectiveness research (e.g., expansion of Section 1013 of the Medicare Prescription Drug, Improvement, and Modernization Act of 2003); the establishment of a stable and independent infrastructure for comparative effectiveness research; funding for public health efforts in support of evidence-based prevention and screening; the acquisition of additional resources for the Food and Drug Administration to conduct postmarketing surveillance after drugs and devices have been approved; greater transparency of cost and quality information, as well as the disclosure of proprietary relationships that may influence treatment recommendations; secure, electronic, interoperable health information exchange; changes to medical school curriculums and continuing education to address quality improvement and application of EBM; reform that aligns payment with performance objectives; funding for a national U.S. subscription to *The Cochrane Library* that would give all residents free access to this resource; and the development of model informed consent statements.

Representation of the consumer-patient perspective on policy-making boards, task forces, and committees to articulate and advance consumer preferences and needs, build capacity within the consumer sector to participate effectively with technical experts, and help professionals understand the essential role of full consumer participation on such bodies.

There is growing recognition of the value of having consumer and patient representation on decision-making and advisory bodies in the healthcare sector, but there are not sufficient numbers of well-trained individuals to fulfill the growing demand for this type of representation.

Consumer organizations acknowledge the importance of enlarging their ranks of qualified consumer-patient spokespeople. To effectively represent consumer and patient views in policy development, the design of research agendas, and the implementation of public policies, train-the-trainer and train-the-advocates programs are needed to enlarge the consumer advocacy base. Such programs should include training on the fundamental concepts of the research disciplines and areas of policy that consumers seek to influence. For example, Consumers United for Evidence-Based Healthcare has developed online modules to provide consumer advocates with critical appraisal skills. The National Breast Cancer Coalition (NBCC) developed Project LEAD, a family of science courses for consumer activists that has trained almost 1,300 individuals. The NBCC courses cover basic science, epidemiology, biostatistics, concepts of evidence-based health care, and consumer advocacy. There are advanced courses in clinical trials and quality care. Faculty members are researchers and experts in adult learning. These training efforts have enabled the meaningful participation of consumers at all levels on research programs, most notably, the U.S. Department of Defense Breast Cancer Research Program, collaborations on specific clinical trials, and patient-led strategic consensus processes.

Development and dissemination of valid and reliable information that is publicly available, provided by trusted sources, and disseminated either directly or through intermediaries.

In general, information should be meaningful and useful for end users (consumers, purchasers, etc.). The content should help consumers understand risk and uncertainty and how to use complex systematic reviews and treatment guidelines; information on the benefits and harms of preventive, diagnostic, monitoring, and therapeutic interventions; and the evidence behind standards of care. Such information should help inform patient decisions and activate them so that they can establish an effective partnership in their care. Information should address condition-specific inventories of (1) evidence that is ready to be implemented, (2) disproven practices, (3) practices with trade-offs that should be carefully weighed, and (4) effective practices with few or no known harms.

Experts advise that the manner of presentation can be as important as the content itself (Hibbard et al., 2003). Materials need to use plain English (and other languages, as appropriate) in easily understandable and evaluable formats. Health literacy and numeracy levels need to be assessed and taken into account when information is designed, as do the cultural and socioeconomic factors that may affect a target audience.

It is generally understood that it is most efficient and effective to take advantage of the multiple opportunities to influence consumer decision making at the time of greatest impact—the "teachable moment." These moments typically occur when people are contemplating the choice of health plans, health professional, hospital, skilled nursing facilities, and so forth; at the time of a diagnosis when the selection of a treatment option is required; when self-management techniques are presented; when a patient is considering whether or not to participate in a clinical trial; and as patients contemplate healthy lifestyle changes, such as changes to their diet or to their exercise and physical activity patterns, smoking cessation, and substance abuse prevention and treatment. For pregnant women, the 9-month prenatal period offers a window of opportunity to provide them with information based on the best available evidence to help them make informed decisions about maternity and newborn care.

In reaching out to educate consumers about EBM, it is necessary to communicate with general consumer audiences as well as consumer groups that represent specific health conditions and specific populations on the basis of socioeconomic or demographic characteristics. To achieve the maximum impact, communications specialists advise the appropriate segmentation of target audiences. Research should be conducted to identify these segments (on the basis of, for example, patient characteristics, health status, disease, decision-making skill, or health literacy level) so that materials can be customized for different audiences. Studies are needed to identify and evaluate effective dissemination approaches. The research agenda should test print formats (e.g., different lengths, fonts, colors, and graphics), refine assessment tools to determine individuals' health literacy skills, test formats and content in different languages, determine whether different media are more effective, and identify those who are the most trusted and effective intermediaries. Finally, as noted earlier, decision aids are valuable tools that can be used to support evidenced-informed decisions. Therefore, an important research focus should be the expansion of evidence-based decision aids.

There are many good examples of effective dissemination approaches that adapt conventional educational vehicles to advance evidence-based frameworks. For example, Childbirth Connection makes relevant evidence-based resources accessible to health professionals by specialty area in the health professional area of its website, where it maintains an Evidence-Based Maternity Care Resource Directory; Childbirth Connection also has, since 2003, contributed a quarterly column, Current Resources for Evidence-Based Practice, that is published simultaneously in the official journals of the leading U.S. maternity nurses association and of the leading U.S. midwifery association. Information can be disseminated in waiting rooms; on pharmacy counters; in libraries and schools; and through community organizations (e.g., senior organizations), health insurance plans, pharmacy benefit managers, and employers and human resources departments. Specialized websites help consumers obtain the most accurate, reliable information.

Public education efforts to focus on building broad public awareness of quality issues using multiple, segment-appropriate media (e.g., newspapers and magazines, public service announcements, brochures, television, and radio).

It may be instructive to examine other public-interest initiatives to determine whether lessons may be learned from public campaigns on smoking, drunk driving, human immunodeficiency virus transmission and safe sex, and so forth or from the efforts of the Partnership for a Drug-Free America. It may also be instructive to consider the regulation of commercial advertising and marketing practices in support of EBM. Equally important are education messages and tools tailored for caregivers, such as family members, who may need to have such information to assist their loved ones with navigating complex healthcare choices.

An important component of public education is education of members of the mainstream media on how to report on sophisticated medical research to a general audience and improvement of the accuracy of medical reporting and the presentation and evaluation of evidence and new healthcare interventions. (See, for example, www.healthnewsreview. org; the Kaiser Family Foundation health policy journalism fellowships may serve as a model that can be used to promote better reporting and to stimulate journalists' interest in this area.)

Finally, education initiatives should not overlook opportunities to train clinicians to communicate more effectively with patients, enhance clinician awareness of the wide range of health literacy and decision-making skills among consumers, as well as train clinicians on the need to respond appropriately to consumer cultural and language preferences. Ultimately, medical education and training need to be revamped to become more patient focused, to incorporate courses on patient communication to teach physicians how to foster patient autonomy and self-management, and to encourage patient engagement in decision making.

Consumer participation in research and research design is important to ensure that the research is transparent, is clinically important, reflects consumers' interests and preferences, and helps answer questions of clinical relevance to patients (e.g., does the use of magnetic resonance imaging for breast cancer screening among certain at-risk populations lead to decreased mortality or just to more diagnoses?) For example, Childbirth Connection commissions and conducts research to fill priority gaps in knowledge of special interest to consumers. It involves consumers from North America on the Cochrane Pregnancy and Childbirth Group's Consumer Panel. These consumers act as referees of draft systematic reviews to help improve the quality of the reviews and ensure that they meet the needs of consumers.

Environmental Scan

Public Views on Quality

In 2006, only 13 percent of Americans thought that the healthcare system was working well, although the vast majority did not believe that it had reached a state of crisis (Blendon et al., 2006). It is noteworthy that whether or not one has comprehensive and secure health insurance coverage affects public attitudes. In addition, despite their dissatisfaction with the healthcare system, 84 percent rated the medical care that they received as either "excellent" or "good."

Perceptions of Quality

Experts generally agree that consumer perceptions are a valid and important dimension in assessing healthcare quality. The Agency for Healthcare Research and Quality (AHRQ) has funded the development of a suite of consumer surveys (Consumer Assessment of Healthcare Providers and Systems [CAHPS]) designed to probe aspects of care (1) about which consumers and patients are the best source of information and (2) that consumers and patients have identified as being important. The National CAHPS Benchmarking Database (Agency for Healthcare Research and Quality, 2007), the national repository for data from the CAHPS family of surveys, is an important resource for survey sponsors, researchers, and others interested in using comparative CAHPS survey results and detailed benchmark data. Other patient surveys also assess patients' experiences with their care, including Childbirth Connection's national Listening to Mothers surveys, which elicit women's childbearing experiences and evaluations of their care (Declerqc et al., 2006), and the Experience of Care and Health Outcomes Survey, which assesses patients' experiences with behavioral health services in managed care plans and behavioral healthcare organizations.

Information Preferences

The type of information that consumers request is often different from the types of information most typically available. *CheckBook* magazine, published by the nonprofit Center for the Study of Services, found that the type of physician rating information that its subscribers prefer to have first is how the surveyed doctors rated other doctors when the surveyed doctors were asked which doctors they would consider to be the most desirable as the provider of care of a loved one (as opposed to, for example, information about how doctors rated when various healthcare system records were used to measure how well doctors keep costs down) (Krughoff, 2007). *CheckBook* magazine also confirms other research that consumers value information about how well their doctors communicate (listening and explaining to patients).

Although the proportion of consumers who use information about healthcare quality for decision making is growing, in 2006, only about 20 percent reported that they had seen information about health insurance plans, hospitals, or doctors and then factored such information into a decision (Kaiser Family Foundation/Agency for Healthcare Research and Quality, 2006). An earlier Kaiser Family Foundation/AHRQ study found that those who had seen information did not use the quality information because the information that they saw was not specific to their personal health conditions or concerns; factors other than quality, such as location or cost, were more important to their decision making; and the information that they saw about quality was confusing or difficult to understand (Kaiser Family Foundation/Agency for Healthcare Research and Quality/Harvard School of Public Health, 2004). Finally, with respect to medical errors, the vast majority of patients (87 percent) believe that physicians should be required to tell patients if a preventable medical error resulting in serious harm was made in their care.

Decision Making

Many people have difficulty managing the volume of information that they receive and identifying which information will best promote their values and preferences. Evidence shows that people can process and use only a limited number of variables and that having to differentially weight multiple factors in making trade-offs increases the cognitive burden in decision making (Hibbard et al., 2003). Furthermore, many consumers, particularly some older individuals, are burdened by having to make choices and are likely to need assistance (Hibbard et al., 2000). Therefore, in developing communication strategies, the research findings that describe how consumers use information must be built on and the decision-making skills of target audiences must also be considered by employing methods that lower the cognitive effort required to make decisions. Effective techniques include summarizing and interpreting information for users and helping them apply the information to their personal situations through the use of narratives or testimonials (Demchak, 2007b).

A 2004 national survey found that although most people want to be asked whether they prefer to be offered choices and asked their opinions by their doctors, preferences for participation in decision making vary by age, ethnicity, and gender. Women and those who are healthier and better educated prefer to be involved, whereas respondents who are African American, Hispanic, or over age 45 years are more likely to prefer that their physicians make the decisions (Levinson et al., 2005). The authors of the study conclude, "While a collaborative model of decision making is popular and may be desirable, it is by no means universally held by the public" (Levinson et al., 2005). However, other research finds that among those who do prefer to collaborate in their care, less than half achieve their preferred level of participation in their own care (Fraenkel and McGraw, 2007).

Patient Engagement

Patients who are more engaged, confident, and informed make better healthcare decisions. Using a tool (Hibbard et al., 2004) that she and her colleagues developed to assess patient knowledge, skill, and confidence for self-management, Judith Hibbard of the University of Oregon estimates that in a national sample of adults ages 45 years and older, approximately 40 percent score in the low end of the activation measure, which indicates that they do not recognize their need to play an active role in their own care; individuals who are sicker tend to have lower scores than the general population.[1] However, the degree of patient activation can be modified with strategies designed to encourage engagement (Demchak, 2007b).

Health Literacy and Numeracy

Health literacy is the "degree to which individuals have the capacity to obtain, process, and understand basic health information and services needed to make appropriate health decisions" (Institute of Medicine, 2004). More than 47 percent of adults in the United States have difficulty locating, matching, and integrating information in texts (Institute of Medicine, 2004). The capacity to navigate successfully in the healthcare system requires patients to have adequate health literacy skills. It is important to recognize that the level of health literacy required is situation specific: more complex and complicated healthcare situations require higher, more advanced skills. Thus, even if an individual is able to read materials whose content is familiar, unfamiliar subjects or concepts may be more difficult to understand. The level of functional health literacy has been found to be "markedly lower" among older individuals, even after adjustment for the higher prevalence of dementia or other cognitive impairment, chronic disease, or other health conditions in that population (Dubow, 2004). An analysis of the content of English- and Spanish-language healthcare-related websites indicated that, as written, the sites required a high school or higher level of reading ability (Berland et al., 2001).

Studies that seek to determine whether information presentation methods differentially influence consumers with different numeric skills find that "less is more," particularly for those with lower numeracy skills (Peters et al., 2007). Of course, all materials should be written clearly and precisely so that they are understood by their intended audiences, including culturally diverse population groups. It is also important to assess the content and format for their appropriateness for older consumers. AHRQ's website Talking Quality.gov provides guidance on presenting information on healthcare quality to consumers and includes guidance on designing materials. Similarly, www.usability.gov, a website maintained by the U.S. Department of Health and Human Services, provides guidance on creating websites that are usable and useful and that contains an automated usability tool, the Usability Test Environment, to allow federal website managers to

---

[1]Personal communication, J. Hibbard and J. Dubow, AARP Public Policy Institute, Washington, DC, 2007.

design their websites in citizen-centric formats (U.S. Department of Health and Human Services, 2007).

Health Information Technology

Health information technology (HIT) is a critical enabling tool that can advance quality improvement and safety and, eventually, achieve savings through better decision support for clinicians and patients, as well as enhance physician-patient communication. The vast majority of consumers believe that personal health records will improve the quality of health care (Markle Foundation, 2005). About one-third of adults report creating their own set of medical records so that their providers can have access to the information that the patients consider important (Kaiser Family Foundation/Agency for Healthcare Research and Quality, 2006).

Consumers support the creation of a nationwide health information exchange for doctors and hospitals (Markle Foundation, 2005). A recent survey conducted for eHealth Initiative offers guidance on how healthcare providers should communicate to consumers about health information exchange: the message that appears to be the most salient to consumers is "having access to information in an emergency medical situation" (eHealth Initiative, 2007). In addition, they respond favorably to messages from their doctors about the importance of electronic information exchange.

Nevertheless, consumers are concerned about the privacy of their personal health information. It is noteworthy that 73 percent of racial and ethnic minority respondents and 67 percent of those with a chronic illness expressed such concerns in a 2005 nationwide survey on health privacy (California HealthCare Foundation, 2005). Underscoring the value that they place in participating in HIT policy development, consumer organizations have set forth a set of principles to guide electronic information sharing that address transparency, access to and the use of personal health information, individual control, data security, and the enforcement of privacy protections (Detmer and Steen, 2006). In addition, although consumer advocates appreciate the potential for HIT to facilitate data sharing, a broad consensus on the secondary uses of health information data remains to be achieved. In support of the more widespread adoption of HIT and in recognition of the criticality of consumer confidence in the system's ability to protect personal health information, consumer organizations have been advocating for an overarching set of privacy and data security policies to govern federally funded and sanctioned HIT efforts.

Knowledge of EBM

As noted earlier in this chapter, there are widespread challenges to the adoption of evidence-based health care. The American Institutes for Research (AIR) conducted focus groups on communication about EBM and found that improved safety and transparency are salient to consumers, although the terminology, in general, is not (Shore and Carman, 2006). A 2004 AARP survey of a nationally representative sample of Americans ages 50 years old and over found that the majority of respondents said that it was very important to them to have access to information that allows them to evaluate different prescription drugs on their effectiveness, safety, and cost (AARP, 2004). More than 80 percent also said that it was very important that pharmaceutical companies be required to publish information about the effectiveness of their medications for the treatment of specific conditions. A 2005 AARP survey of Hispanic New York City dwellers 18 years of age and older found that 90 percent said that it was "very important" (70 percent) or "somewhat important" (20 percent) for the state to provide access to information that compares the safety and effectiveness of prescription drugs (AARP, 2006).

AIR's work suggests that targeting certain types of consumers is a reasonable strategy because patients with chronic diseases are more likely to seek evidence than others. Effective messengers should thus be used to target certain types of consumers. Effective messengers are those who are considered objective and credible, as well as peers who share demographic characteristics or the same condition. In addition, organizations that are perceived to have a stake in the outcome (e.g., employers) should partner with other organizations to convey information on EBM.

LEADERSHIP COMMITMENTS AND INITIATIVES

Transformational Opportunities Through Collaboration

Because multiple factors deter informed decision making, these obstacles must be removed to achieve reform. Most consumers do not have access to "good" information on treatment options or provider performance on which to base their healthcare decisions and rarely have enough information to make informed decisions (Demchak, 2007a). Even if information were available, many consumers do not have the requisite skills to apply it in their own best interest. Transformation from the status quo, in which health care is fragmented and provider focused, to a system of care that is coordinated and designed with the patient at its center will require major changes in every sector. By their very nature, the transformational opportunities necessitate collaborative engagement and shared accountability. Acting alone, no stakeholder will likely attain the desired outcomes.

First, to achieve the Roundtable's objective of transforming the way in which evidence on clinical effectiveness is generated and used to improve health and health care, consumer organizations will have to join with other stakeholders to advocate for the establishment of an independent, public-private entity tasked with coordinating comparative effectiveness research whose analyses are objective and fully transparent. This will involve achieving consensus on the structure and purpose of such an entity.

Second, although there is already agreement among stakeholder groups for the need to promote an accountability and transparency agenda (initially, using the existing body of evidence) that makes evidence-based information on cost and quality publicly available, more work needs to be done to improve the type and level of information. HIT—an essential enabling tool—will be integral to this transformation to facilitate access to and the dissemination of valuable information that is not now readily available. Promoting the widespread adoption of HIT with appropriate and effective protections for personal health information presents yet another opportunity for broad collaborative initiatives.

Less advanced are efforts to support informed patient decision making. A transformation to a well-informed, highly motivated patient as the norm rather than the exception rests on helping patients become more active partners in their health, improving patient-physician communication, and revamping medical education curriculums to help providers recognize the need for them to become better aware of their patients' decision-making skills and preferences. Medical education also needs to help physicians and other health professionals acquire motivational communications skills to increase consumer and patient engagement.

Hibbard and colleagues (2004) have identified approaches to improving patient activation. These include participatory rather than didactic programs, family involvement, and the deployment of multiple rather than single strategies (Demchak, 2007b). Customized patient support programs that recognize an individual's level of activation help people achieve self-efficacy through incremental successes. Providers can foster success by identifying their patients' levels of activation and then tailoring their coaching and support for patient self-management. Continued research to develop and test decision support tools for patients and educational and screening approaches for providers are needed and are areas ripe for cross-sector collaboration.

Finally, the ultimate transformation to a healthcare system that is patient focused, better integrated, and better coordinated will require not only changes in the delivery of care but also the realignment of the provider payment system. To effect genuine change, payment must be aligned with the desired outcomes. Ideally, reimbursement approaches will be episode based to reflect how patients actually experience care.

NEXT STEPS

Opportunities for Cross-Sector Collaborations

The goal of this sector group is to ensure that health care is evidence based and that consumers benefit from a healthcare system that is continuously learning through clinical research. The desire is to foster improved communication between the physician and the patient to ensure that care is informed by the best evidence and that resources are allocated to research to expand the evidence base. Activities should build toward giving providers and patients a better understanding of the value of EBM and its contribution to patient outcomes and improved quality. However, to enhance the likelihood of achieving success, it is important to have realistic expectations of the challenges of educating the public and to be mindful that, as yet, EBM is not well understood or widely accepted by consumers.

Going forward, it is critical to ensure that patients are at the table during all activities, including setting priorities, formulating research questions, establishing the study design, and peer review of proposals. An agenda of transparency and public accountability among providers at all levels of the system must continue to be promoted, and the publication and dissemination of information on comparative cost and quality must be continued. To better understand how the desired audiences may be reached, a more refined understanding of the audience segments is required, including the identification of criteria for prioritizing the audiences and the patient populations to be targeted for outreach and education. Further research on communication approaches to reach mass audiences would help. Several recent communication initiatives may inform the development of the core messages, including the AHRQ and Ad Council campaign Questions Are the Answer, and several efforts by health plans (Aetna), the Joint Commission (Speak Up), and others. Communication and media specialists should advise on the development of a campaign strategy. The Roundtable has convened a workgroup to convene experts to offer guidance on how to proceed and is a useful and necessary point of departure. Consumers and patients will not fully accept HIT unless their privacy concerns are resolved. Finally, it will be necessary to identify and resolve issues of trust among collaborating stakeholders, perhaps working with neutral third parties to convene conversations among drug and device makers and consumer advocates to develop better communication and collaboration and to clarify areas of agreement and disagreement.

In summary, consumer organizations have identified several areas in which cross-sector collaboration would accelerate change and in which each sector has an appropriate role to play. These include advocacy for

- an enhanced research capacity (including funding and training) to determine the comparative effectiveness of all types of treatment and pharmaceutical interventions under different circumstances;
- greater transparency and the availability of comparative performance information across all settings and collaboration with providers, plans, and employers to develop quality and efficiency measurement for public reporting;
- improved means of capturing clinical data to accelerate evidence development, particularly on late effects and the effect on the general population after the initial demonstration of efficacy in controlled clinical trials; and
- the more widespread adoption of HIT that ensures secure data sharing while protecting patient privacy.

In addition, there are opportunities for consumers-employees to work with employers and purchasers to reach a consensus on the mutually acceptable use of EBM in benefit design, benefit tiering, and cost sharing and to collaborate with researchers on the design and testing of decision support tools to ensure that they meet consumer needs. Finally, work should be initiated to enlist increased media attention and engagement in EBM issues.

REFERENCES

AARP. 2004. *Telephone survey.* October. Washington, DC.
———. 2006. *Survey of Hispanic New Yorkers, prescription drug affordability.* Washington, DC.
Agency for Healthcare Research and Quality. 2007. *The national CAHPS benchmarking database.* https://www.cahps.ahrq.gov/content/ncbd/ncbd_Intro.asp?p=105&s=5 (accessed November 2007).
Alliance for Better Health Care. 2007. U.S. House, Ways and Means Committee, Subcommittee on Health. *Alliance for Better Health Care statement for the record on strategies to increase information on comparative clinical effectiveness,* June 12.
AQA Alliance. 2006. *AQA principles for public reports on health care,* April. http://www.aqaalliance.org/files/ConsumerPrinciplesMay06.doc (accessed November 2007).
Berland, G., L. S. Morales, M. N. Elliott, J. I. Algazy, R. L. Kravitz, M. S. Broder, D. E. Kanouse, J. A. Munoz, J. Hauser, M. Lara, K. Watkins, H. Yang, J. A. Puyol, L. Escalante, J. Hicks, A. Griffin, K. Ricci, R. H. Brook, E. A. McGlynn. 2001. *Proceed with caution: A report on the quality of health information on the Internet.* Oakland, CA: California HealthCare Foundation and RAND Health.
Blendon, R. J., M. Brodie, J. M. Benson, D. E. Altman, and T. Buhr. 2006. Americans' views of health care costs, access, and quality. *Milbank Quarterly* 84(4):623-657.
Brownlee, S. 2007. Giving patients a larger voice. *The Washington Post,* October 23, p. F4.

California HealthCare Foundation. 2005. *National consumer health privacy survey—2005.* Oakland, CA.

Centers for Medicare and Medicaid Services. 2007. *National health expenditure accounts: Definitions, sources, and methods used in the NHEA 2004.* http://www.cms.hhs.gov/NationalHealthExpendData/downloads/dsm-04.pdf (accessed September 2007).

Davis, K., C. Schoen, S. Guterman, T. Shih, S. C. Schoenbaum, and I. Weinbaum. 2007. *Slowing the growth of U.S. health care expenditures: What are the options?* New York: Commonwealth Foundation. http://www.commonwealthfund.org/publications/publications_show.htm?doc_id=449510 (accessed November 2007).

Declerqc, E., C. Sakala, M. Corry, and S. Applebaum. 2006. *Listening to mothers 2: Report of the second national survey of U.S. women's childbearing experiences.* New York: Childbirth Connections.

Demchak, C. 2007a. *Choice in medical care: When should the consumer decide?* Issue brief 5. Washington, DC: AcademyHealth.

———. 2007b. *The elusive health care consumer: What will it take to activate patients?* Issue brief 2. Washington, DC: AcademyHealth.

Detmer, D., and E. Steen. 2006. *Learning from abroad: Lessons and questions on personal health records for national policy.* Washington, DC: AARP. http://www.esi-bethesda.com/ncrrworkshops/clinicalResearch/pdf/2006_10_phr_abroad_DED_AARP.pdf (accessed November 2007).

Dubow, J. 2004. *Adequate literacy and health literacy: Prerequisites for informed health care decision making.* Washington, DC: AARP Public Policy Institute.

eHealth Initiative. 2007. *A majority of consumers favor secure electronic health information exchange.* Washington, DC.

Fraenkel, L., and S. McGraw. 2007. What are the essential elements to enable patient participation in medical decision making? *Journal of General Internal Medicine* 22(5):614-619.

Health Care Quality Leaders Join Forces. 2006. *AQA and HQA collaborate to expedite national quality strategy.* Press release. Washington, DC: Agency for Healthcare Research and Quality. http://www.ahrq.gov/news/press/pr2006/aqahqapr.htm (accessed November 2007).

Hibbard, J., P. Slovic, E. Peters, and M. Finucane. 2000. *Older consumers' skill in using comparative date to inform health plan choice: A preliminary assessment.* Washington, DC: AARP Public Policy Institute.

Hibbard, J., J. Dubow, and E. Peters. 2003. *Decision making in consumer-directed health plans.* Publication 2003-05. Washington, DC: AARP Public Policy Institute.

Hibbard, J. H., J. Stockard, E. R. Mahoney, and M. Tusler. 2004. Development of the patient activation measure (PAM): Conceptualizing and measuring activation in patients and consumers. *Health Services Research* 39(4 Pt 1):1005-1026.

Institute of Medicine. 2001. *Crossing the quality chasm: A new health system for the 21st century.* Washington, DC: National Academy Press.

———. 2004. *Health literacy: A prescription top end confusion.* Washington, DC: The National Academies Press.

Kaiser Family Foundation/Agency for Healthcare Research and Quality/Harvard School of Public Health. 2004. *National survey on consumers' experiences with patient safety and quality information.* Menlo Park, CA: Author.

Kaiser Family Foundation/Agency for Healthcare Research and Quality. 2006. *Update on consumers' views of patient safety and quality information.* Menlo Park, CA: Author.

Kaiser Family Foundation/Health Research and Educational Trust. 2007. *Survey of employer health benefits.* http://www.kff.org/insurance/7527/upload/7527.pdf (accessed September 2007).

Kasper, J. F., A. G. Mulley, Jr., and J. E. Wennberg. 1992. Developing shared decision-making programs to improve the quality of health care. *Quality Review Bulletin* 18(6):183-190.

Krughoff, R. 2007. Advancing value-driven health care. Paper presented at Third Annual Incentive and Rewards Symposium, Philadelphia, PA, May 15.

Learning What Works Best. 2007. *The nation's need for evidence on comparative effectiveness in health care.* http://www.iom.edu/Object.File/Master/43/390/Comparative%20Effectiveness%20White%20Paper%20(F).pdf (accessed November 2007).

Levinson, W., A. Kao, A. Kuby, and R. A. Thisted. 2005. Not all patients want to participate in decision making. A national study of public preferences. *Journal of General Internal Medicine* 20(6):531-535.

Markle Foundation. 2005. *Attitudes of Americans regarding personal health records and nationwide electronic health information exchange: Key findings from two surveys of Americans.* New York, NY.

O'Connor, A. M., F. Legare, and D. Stacey. 2003. Risk communication in practice: The contribution of decision aids. *BMJ* 327(7417):736-740.

Office of New York State Attorney General Andrew M. Cuomo. 2007. *Attorney general Cuomo announces agreement with Cigna creating a new national model for doctor ranking programs.* Press release. Albany, NY.

Peters, E., N. Dieckmann, A. Dixon, J. H. Hibbard, and C. K. Mertz. 2007. Less is more in presenting quality information to consumers. *Medical Care Research and Review* 64(2):169-190.

Pronovost, P. J., M. Miller, and R. M. Wachter. 2007. The gap in quality measurement and reporting. *JAMA* 298(15):1800-1802.

Regenstreif, D. I. 2005. Medicare's cost crisis: Solutions are within our grasp. *Health Affairs* 24(Suppl 2):W5R90-W5R93.

Robert Wood Johnson Foundation. 2007. *Quality/equality survey results.* Washington, DC: Lake Research Partners.

Robert Wood Johnson Foundation-Aligning Forces for Quality. 2007. *The regional market project—healthy markets, healthy people: Accelerating change.* http://www.forces4quality.org/pdf/678.AF4QMeetingReport.finaldraft.pdf (accessed November 2007).

Schoen, C., R. Osborn, M. M. Doty, M. Bishop, J. Peugh, and N. Murukutla. 2007. Toward higher-performance health systems: Adults' health care experiences in seven countries, 2007. *Health Affairs* 26(6):w717-w734.

Shore, K., and K. Carman. 2006. *Communicating about evidence-based health care decisionmaking.* Washington, DC: American Institutes for Research.

Shortell, S. M., T. G. Rundall, and J. Hsu. 2007. Improving patient care by linking evidence-based medicine and evidence-based management. *JAMA* 298(6):673-676.

Smith, R. 1991. Where is the wisdom . . .? *BMJ* 303(6806):798-799.

U.S. Census Bureau. 2007. *Health insurance.* http://www.census.gov/hhes/www/hlthins/hlthin06/hlth06asc.html (accessed September 5, 2007).

U.S. Department of Health and Human Services. 2007. *Automated usability test environment (UTE) tool fact sheet.* http://www.usability.gov/refine/UTEfactsheet.html (accessed November 2007).

U.S. House Committee on Appropriations, Subcommittee on Military Construction, Veterans Affairs, and Related Agencies. 2007. *Health care spending: Public payers face burden of entitlement program growth, while all payers face rising prices and increasing use of services.* Report GAO-07-497T. Washington, DC: Government Accountability Office, February 15.

6

Healthcare Professionals

Coordinator

Rae-Ellen W. Kavey, National Heart, Lung, and Blood Institute

Other Contributors

Frank Ascione, University of Michigan; Lisa Bero, University of California, San Francisco; Linda Burns-Bolton, U.S. Department of Veterans Affairs; Barry Carter, University of Iowa; Gray Ellrodt, University of Massachusetts; Pat Ford-Roegner, American Academy of Nursing; Arthur Garson, Jr., University of Virginia; Ada Sue Hinshaw, University of Michigan; Cato T. Laurencin, University of Virginia; Rona F. Levin, Pace University; Daniel Malone, University of Arizona; Bernadette Melnyk, Arizona State University; Nancy H. Nielsen, American Medical Association; Kimberly Rask, Emory University; Jon Schommer, University of Minnesota; Glen Schumock, University of Illinois at Chicago; Cary Sennett, American Board of Internal Medicine; Lee Vermeulen, University of Wisconsin; Lynda Welage, University of Michigan

SECTOR OVERVIEW

Evidence-based practice (EBP) has been defined as "the integration of individual clinical expertise and patient preferences and values with the best available external clinical evidence from systematic research" (Sackett et al., 2000). Although healthcare professionals may believe that this is how they have always practiced, performance assessments indicate that this is not the case (McGlynn et al., 2003). A growing literature recommends the use of evidence-based management practices, but such recommendations are not consistently implemented. The behavior of healthcare professionals represents the critical juncture between the theory of evidence-based medicine (EBM) and actual EBP. Effective mechanisms that link knowledge development to the diffusion and adoption of that knowledge will be essential to promoting the use of EBM in clinical decision making.

In 2003, the Institute of Medicine (IOM) Committee on the Health Professions Education Summit developed a new vision for clinical education in the healthcare professions. The overarching goal is that "all health professionals will be educated to deliver patient-centric care as members of an interdisciplinary team, emphasizing EBP, quality improvement approaches, and informatics" (Institute of Medicine, 2003). The goal of this health professional sectoral strategy process is to support that vision, as it applies specifically to increasing use of EBM in clinical practice. The focus is on the delineation of strategies that will shift healthcare delivery away from the traditional physician-dominated practice and toward a concept of practice performed by interdisciplinary teams empowered to seek out and implement the best evidence for patient care. Such teams will have both the ability and expectation to continuously learn and change, through informed access to evidence-based clinical decision support, informatics, and clinical data repositories.

The potential scope of the sector includes all healthcare professionals. A minimal list would include physicians, nurses, nurse practitioners, physician's assistants, pharmacists, social workers, dietitians, physical and occupational therapists, and medical technologists. This discussion uses physicians, nurses, and pharmacists as representatives of the healthcare professional sector; but the concepts articulated here are intended for potential application to all healthcare professionals. The remainder of this chapter describes the current state of EBP, identifies key activity categories, and proposes potential transformative initiatives for each of these three types of healthcare professionals.

Physicians

The vision of physicians as members of teams in which each participant is empowered to seek out the best evidence for care is a new and powerful image. Achieving this vision will require profound change, but evidence-based health care will not occur without that change. Effective mechanisms that link knowledge development to the diffusion and adoption of that knowledge will be critical components in promoting the active use of EBM in clinical care. The broader dissemination of technologies that support the delivery of evidence-based care will clearly be essential; but the information collected for this report—summarized in the paragraphs below—suggests that the main issue here is not only technical but also cultural: commitment to the principles of evidence-based, team-directed, patient-centered care will require a fundamental change in what physicians understand to be their primary obligations as healthcare professionals. That change in culture and professional norms—from an emphasis on the physician as the knowledge expert to an emphasis on the physician as a team member whose role is to access and interpret relevant, timely, and appropriate information for delivery to the patient in conjunction with all members of the healthcare team—will drive the acquisition of the tools required to implement a vision of evidence-based care.

The primary construct of patient-centric care—that patients themselves are central to the process and are actively engaged in self-education and management—is one that necessitates a major shift in how physicians are trained and how they practice. Without such changes in culture and professional norms, physicians will fail to capitalize on opportunities to acquire and deploy the knowledge and technologies essential to achieving that vision of patient-centric care.

The implementation of any process requires an assessment of the existing state of the field. The current practicing physician population in the United States includes just less than 600,000 individuals; 86 percent of physicians are primarily involved in clinical practice, with 50 percent in practices with four colleagues or fewer, and of that 50 percent, 20 percent are in solo practice (American College of Physicians, 2005). Active practitioners range from those who have just completed training to those whose formal education occurred as long as 40 years ago. Actualization of the concepts of both EBM and practice quality assessment is also closely linked to access to information technology (IT). The rate of use of IT support systems, from handheld computers to completely electronic medical record (EMR) systems, is continuously increasing in medical practice; but less than 25 percent of physicians currently use some kind of EMR and 40 percent use a handheld computing device to support their practice (Gans et al., 2005; Garritty and El Emam, 2006; Jha et al., 2006). Of note, the rate of EMR adoption is the lowest among physicians in smaller practices. In addition, training in EBP is also a relatively new concept, with the time dedicated to training in EBM varying with the specialty and the training program (Green, 2000). With such diverse ranges of individuals, baseline knowledge, technical support systems, and practice settings, any recommendations for change must be broad, flexible, and incremental.

What is less well known but what can perhaps be inferred from data on behavior is how physicians perceive the technologies that are relevant to the implementation of EBM, that is, whether they perceive them to be important to their efforts to improve patient care. Clearly, one must be concerned that the slow adoption of healthcare IT—and the push back that has been apparent among leaders in the healthcare professions regarding efforts to promote quality measurement and industrial approaches to quality improvement based on that measurement—reflects a prevalent attitude that the adoption of healthcare IT is not necessarily in the best interests of patient care (Audet et al., 2005). The shift to electronically based practice is expensive, particularly in a solo or small group practice setting. The implementation of many IT practices can require major changes in clinical processes that can slow the delivery of care, especially during the early stages of their adoption. Promoting the use of technologies believed to be fundamental to the implementation of evidence-based care will have to address these issues to overcome practitioner resistance. Again, the most important set of activities in which the healthcare professional sector may have to engage may be related to changing that attitude.

Medical School Education

The process of integrating EBM into medical school education is already well under way. In 1999, the American Association of Medical Colleges identified the concepts of EBM as a critical objective for medical education (Medical School Objective Project Writing Group, 1999). As an intrinsic part of medical education, training in EBM provides individual physicians with critical search and appraisal skills for review of the medical literature, introduces the concept of continuous quality assessment as a routine of medical practice, and provides the basis for effective lifelong learning directly linked to patient care. Adoption of evidence-based recommendations optimizes the diagnosis and management of clinical conditions for which an evidence-based approach has been developed. One aspect of EBM that should make its adoption easier for current medical students is their nearly universal facility with IT as a routine part of daily life; maximizing this advantage should be considered in the development of changes in the medical school curriculum. From these precepts, medical school educators have introduced EBM into the medical school curriculum in a variety of ways. For example, innovative courses have transformed basic classes in epidemiology and statistics into intensely participatory discussions of cases designed to illustrate the principles of population health (Marantz et al., 2003). Preventive medicine has been integrated into clinical clerkships, and evidence-based decision making has become relatively standard during internal medicine rotations (Carey, 2000; Green, 2000). Evidence of the increased knowledge and use of EBM concepts in the first 3 years after medical school graduation is beginning to be reported; but as yet, there are few, if any, reports evaluating the use of EBM in posttraining clinical practice (Davidson et al., 2004; Dorsch et al., 2006).

Finally, assessment of medical students' knowledge of population health and evidence-based decision making needs to be a requirement for medical school graduation. A review of content outlines and sample questions from the National Board of Medical Examiners published in 2003 indicates no formal content of this kind (National Board of Medical Examiners, 2003).

Graduate Training

Beginning in 1999, the Accreditation Council for Graduate Medical Education (ACGME) Outcomes Project redesigned the curriculum for residency and fellowship training after graduation from medical school to focus on the outcomes of the training rather than program process measures (ACGME, 1999). The project defined six basic core competencies: medical knowledge, patient care, systems-based practice, professionalism, interpersonal/communication skills, and practice-based learning and improvement. Achievement of the last competency explicitly requires exposure to "investigation and evaluation of patient care practices, appraisal and assimilation of scientific evidence, and continuous improvement of patient care practices." There is a timeline for implementation of this new approach to resident education: at this time, all residency training programs must have begun to provide learning opportunities in the six defined competency domains, with the requirement for full integration of the training in the competencies and their assessment by June 2011 (ACGME, 1999).

The ACGME standards set a critical goal to provide residents with a practical working knowledge of EBP during their residency training that will allow them to provide optimal patient care on the basis of the best available evidence. Reports of early approaches to meeting the ACGME standards provide models of how evidence-based theory and EBP can be integrated into residency training; these approaches include exposures in multiple disciplines (Bradt and Moyer, 2003; Rucker and Morrison, 2000).

Ross and Verdieck (2003) have validated that this kind of educational exposure increases residents' knowledge of EBM and their use of EBM principles in practice during their residency training. Proof that this kind of training will be sustained into postresidency practice is not yet available, nor is evidence that such training will improve patient outcomes.

Education of Practicing Physicians

The challenge of increasing the practice of EBM among physicians in practice is formidable. Physicians represent a diverse group of individuals, not least because of the wide range of time from the completion of medical training to the present. For example, 18 percent of practicing physicians are between 55 and 64 years of age and completed medical school an average of 30 to 40 years ago (U.S. Department of Health and Human Services, 2003). Not surprisingly, the time that a physician has been out of residency training has been shown to correlate with a lower rate of adherence to evidence-based management and the greater use of tests and therapies with no proven benefit (Conway et al., 2006). Despite continuing medical education (CME), there will be many for whom the formal concept of EBM is completely unknown. Nonetheless, winning the minds and hearts of practicing physicians will be essential in achieving universal EBP. One potential mechanism for achieving this is CME, the standard approach to continuous learning for healthcare professionals. Currently, physicians are required to accrue a defined number of CME credits annually to maintain hospital privileges, qualify for relicensure, or maintain specialty certification. However, despite the clear demonstration that the pure dissemination of information has a limited impact on behavior change among physicians, traditional lecture formats persist as the most common form of CME. Randomized controlled trials of educational interventions have shown that for physicians automated reminders, patient-mediated interventions, outreach visits, and the use of opinion leaders are more effective behavior change strategies than CME. Training on quality assessment in practice based on EBM-based quality assessment with pre- and posttraining practice audits has also been used effectively to increase knowledge and the rate of implementation of EBM (Dexter et al., 2001; Hunt et al., 1998; Kuperman et al., 1996). With this uneven landscape as the starting point, flexible innovative approaches to increasing evidence-based clinical practice will be essential.

Although current medical school students and trainees have high levels of access to and comfort with computers and IT, these levels are highly variable among all medical practitioners (Gans et al., 2005; Garrity and El Emam, 2006; Jha et al., 2006). To remain up-to-date with recent evidence for optimal care, physicians need easy and immediate access to Internet-based knowledge repositories. A variety of computer-based clinical decision support systems have been shown to improve clinician performance and patient outcomes (Hunt et al., 1998; Kuperman et al., 1996) and to specifically increase the rate of use of evidence-based guidelines (Dexter et al., 2001). However, physicians currently have limited access to such systems, and the initial investment and the technological support necessary to establish and maintain them are substantial (Maviglia et al., 2003).

Even with adoption of EMR systems, there is wide variation in the technical capabilities of these systems, with only 65 percent of the systems providing immediate access to clinical guidelines and protocols, and most of these have limited decision support capabilities. In addition, many of these systems do not include the essential ability to interrogate patient records for quality assessment and research (Gans et al., 2005).

Although the use of such systems may eventually become universal and the functional capacities of physicians are likely to improve, the transition to EMR alone does not increase the rate of use of EBP. It does, however, provide the critical infrastructure needed to facilitate EBP. Given the financial limitations inherent in small practice settings and the dominance of this mode of practice, external support will be needed to facilitate IT-supported practice for the majority of healthcare professionals. Therefore, at a minimum, proposals to increase the rate of adoption of EBP must address both computerized and noncomputerized practice settings.

Finally, regulatory oversight for practicing physicians needs to be expanded to include standards of EBM practice, quality assessment and improvement, and continuous learning, which should be mandatory for maintenance of certification. This oversight is beginning to occur, especially in internal medicine, in which the American Board of Internal Medicine has developed evidence-based clinical performance measures for physi cians (LaBresh et al., 2004). There are several different practice assessment options, each of which includes a World Wide Web–based self-evaluation as well as some form of formal practice assessment; successful completion of an assessment results in credits for both the maintenance of certification and CME.

Nurses

Nursing is the largest of the healthcare professions, with nearly 3 million nurses in the United States, the majority of whom are practicing in hospital settings (U.S. Department of Labor, 2006). Registered nurses (RNs) are educated at various levels and receive associate degrees, hospital program-based diplomas, and baccalaureate degrees. Advanced-practice nurses (e.g., nurse practitioners and clinical nurse specialists) are educated through master's degree and clinical doctoral programs, whereas nurse researchers are educated in doctor of philosophy and nursing science doctoral programs that place an emphasis on the learning of the knowledge and skills required to conduct rigorous studies that extend science and produce evidence to guide best clinical practices.

Nurses assume vital roles in the healthcare system, such as (1) providing high-quality direct patient care across the care continuum; (2) assessing and monitoring patients' health status and outcomes; (3) planning, tailoring, implementing, and evaluating clinical interventions; (4) facilitating self-management strategies so that individuals achieve the highest level of health and adhere to prescribed treatments; and (5) promoting physical and mental health through patient education and anticipatory guidance. In addition, nurses are clinical researchers/scientists who lead interdisciplinary research teams in generating new knowledge and evidence to guide best clinical practices. They are also healthcare leaders and administrators who spearhead organizational change and systems improvements and teachers and mentors who prepare the next generation of direct care providers, educators, and nurse scientists.

Although federal agencies, professional organizations, healthcare leaders, and insurers have emphasized EBP as a key strategy for improving the quality of health care and patient outcomes, the majority of nurses do not deliver evidence-based care (Institute of Medicine, 2003; Melnyk et al., 2005). A recent descriptive survey with a random sample of 1,097 randomly selected RNs from across the United States found that (1) almost half were not familiar with the term "evidence-based practice"; (2) more than half reported that they did not believe that their colleagues use research findings in practice; (3) only 27 percent of the survey participants had been taught how to use electronic databases; and (4) most reported that they did not search information databases (e.g., Medline and Cumulative Index to Nursing and Allied Health Literature [CINAHL]) to gather practice information, and those who did search these resources did not believe that they had adequate search skills (Pravikoff et al., 2005).

Numerous studies have identified major barriers to the use of EBP, including (1) inadequate education and knowledge in EBP, including IT; (2) weak beliefs about the value of EBP; (3) negative attitudes toward research; (4) misperceptions about EBP (e.g., a perceived lack of time to implement EBP); (5) a non-EBP culture in healthcare settings and few resources at the point of care, including appropriate tools and a formal structure; (6) competing priorities; (7) a lack of administrative support and incentives to change practice; (8) insufficient numbers of advanced-practice nurses to serve as EBP mentors to direct care staff; (9) various levels of educational preparation; and (10) the omission of EBP as a responsibility and a lack of accountability in clinical practice (Fineout-Overholt et al., 2005; Melnyk and Fineout-Overholt, 2005; Pagoto et al., 2007).

Recent anecdotal reports indicate that when nurses and healthcare professionals implement EBP, they feel more empowered and more satisfied in their roles as healthcare providers (Maljanian et al., 2002; Strout, 2005). These are important findings, because the nursing profession is facing the most severe personnel shortage in its history, with the current vacancy rate for RNs reported to be 8.5 percent (American Hospital Association, 2006). The demands on nurses as a result of this shortage have led to increasing reports of job dissatisfaction and an intent to leave the profession (Bowles and Candela, 2005). In a recent study, 23 percent of nurses intended to leave the profession, with another 37 percent uncertain of their future (Larrabee et al., 2003). Another recent report noted that the national average turnover rate for new nursing graduates is 35 to 60 percent (Zucker et al., 2006). High turnover rates are costly to the healthcare system and negatively affect patient outcomes (Aiken et al., 2003). Furthermore, an IOM paper, Keeping Patient's Safe: Transforming the Work Environment of Nurses, stressed the importance of the simultaneous use of EBPs and the removal of the inefficient work of nurses as key strategies to obtaining a safe and satisfying practice environment (Institute of Medicine, 2004). Thus, in addition to improving the quality of care and patient outcomes, EBP may be a key factor in increasing job satisfaction and reducing nurse turnover rates.

Although RNs receive their foundational preparation through a variety of educational mechanisms (i.e., associate degrees, hospital program-based diplomas, and baccalaureate degrees), all educational programs need to cultivate a spirit of inquiry in their students and prepare them to be clinicians who practice EBM, appropriately leveling EBP-related knowledge, skills, and competencies on the basis of the level of educational preparation. A meta-analysis conducted in the late 1980s indicated that nursing interventions based on scientific evidence rather than steeped in tradition achieved better patient outcomes (Heater et al., 1988). Despite the findings from that meta-analysis, academic programs in nursing have been slow to incorporate the teaching of EBP. Nursing education at both the baccalaureate and the master's levels has historically focused on preparing graduates to be the generators of research instead of the users of evidence who can efficiently translate research findings into practice to improve care, even though the American Association of Colleges of Nursing contends that nursing education is to prepare students to "use scientific knowledge in their practice" (American Association of Colleges of Nursing, 2004).

Research in nursing academic programs has also traditionally been taught in isolation and not as part of other nursing courses, and thus, students have failed to see the application of research findings to clinical practice (Burke et al., 2005). The tedious nature of the methods used to teach research and a lack of relevancy to real-time clinical situations have contributed to the pervasive negative attitudes toward research by practicing nurses and misperceptions that EBP is not feasible because of today's healthcare environment and nursing shortage.

To prepare nursing graduates to be evidence-based clinicians, nursing school faculty must have the in-depth knowledge and skills needed to teach and model EBP. In a recent descriptive survey of 79 nurse practitioner educators from the National Organization of Nurse Practitioner Faculties and the Association of Faculties of Pediatric Nurse Practitioners, participants' self-reported knowledge of EBP was high and they believed in the benefits of EBP as well as the need to integrate it into academic curriculums. However, the faculty responses on the survey indicated a knowledge gap in EBP teaching strategies. Furthermore, few of the faculty's academic programs offered a foundational course in EBP. Additional findings from that study indicated significant relationships among educators' knowledge of EBP and (1) their beliefs that EBP improves clinical care, (2) their beliefs that teaching EBP will advance the profession, (3) how comfortable they feel in teaching EBP, and (4) whether clinical competencies in EBP are incorporated into clinical specialty courses (Melnyk and Fineout-Overholt, 2008). Therefore, there is a tremendous need to equip academic faculty with in-depth knowledge and skills in EBP so that they can teach and model it for their students. A recent position statement from the National League for

Nursing (NLN) calls for new models of nursing education that will address demands for competencies in EBP. In that statement, the NLN reports that the "wide-scale transformation of education continues to be slow to materialize" (National League for Nursing, 2007).

Finally, the findings from a recent systematic review indicated that stand-alone classroom teaching of EBP or critical appraisal courses improved students' knowledge of EBP but that only clinically integrated teaching improved their EBP-related skills, attitudes, and behaviors. Therefore, the consistent integration of EBP in the curriculum and skills building in EBP through an interdisciplinary approach to learning, including healthcare IT, throughout educational programs are necessary to prepare clinicians who will deliver evidence-based care upon entry into practice and throughout their careers (Coomarasamy and Khan, 2004).

In the current healthcare climate, nurses are challenged with heavy patient caseloads and understaffing in nearly all types of healthcare systems, including acute-care hospitals, home health care, primary care, correctional facilities, and long-term care settings. The typical profile for a practicing nurse as well as a faculty member in the new millennium is a 47-year-old individual who has not been educated in EBP or healthcare IT as part of his or her basic nursing curriculum (U.S. Department of Health and Human Services, 2004). These factors create substantial challenges for the rapid advancement of EBP in the nursing profession. Additionally, continuing education for nurses is not mandated in many states. In those states in which continuing education is required for relicensure, it is typically less than 25 contact hours every 2 years. Therefore, rigorous initiatives are necessary to transform and sustain an evidence-based approach to clinical care, including education in and access to healthcare IT, tools that enhance EBP, and a culture that supports this type of practice.

Even if healthcare providers are educated in and have the skills needed to implement EBP, without a culture that supports and provides the necessary resources for this type of practice, it is unlikely that EBP will be sustained. Leaders within healthcare organizations (e.g., chief medical and nursing officers), with the input of interdisciplinary healthcare professionals, need to create an exciting vision and strategic plan for EBP, as well as provide the culture and necessary resources to support it (Melnyk and Fineout-Overholt, 2005). The strategic plan must then be clearly communicated to all interdisciplinary healthcare professionals. Expectations for EBP should be set and integrated throughout the healthcare system's philosophy and performance standards, with staff having accountability and incentives for meeting those standards.

Findings from previous studies have indicated that there are a number of facilitators of EBP in healthcare systems, including (1) healthcare providers' knowledge and skills in EBP, (2) healthcare providers' beliefs that

EBP improves care and patient outcomes, (3) healthcare providers' beliefs in their ability to implement EBP, (4) EBP mentors who are skilled in EBP and organizational change, (5) administrative/organizational support, and (6) journal clubs and EBP fellowship programs (Fineout-Overholt et al., 2005a,b; Levin et al., 2007; Melnyk and Fineout-Overholt, 2005; Pagoto et al., 2007). Evidence from a recent survey also indicates that healthcare professionals who rate themselves higher on knowledge and beliefs about EBP are more likely to teach it to others (Melnyk et al., 2003). Therefore, to advance EBP, healthcare systems should implement educational and fellowship programs to enhance the EBP-related knowledge, beliefs, and skills of its staff; provide EBP mentors who can work directly with staff to implement EBP initiatives, such as journal clubs and EBP implementation/ outcomes management projects; and provide the necessary administrative support and resources, including computers for the use of EBP at the point of care and healthcare IT systems that are user friendly.

Several conceptual models can guide the implementation of EBP in healthcare systems. Some models provide process frameworks for the implementation of EBP by individual practitioners. These include (1) the model of Stetler (2001), (2) the EBP model of DiCenso and colleagues (2005), and (3) the Clinical Scholar Model (Schultz, 2005). Other models are focused on the systemwide implementation of EBP, including (1) the Iowa Model (Titler, 2002), (2) the model of Rosswurm and Larabee (1999), and (3) the model of advancing research and clinical practice through close collaboration (Fineout-Overholt et al., 2005a,b; Melnyk and Fineout-Overholt, 2002). However, evidence has yet to be generated in the form of model testing or full-scale randomized clinical trials to support the majority of these models. Thus, studies of this nature are greatly needed.

Outcomes management is another key substantive area within EBP. The measurement of outcomes related to practice changes based on evidence is the final step of EBP and provides empirical support for the impacts that these changes have on patient outcomes and healthcare systems. The measurement of outcomes is key to influencing healthcare policy and facilitating the widespread adoption of best practices across healthcare systems.

Pharmacists

Historically, the pharmacist's role focused on the preparation, formulation, and distribution of drug products to the public. As drug formulations became more standardized and the manufacture of drug products gradually became the responsibility of the pharmaceutical industry, the role of the pharmacist shifted more to the safe distribution of the drug product, ensuring that the patient received the right drug in a timely manner. Over the years, the pharmacy profession has continued to evolve to one that is responsible for drug use control and as a knowledge system focused on the distribution of drug products, resulting in the concept of "pharmaceutical care." Pharmaceutical care involves the process through which a pharmacist cooperates with a patient and other healthcare professionals in designing, implementing, and monitoring a therapeutic plan that will produce specific therapeutic outcomes for the patient (Hepler and Strand, 1990).

Overall, the reorganization of pharmacy under the constructs of pharmaceutical care/medication therapy management has extended the roles of pharmacists. These new roles include the provision of medication therapy management and patient-focused services that are aimed at improving the therapeutic outcomes for Medicare beneficiaries who have multiple chronic diseases and who are receiving multiple medications (Bluml, 2005); the provision of disease state management; monitoring of drug therapies; participation in multidisciplinary clinical care teams; the provision of consultation on drug use; the provision of drug information and patient education; formulary management; and the provision of smoking cessation programs, disease awareness and education programs, and immunization programs (American College of Clinical Pharmacy, 2000; Bluml, 2005; Bluml et al., 2000; Bond et al., 2004; Chrischilles et al., 2004; Cranor et al., 2003; Doucette et al., 2006; Ellis et al., 2000; Fahey et al., 2006; Kaboli et al., 2006; Leape et al., 1999; McMullin et al., 1999; Schumock et al., 1996; U.S. Department of Health and Human Services, 2000).

In addition, many recent initiatives have focused on the development of physician-pharmacist collaborative management programs in which pharmacists work directly with physicians to optimize therapy (Hammond et al., 2003). Evidence throughout the literature shows pharmacists' value to the healthcare team through the provision of patient-oriented services, with data showing improved patient outcomes and reductions in overall healthcare expenditures (American College of Clinical Pharmacy, 2000; Bhandari et al., 2004; Bluml, 2005; Bluml et al., 2000; Doucette et al., 2006; Ellis et al., 2000; Fahey et al., 2006; Kaboli et al., 2006; Kaushal and Bates, 2001; Leape et al., 1999; Logemann, 2003; McKenney and Wasserman, 1979; McMullin et al., 1999; Nester and Hale, 2002; Schumock et al., 1996). It is noteworthy, however, that pharmacy is the only healthcare profession reimbursed primarily for a product rather than for the provision of patient-specific services. Thus, it has been a challenge for the profession to implement the services described above more broadly without a payment model for drug therapy management or patient care. Clearly, with the extensive shift to patient-focused services, there is a greater need for pharmacists to use an evidence-based approach to clinical decision making. However, evidence demonstrating that pharmacists are knowledgeable in the constructs of EBP and are able to successfully apply evidence-based principles to the care of patients is lacking.

The implementation of EBP presents many challenges to pharmacists and other healthcare professionals. The majority of evidence on which clinical decisions are based continues to come from individual trials, but the quality of these trials varies. Although meta-analyses and preappraised resources have increased in numbers over recent years, they remain in their infancy. The potential lack of high-quality evidence with which clinically important issues are addressed is compounded by multiple issues, including (1) the priorities of funding agencies; for example, pharmaceutical companies may not align to address clinically important issues in a meaningful manner (i.e., many therapy clinical trials compare new therapies with a less optimal comparator, thus making it difficult to determine the precise role of the new drug in practice); (2) most existing evidence regarding drug therapy assesses efficacy under ideal circumstances rather than effectiveness in the general population; (3) a lack of publication of the negative findings of studies (publication biases), which is common in industry-sponsored trials; and (4) a lack of sufficient meta-analyses or a preappraised literature to facilitate decision making by end users (Bhandari et al., 2004; Feldstein, 2005).

Moreover, even with adequate sources of high-quality evidence and appraisal, the integration of this information into the decision-making process (i.e., the implementation of EBP) to improve patient care is often suboptimal. The literature contains many examples of high-quality systematic reviews, evidence-based guidelines, and so forth that could be used to recommend best practices; however, the implementation and adoption of these practices fail to achieve the desired goals. One such example is that even though evidence-based guidelines recommend that all individuals 50 years of age and older should undergo screening for colorectal cancer, screening rates remain extremely low (~30 percent) (Winawer et al., 2003).

Although many individuals hoped that technology such as computerized alerts would facilitate the implementation of evidence, recent data suggest that such alerts are often inadequate as sole tools to facilitate utilization of the evidence. For example, a recent evidenced-based review of 63 controlled studies of quality improvement interventions for hypertension noted that the median reductions in blood pressure were minimal for individual interventions such as audit/feedback (1.3 mm Hg), facilitate relay of clinical information (4.5 mm Hg), and patient reminder systems (2.8 mm Hg) were minimal compared with those achieved by organizational changes (10.1 mm Hg), which included physician-pharmacist collaborative management (14.1 mm Hg) (Walsh et al., 2006). A unique contribution of pharmacists would be for them to better integrate technology within the organizational structure of the healthcare system and provide EBM to improve patient care (Bailey et al., 2007). Overall, a greater emphasis needs to be placed on knowledge translation. Specifically, additional research is needed to identify the best approaches to promoting the implementation and adoption of the evidence to achieve the desired clinical outcomes (e.g., what strategies improve the use of the evidence? how should patient preferences best be incorporated?). Such information on best approaches should then feed back into the educational paradigm to further promote EBP.

Pharmacy Core Education

The educational response to the expanded role of the pharmacist in health care has been to increase the level of education required for licensure. In 2000, the Doctor of Pharmacy (Pharm.D.) became the entry-level degree into the profession of pharmacy. The process of incorporating EBP training into the pharmacy curriculum is ongoing. For years, pharmacists have received extensive training in drug information as well as appraisal of the literature; and the most recent accreditation standards (July 2007), set forth by the Accreditation Council on Pharmacy Education, explicitly highlight the need to incorporate EBP, quality improvement, and informatics into the professional pharmacy education curriculum (Accreditation Council for Pharmacy Education, 2006). The training of pharmacists in EBP provides individual pharmacists with the critical skills that they need to formulate and revise clinical questions, efficiently and effectively search for information, critically evaluate the information, and integrate the patients' values and preferences into the decision-making process. In addition, EBP introduces the concepts of the scientific method to investigating problems, continuous quality assessment and improvement, as well as lifelong learning.

To practice as a registered pharmacist, graduates from accredited schools of pharmacy must take a pharmacy licensing examination. Assessment of knowledge in evidence-based decision making needs to be a requirement for pharmacy school graduation; however, a review of the blueprint for the North American Licensure Examination indicates that competencies related to EBP or decision making are not included as core elements (National Association of Boards of Pharmacy, 2005). Of note, the Foreign Pharmacy Graduate Equivalency Examination, the licensing examination for pharmacists trained outside the United States, clearly identifies evidence-based decision making as a competency standard in its blueprint (National Association of Boards of Pharmacy, 2007).

Pharmacy Residency Training

Numerous accredited residency and specialty residency programs allow trainees the opportunity to gain additional knowledge and expertise after graduation from pharmacy school. All residency programs accredited or coaccredited by the American Society of Health System Pharmacists include standards regarding EBP. For example, post-graduate year-1 residents must provide evidence-based, patient-centered care and collaborate with other healthcare professionals to optimize patient care (ASHP, 2006).

Graduate Programs and Postdoctoral Fellowship Training

Postdoctoral fellowship training programs, master's degree programs, and doctoral programs in pharmacy emphasize the research skills needed for drug discovery, product development, the translation of basic science into clinical practice, health services research, and postmarketing surveillance research. One important aspect of EBP is the generation of new high-quality evidence. This aspect requires that individuals be adequately trained to conduct rigorous bidirectional translational research of type 1 (from bench to bedside) and type 2 (from bedside to adoption of best practices in the community) (National Institutes of Health Guide for Grants and Contracts, 2005). Pharmacy schools are unique in that they house individuals with an array of clinical and scientific expertise (i.e., expertise in medicinal chemistry, natural products, pharmacology, pharmaceutics, clinical sciences, pharmacoepidemiology, pharmacoeconomics) essential to translating a new drug molecule into a drug that may be used in clinical practice. Pharmacy graduate programs are diverse (e.g., medicinal chemistry, pharmaceutics, social and administrative sciences, pharmacology, and clinical sciences), but they all focus on building strong scientific inquiry skills.

Historically, most clinical pharmacy researchers have been trained through postdoctoral fellowship programs. Over the years several professional organizations (e.g., the American Association of Colleges of Pharmacy [AACP], Research and Graduate Affairs Committee, and the American College of Clinical Pharmacy Research Affairs Committee) have recommended that schools of pharmacy shift from a fellowship model to a graduate degree model for the training of clinical pharmacy scientists (American Association of Colleges of Pharmacy, 2007). In general, fellowships have suffered from a lack of consistent funding and disparate program completion criteria. Recently, the AACP Clinical Scientists Task Force recommended that there could be several pathways to the training of a clinical scientist, such as achievement of the Pharm.D. followed by the completion of a doctoral degree or dual degree programs (Pharm.D. and Ph.D., Pharm.D. and master's degree) (American Association of Colleges of Pharmacy, 2007). Overall, the movement to train new interdisciplinary clinical scientists will facilitate the generation of high-quality evidence in the future and facilitate the translation of this information into clinical practice. In designing new programs for clinical scientists, one should consider the elements described in the next section.

Education of Practicing Pharmacists

Today, pharmacists make up the third largest group of healthcare professionals in the United States, with approximately 200,000 pharmacists in active practice (U.S. Department of Health and Human Services, 2000). The expanded roles of pharmacists plus the additional need to provide medicines to aging patients have resulted in an increasing need for registered pharmacists, the shortage of which is projected to be as high as 157,000 by 2020 (Cooksey et al., 2002; Knapp, 2002; U.S. Department of Health and Human Services, 2000).

Pharmacists represent a diverse group of healthcare professionals. Thus, the challenge of increasing the rate of adoption of EBP by pharmacists is formidable. Pharmacists not only practice in a diverse array of settings but also differ according to their educational backgrounds as well as the time since graduation or postdoctoral training. For example, the U.S. Department of Health and Human Services (2000) estimated that in 2000 approximately 30 percent of pharmacists were between 51 and 65 years of age and had completed their formal pharmacy education about 30 years earlier.

Although pharmacy is practiced in a wide variety of settings, the majority of pharmacists practice in a community setting (U.S. Department of Health and Human Services, 2000). Potential barriers to pharmacist delivery of evidence-based care in these settings include a lack of education and training in EBP; attitudes and misperceptions regarding EBP (i.e., a perceived lack of value or relevance); a lack of administrative and institutional support; insufficient time; a perceived lack of evidence; a lack of relevant patient data; and logistical issues, including a lack of resources to effectively retrieve high-quality evidence or a lack of infrastructure to support EBP (Pagoto et al., 2007). For example, in the community pharmacy setting, most pharmacists face increased patient volumes, increased numbers of prescriptions to be filled, staff vacancies, and increased administrative duties (10 to 20 percent of their time is spent dealing with third-party payers and formulary issues), all of which may detract from EBP (U.S. Department of Health and Human Services, 2000). In addition, pharmacists practicing in the community setting may lack adequate training in EBP, may not have access to searchable databases or preappraised information, and may be constrained by the environment and a lack of privacy to discuss issues and preferences with patients.

Engaging all pharmacists in EBP will require aggressive educational campaigns, which may be accomplished through continuing education (CE) programs as well as by making such training a requirement for existing specialty certifications. Most state boards of pharmacy require practicing pharmacists to undergo CE for licensure; although the precise amount and type of CE varies among the states, it is generally about 30 hours every

2 years. Pharmacists obtain CE through a variety of mechanisms, including through online web-based programs; by reading published CE articles and completing self-assessment questions; and by attending live CE programs often offered or sponsored by professional organizations, pharmaceutical industry, schools of pharmacy, or healthcare organizations. CE for pharmacists is undergoing a shift to a continuing professional development model, which embraces the concept of life-long learning. The continuing professional development model is self-directed, practitioner centered, and outcomes based and emphasizes the importance of practice-based learning. Use of this model may be a strategy by which EBP may be enhanced.

Increasing the adoption of EBP by practicing pharmacists will require extensive educational training. In addition, cultural changes in the delivery of health care will be necessary. The ultimate goal is to enable healthcare professionals to work together as members of an interdisciplinary team to integrate their clinical expertise and patient preferences and values with the best available external clinical evidence from systematic research to optimize clinical decision making.

ACTIVITY CATEGORIES

Cultural Change and Education

The primary shift to EBP will require its integration into the curriculum throughout the following areas of formal education of all future healthcare professionals:

- core education, in partnership with medical schools and the American Association of Medical Colleges, nursing schools, pharmacy schools, and so forth;
- postgraduate training programs and internships, in partnership with academic medical centers and ACGME, plus residency review committees, nursing and pharmacy schools, and so forth; and
- required competency, in partnership with licensing organizations, including the National Board of Medical Examiners, specialty and subspecialty certification boards, and state licensing boards; the National League for Nursing Accrediting Commission; the Commission on Collegiate Nursing Education; and the National Council of State Boards of Nursing.

A multifaceted approach to the education of practicing healthcare professionals to promote the universal adoption of EBP will require

- a national public education campaign to educate all healthcare consumers,
- individually directed continuous learning as an active concept in partnership with professional societies and in existing CME settings,
- the use of improved patient care as the incentive for specific training in the use of evidence-based data,
- regulatory oversight to mandate education in EBP—in partnership with state licensing organizations and specialty and subspecialty boards), and
- interactions with professional organizations to develop educational programs to support evidence-based guidelines.

Systems Change in the Practice Setting

Changes to the healthcare practice setting will be important for the incorporation of EBP into the practices of healthcare professionals. The following describes some of these changes:

- With healthcare professionals being the critical lynchpin in the delivery of evidence-based care, improved user-friendly clinical decision support systems are essential.
- Changes to the healthcare culture are essential to support EBP.
- To involve healthcare professionals in routine EBP, universal rapid access to medical knowledge and clinical practice guideline repositories in all clinical practice settings is necessary.
- Continuous quality improvement mandates the ability to interrogate practice records for self-assessment, quality assurance, and research.
- To realize universal evidence-based care, the use of EMRs must be universal.
- The availability of a common IT vocabulary and interoperable technologies is essential to maximize the benefits of EMRs.

Increased Body of Evidence-Based Knowledge

To achieve the vision of universal EBP, a greatly expanded inventory of evidence-based guidelines and recommendations is needed. This can be done by:

- generating medical evidence with existing patient care data by involving healthcare professionals as data generators as a standard part of care delivery,

- increasing the rate of formal participation of healthcare professionals in practice-based research by making locations for participation readily accessible,
- rigorously evaluating the outcomes of EBP to foster the adoption of evidence-based recommendations, and
- increasing the rate of adoption of evidence-based guidelines by performing research on methods that can be used to enhance the translation of evidence into clinical practice.

LEADERSHIP COMMITMENTS AND INITIATIVES

Proposed Initiatives in Core Education

Critical concept: Incorporate precepts of population health; evidence-based knowledge and skills training; and quality measurement, improvement, and outcomes management.

Preclinical

- evidence-based review methodology,
- principles of epidemiology,
- explicit training in searching the literature and evaluating the evidence found,
- training in database interrogation, and
- training in the basics of clinical research.

Clinical

- the concepts of quality measurement and improvement through the use of routine patient data and through audits and reviews of practice results, as illustrated routinely during clinical rotations;
- continuous access to medical knowledge and clinical guideline repositories;
- modeling of evidence-based decision making by faculty with knowledge and experience in EBP; this will often require faculty to have training and experience in EBP;
- exposure to innovative cross-disciplinary curriculums that train integrated teams of healthcare professional faculty and students;
- routine exposures to interdisciplinary team care; this will require integration with other healthcare professionals;
- the concept of continuous learning, which should be explicit in the curriculum and implicit in clinical rotations, as modeled by faculty;

- explicit training in finding and evaluating materials for patient education;
- exposure to clinical research and opportunities to participate in clinical research; and
- training in the critical appraisal of the medical literature.

The vertical integration of accreditation organizations should be addressed so that core competencies in EBM are specifically reinforced in clinical training. In addition, healthcare professional students should be assessed for their competence in preventive medicine and evidence-based knowledge and decision making before they graduate.

Proposed Initiatives in Graduate Clinical Education

As part of their graduate clinical education, students should routinely be exposed to interdisciplinary healthcare teams that use evidence-based methods to deliver care. Means of accomplishing this are described below.

- Based on defined competencies, support training in EBP as a core competency in all clinical training programs.
- Make best practices from programs like education innovation projects available as models for training programs.
- Work with certification boards to introduce the skills necessary for EBP. This work should be aligned with expectations in the postgraduate period for the demonstration of competency in EBP.
- Integrate the concept of continuous learning in the curriculum for clinical training both explicitly and implicitly, as modeled by the faculty.
- Integrate and model the concepts of quality measurement and improvement, systems-based practice, and team-based care into clinical training.
- Evaluate the students' knowledge of evidence-based decision making in certifying examinations and state licensure standards.

Proposed Initiatives in Postgraduate Education and Culture Change

Critical Concept: Changing the way health care is delivered will require broad educational initiatives that include the general public as well as practicing healthcare professionals.

Public Education Campaign: Use the media to introduce the concept and benefits of EBP to the public in general and practicing health professionals, in particular:

- Educational segments in the media and packaged for healthcare settings should feature health professionals in the educational role.
- Studies indicate that a majority of Americans get their health information from the media; questions from patients will represent a powerful reinforcement of EBP.

For healthcare professionals, continuous learning can be achieved in a variety of ways:

- Use healthcare professional leaders and professional organizations to establish lifelong learning as a professional obligation.
- Interact with professional societies to educate the membership about EBP through society journals, meetings, and educational programs.
- Develop and market a model CME program for use at the community level to introduce the principles of EBP. The program will include (1) the concepts of evidence-based decision making, (2) examples of healthcare professional and patient tools that facilitate EBP, and (3) a project for CME credit consisting of a self-scoring assessment of practice adherence to best practice recommendations. The program can be made available to hospitals, medical centers, practice groups, and professional organizations.
- Expand traditional CME and continuing education units to include the use of web-based EBP training by providing extra credit CME for EBM training to increase exposure.
- Support incentives to increase the rate of implementation of EBM.
- Provide oversight by
  - requiring licensure standards to include knowledge of EBM;
  - assessing a healthcare professional's knowledge of EBM in specialty and subspecialty board examinations as a component of the initial certification and the maintenance of certification; and
  - including specific training in EBM and reporting of EBM as a performance standard for licensure and maintenance of certification.

Proposed Initiatives in Practice Setting Systems Change

Table 6-1 provides examples of some of the initiatives already in place in the clinical practice setting. The following describe other means of changing the practice setting:

- Endorse the investments made by government agencies, insurers, and hospitals in the acquisition of EMRs in hospitals, medical

TABLE 6-1 Sample Initiatives Already in Place

Competency	Initiative	Roles	Model
Practice support	Interoperable technology to support implementation of EBP	MD, RN, NP, LPN, Pharm.D.	The Veterans Health Administration provides care for 5.3 million patients at 1,400 care sites and provides systemwide access to EMR. To increase adherence to evidence-based guidelines for decision making, performance profiles based on EBM-defined risk markers were created for all care providers. Self-comparisons of performance resulted in serial improvement in all markers of diabetes care (Kupersmith et al., 2007).
Continuous learning and practice support	Web-based training included with roll-out of evidence-based guidelines	MD, RN, NP, LPN, Pharm.D.	The American Heart Association created Get with the Guidelines program to increase the rates of physician adherence to secondary prevention guidelines after myocardial infarction. Physicians use a web-based management tool for data collection and online feedback. Twenty-four hospitals collaborated in a pilot study; after 12 months, clinically and statistically significant increases in the use of four of seven measures from the baseline were demonstrated, with a high rate of baseline use maintained for the other measures (LaBresh et al., 2004).
	Online distance education and immersion workshops	MD, RN, NP, LPN, Pharm.D.	The Center for the Advancement of EBP at Arizona State University offers a 17-credit online distance education graduate/post-master's degree certificate in EBP plus week-long EBP multidisciplinary immersion workshops for healthcare professionals.
CME and regulatory oversight	Inclusion of physician-specific EBM training and reporting for maintenance of certification	MD	The American Board of Internal Medicine Physician Consortium for Performance Improvement has developed three different practice assessment options. Each includes a web-based self-evaluation as well as some form of formal practice assessment. Successful completion results in credits for both maintenance of certification and CME (American Board of Internal Medicine, 2007).

NOTE: LPN = licensed practical nurse; NP = nurse practitioner.

centers, and practices as a way to jump-start their adoption by healthcare professionals.

- Establish healthcare cultures that support the systemwide implementation and the sustainability of EBP, including resources at the point of care, EBP mentors, and time for healthcare professionals to engage in EBP as routine.
- Support the development and implementation of a common vocabulary and interoperable technology to optimize the use of patient data both in practice and for assessment of evidence-based guideline implementation, and provide feedback to healthcare professionals.
- Recommend the provision of EBM guidelines in an IT format compatible with all forms of EMR as well as in paper versions for healthcare professionals who do not yet routinely use electronic technologies.
- Work with professional practice organizations to develop guideline implementation packages, including clinical practice and patient education tools, to be released with all major guidelines.
- Support the provision of add-on modules (electronic and paper based) to efficiently update existing evidence frameworks.
- Support the study of regionalized processes for the provision of IT support to small practices, such as collaborative practice models, virtual large group practices, public health-based support, or regionalization through interaction with academic medical centers.
- Involve healthcare professionals in the design and development of IT support systems to reduce redundant data entry, screen changes, and forced recommendation practices. This will serve the dual role of making such systems directly responsive to the needs of practicing healthcare professionals and of creating leaders who will advocate for EBM and IT-supported care in their home communities.

Proposed Initiatives in Use of Medical Evidence Generation as Standard Care

- Educate healthcare professionals about how existing information from patient care can be used as clinical research data.
- Increase opportunities to participate in practice-based research to expose healthcare professionals to the means of generating the science base from which evidence-based recommendations are developed.
  - Involve practicing healthcare professionals in the development of research questions with direct clinical practice.
  - Provide specific opportunities for solo and small group practice and community hospital settings to participate in clinical practice research networks.

- Support formal evaluations of the impact of EBP on clinical outcomes.
- Seek mechanisms for financial support of participation in registries and research databases, for example, the American College of Surgeons National Surgical Quality Improvement Program.
- Support EMR development to allow inquiries of the patient database for clinical research.

Collaboration of Healthcare Professionals Sector with Other Sectors

Clinical Investigators

- Interact to expand the clinical base from which evidence is generated to include a wide range of practice settings and observational data.
- Support the federal funding of research on outcomes from the implementation of EBP.
- Encourage research on the dissemination of EBP and the implementation of best practices.
- Release major new guidelines simultaneously with the findings of a funded research trial for evaluation of defined practice outcomes.
- Support the development of evidence-based guidelines in areas in which few or none exist (e.g., for patients with multisystem diseases and for the screening and treatment of children and adolescents for whom the chances of positive outcomes of a disease process are remote).
- Several systematic reviews have documented the relatively small number of studies and the poor quality of research evaluating the effectiveness of interventions to increase the rate of use of EBP. Support for research into innovative approaches to changing the behavior of healthcare professionals with rigorous outcome evaluation is essential.

Information Technology

- Work with IT developers to develop a common vocabulary and interoperable technologies to allow information sharing.
- Interact with IT developers to improve EBM guideline interfaces to reduce redundant data entry and to screen changes and forced recommended practices, and provide areas for documentation for exceptions.
- Include healthcare practitioners in the design and development of IT support systems.

Consumer-Patient

- Support the concept of the use of observational patient data as evidence for the healthcare system.
- Encourage the development of patient materials to support consumer adoption of evidence-based health concepts and practice.
- Support the development of robust methods to include patient values and preferences in complex decision making.

Insurers

- Encourage the use of performance feedback to adjust rates.
- Endorse industry support of a transition to EMR with robust decision support at the point of care.
- Support payer endorsement and the support of professional efforts to promote changes to the medical culture.

NEXT STEPS

The adoption of EBP, including the shift to patient-centric care, will require nothing short of a transformation of current medical practice. In this transformation, healthcare professionals can be described as the critical transition point between current healthcare practice and the delivery of evidence-based care. This chapter on the healthcare professionals sector has identified a number of model initiatives that are already under way in a variety of settings to support this process. The chapter has also highlighted key actionable items that will further support the initiation of change. However, to truly make this kind of culture change possible, sustained effective leadership will be essential. To that end, we propose the appointment of an EBM Interdisciplinary Healthcare Professionals Advisory Panel to interact with the leadership at the IOM. The panel would serve as the voice of the healthcare professionals sector in education, practice, and regulatory oversight. The panel would be charged with establishing critical initial steps; identifying benchmarks to define progress; and developing future initiatives in education, practice, and regulatory oversight to sustain the process of adoption of EBM as it evolves. The creation of this panel would represent a new coordinated starting point for an integrated shift to EBP for the healthcare professionals sector.

Proposed Panel Format

We propose that the members of the panel play roles in education and in the practice setting and that they also have an oversight role. In the area of education, leaders in the undergraduate and postgraduate education of healthcare professionals would be charged with the development and implementation of a coordinated set of strategies that would support lifelong learning in EBP throughout the healthcare professions' education. Their initial role would be to consult in development of the EBM public education campaign. Proposed members could come from among the following groups: ACGME; American Academy of Nursing; American Association of Medical Colleges, including the Council of Deans; American Boards of Internal Medicine, Pediatrics, Family Practice, Surgery, and so forth; Commission on Collegiate Nursing Education; National Council of State Boards of Nursing; National League for Nursing; National Organization of Nurse Practitioner Faculties; and professional societies such as the American Academy of Pediatrics, American Association of Colleges of Nursing American College of Cardiology, American College of Pharmacy, American College of Surgeons, and Society of Thoracic Surgeons. IT developers, health practitioners, and leaders from the whole range of healthcare settings and professional organizations would be charged with working together on the design and development of support for EBP, including the development of a culture that supports EBP. Health insurance providers and healthcare regulators would be charged with the development of incentives to facilitate practice change.

Representatives from all those groups involved in the regulation and oversight of competence at all levels of healthcare professional training and practice would be charged with ensuring the vertical integration of competencies in EBM throughout basic and clinical training and postgraduate certification. Regulatory groups from which potential members would be selected include the National Board of Medical Examiners; ACGME; specialty and subspecialty boards; and state medical licensing systems for physicians, nurses, and pharmacists.

Summary: Healthcare Professionals

This chapter has outlined a strategy that can be used to increase the training of new healthcare professionals and those already in practice in EBP, improve IT support for EBP, enhance healthcare system cultures that support EBP, and increase the rates of participation of healthcare professionals in medical evidence generation as standard care. The chapter has also described specific initiatives that address this dual strategy at each stage of training or practice and has provided examples of benchmark programs that address aspects of these priorities. The use of a public information campaign as a way of introducing all practicing healthcare professionals and the American public simultaneously to the concepts of EBP, with reinforcement by the use of CME, educational incentives, and feedback from inquiring patients and the development of partnerships with existing educational, IT, and practice research organizations will be important steps in supporting routine EBP, something that is already under way in many settings.

This review indicates that current models of excellence can be used to increase the rate of implementation of EBM. Whenever possible, these should be used to enhance this process. A combination of support for the required technology, the provision of rewards for improved performance, the provision of regulatory oversight, and increased participation in the generation of clinical research data are proposed as the most effective ways to sustain progress toward this important goal. Finally, appointment of an EMB Interdisciplinary Healthcare Professionals Advisory Panel is recommended as the critical first step in providing sustained leadership for initiation of the process needed to maximize the adoption of EBM in clinical practice.

REFERENCES

Accreditation Council for Pharmacy Education. 2006. *Accreditation standards and guidelines for the professional program in pharmacy leading to the doctor of pharmacy degree.* http://www.acpe-accredit.org/pdf/ACPE_Revised_PharmD_Standards_Adopted_Jan152006.pdf (accessed July 10, 2007).

ACGME (Accreditation Council for Graduate Medical Education). 1999. *ACGME Outcomes Project. Common program requirements: General competencies.* http://www.acgme.org/outcome/comp/compMin.asp (accessed April 18, 2007).

Aiken, L. H., S. P. Clarke, R. B. Cheung, D. M. Sloane, and J. H. Silber. 2003. Educational levels of hospital nurses and surgical patient mortality. *JAMA* 290(12):1617-1623.

American Association of Colleges of Nursing. 2006. *Position statement on nursing research.* http://www.aacn.nche.edu/Publications/positions/NsgRes.htm (accessed May 28, 2007).

American Association of Colleges of Pharmacy. 2007. Report of the AACP educating clinical scientists task force. Paper read at AACP Annual Meeting, July 2007, Orlando, FL.

American Board of Internal Medicine. 2007. *Maintenance of certification.* http://www.abim.org/moc/default.aspx (accessed April 23, 2007).

American College of Clinical Pharmacy. 2000. AACP white paper. A vision of pharmacy's future roles, responsibilities, and manpower needs in the United States. *Pharmacotherapy* 20(8):991-1020.

American College of Physicians. 2005. Physician employment trends. In *Trends in medicine and health.* Philadelphia, PA: Office of Research, Planning and Education, American College of Physicians.

American Hospital Association. 2006. *The state of America's hospitals: Taking the pulse. Findings from the 2006 AHA survey of hospital leaders.* http://www.ahapolicyforum.org/ahapolicyforum/resources/content/StateHospitalsChartPack2006 (accessed May 21, 2007).

ASHP (American Society of Hospital Pharmacists). 2006. *Regulations on accreditation of pharmacy residencies.* http://www.ashp.org/s_ashp/cat1c.asp?CID=3531&DID=5558 (accessed July 10, 2007).

Audet, A. M., M. M. Doty, J. Shamasdin, and S. C. Schoenbaum. 2005. Measure, learn, and improve: Physicians' involvement in quality improvement. *Health Affairs* 24(3):843-853.

Bailey, T. C., L. A. Noirot, A. Blickensderfer, E. Rachmiel, R. Schaiff, A. Kessels, A. Braverman, A. Goldberg, B. Waterman, and W. C. Dunagan. 2007. An intervention to improve secondary prevention of coronary heart disease. *Archives of Internal Medicine* 167(6):586-590.

Bhandari, M., J. W. Busse, D. Jackowski, V. M. Montori, H. Schunemann, S. Sprague, D. Mears, E. H. Schemitsch, D. Heels-Ansdell, and P. J. Devereaux. 2004. Association between industry funding and statistically significant pro-industry findings in medical and surgical randomized trials. *Canadian Medical Association Journal* 170(4):477-480.

Bluml, B. M. 2005. Definition of medication therapy management: Development of profession-wide consensus. *Journal of the American Pharmacists Association* 45(5):566-572.

Bluml, B. M., J. M. McKenney, and M. J. Cziraky. 2000. Pharmaceutical care services and results in project impact: Hyperlipidemia. *Journal of the American Pharmaceutical Association* 40(2):157-165.

Bond, C. A., C. L. Raehl, and R. Patry. 2004. Evidence-based core clinical pharmacy services in United States hospitals in 2020: Services and staffing. *Pharmacotherapy* 24(4):427-440.

Bowles, C., and L. Candela. 2005. First job experiences of recent RN graduates: Improving the work environment. *Journal of Nursing Administration* 35(3):130-137.

Bradt, P., and V. Moyer. 2003. How to teach evidence-based medicine. *Clinics in Perinatology* 30(2):419-433.

Burke, L. E., E. A. Schlenk, S. M. Sereika, S. M. Cohen, M. B. Happ, and J. S. Dorman. 2005. Developing research competence to support evidence-based practice. *Journal of Professional Nursing* 21(6):358-363.

Carey, J. C. 2000. Integrating prevention into obstetrics/gynecology. *Academic Medicine* 75(7 Suppl):S72-S76.

Chrischilles, E. A., B. L. Carter, B. C. Lund, L. M. Rubenstein, S. S. Chen-Hardee, M. D. Voelker, T. R. Park, and A. K. Kuehl. 2004. Evaluation of the Iowa Medicaid pharmaceutical case management program. *Journal of the American Pharmacists Association* 44(3):337-349.

Conway, P. H., S. Edwards, E. R. Stucky, V. W. Chiang, M. C. Ottolini, and C. P. Landrigan. 2006. Variations in management of common inpatient pediatric illnesses: Hospitalists and community pediatricians. *Pediatrics* 118(2):441-447.

Cooksey, J. A., K. K. Knapp, S. M. Walton, and J. M. Cultice. 2002. Challenges to the pharmacist profession from escalating pharmaceutical demand. *Health Affairs* 21(5):182-188.

Coomarasamy, A., and K. S. Khan. 2004. What is the evidence that postgraduate teaching in evidence based medicine changes anything? A systematic review. *BMJ* 329(7473):1017.

Cranor, C. W., B. A. Bunting, and D. B. Christensen. 2003. The Asheville project: Long-term clinical and economic outcomes of a community pharmacy diabetes care program. *Journal of the American Pharmaceutical Association* 43(2):173-184.

Davidson, R. A., M. Duerson, L. Romrell, R. Pauly, and R. T. Watson. 2004. Evaluating evidence-based medicine skills during a performance-based examination. *Academic Medicine* 79(3):272-275.

Dexter, P. R., S. Perkins, J. M. Overhage, K. Maharry, R. B. Kohler, and C. J. McDonald. 2001. A computerized reminder system to increase the use of preventive care for hospitalized patients. *New England Journal of Medicine* 345(13):965-970.

DiCensco, A., N. Cullum, D. Ciliska, and G. Guyatt. 2005. Introduction to evidence-based nursing. In *Evidence-based nursing. A guide to clinical practice*, edited by A. DiCensco, N. Cullum, D. Ciliska, and G. Guyatt. Philadelphia, PA: Elsevier. Pp. 3-19.

Dorsch, J., M. K. Aiyer, K. Gumidyala, and L. E. Meyer. 2006. Retention of EBM competencies. *Medical Reference Services Quarterly* 25(3):45-57.

Doucette, W. R., D. H. Kreling, J. C. Schommer, C. A. Gaither, D. A. Mott, and C. A. Pedersen. 2006. Evaluation of community pharmacy service mix: Evidence from the 2004 national pharmacist workforce study. *Journal of the American Pharmacists Association* 46(3):348-355.

Ellis, S. L., B. L. Carter, D. C. Malone, S. J. Billups, G. J. Okano, R. J. Valuck, D. J. Barnette, C. D. Sintek, D. Covey, B. Mason, S. Jue, J. Carmichael, K. Guthrie, R. Dombrowski, D. R. Geraets, and M. Amato. 2000. Clinical and economic impact of ambulatory care clinical pharmacists in management of dyslipidemia in older adults: The Improve Study. Impact of managed pharmaceutical care on resource utilization and outcomes in Veterans Affairs medical centers. *Pharmacotherapy* 20(12):1508-1516.

Fahey, T., K. Schroeder, and S. Ebrahim. 2006. Interventions used to improve control of blood pressure in patients with hypertension. *Cochrane Database Systematic Review* (4):CD005182.

Feldstein, D. A. 2005. Evidence-based practice: What a start and "oh, the possibilities." *World Medical Journal* 104(3):14-17.

Fineout-Overholt, E., R. Levin, and B. Melnyk. 2005a. Strategies for advancing evidence-based practice in clinical settings. *Journal of New York State Nurses Association* 35(2):28-33.

Fineout-Overholt, E., B. M. Melnyk, and A. Schultz. 2005b. Transforming health care from the inside out: Advancing evidence-based practice in the 21st century. *Journal of Professional Nursing* 21(6):335-344.

Gans, D., J. Kralewski, T. Hammons, and B. Dowd. 2005. Medical groups' adoption of electronic health records and information systems. *Health Affairs* 24(5):1323-1333.

Garritty, C., and K. El Emam. 2006. Who's using PDAs? Estimates of PDA use by health care providers: A systematic review of surveys. *Journal of Medical Internet Research* 8(2):e7.

Green, M. L. 2000. Evidence-based medicine training in internal medicine residency programs: A national survey. *Journal of General Internal Medicine* 15(2):129-133.

Hammond, R. W., A. H. Schwartz, M. J. Campbell, T. L. Remington, S. Chuck, M. M. Blair, A. M. Vassey, R. M. Rospond, S. J. Herner, and C. E. Webb. 2003. Collaborative drug therapy management by pharmacists—2003. *Pharmacotherapy* 23(9):1210-1225.

Heater, B. S., A. M. Becker, and R. K. Olson. 1988. Nursing interventions and patient outcomes: A meta-analysis of studies. *Nursing Research* 37(5):303-307.

Hepler, C. D., and L. M. Strand. 1990. Opportunities and responsibilities in pharmaceutical care. *American Journal of Hospital Pharmacy* 47(3):533-543.

Hunt, D. L., R. B. Haynes, S. E. Hanna, and K. Smith. 1998. Effects of computer-based clinical decision support systems on physician performance and patient outcomes: A systematic review. *JAMA* 280(15):1339-1346.

Institute of Medicine. 2003. *Health professions education: A bridge to quality.* Washington, DC: The National Academies Press.

———. 2004. *Keeping patients safe: Transforming the work environment of nurses.* Washington, DC: The National Academies Press.

Jha, A. K., T. G. Ferris, K. Donelan, C. DesRoches, A. Shields, S. Rosenbaum, and D. Blumenthal. 2006. How common are electronic health records in the United States? A summary of the evidence. *Health Affairs* 25(6):w496 w507.

Kaboli, P. J., A. B. Hoth, B. J. McClimon, and J. L. Schnipper. 2006. Clinical pharmacists and inpatient medical care: A systematic review. *Archives of Internal Medicine* 166(9):955-964.

Kaushal, R., and D. W. Bates. 2001. *The clinical pharmacist's role in preventing adverse drug events. Making healthcare safer: A critical analysis of patient safety.* Rockville, MD: Agency for Healthcare Research and Quality.

Knapp, D. A. 2002. *Professionally determined need for pharmacy services in 2020.* Report of a conference sponsored by the Pharmacy Manpower Project, Inc.: National Association of Chain Drugstores. http://www.ajpe.org/legacy/pdfs/aj660414.pdf (accessed July 10, 2007).

Kuperman, G. J., J. M. Teich, D. W. Bates, F. L. Hiltz, J. M. Hurley, R. Y. Lee, and M. D. Paterno. 1996. Detecting alerts, notifying the physician, and offering action items: a comprehensive alerting system. In *Proceedings of the American Medical Informatics Association Annual Fall Symposium.* Washington, DC. Pp. 704-708.

Kupersmith, J., J. Francis, E. Kerr, S. Krein, L. Pogach, R. M. Kolodner, and J. B. Perlin. 2007. Advancing evidence-based care for diabetes: Lessons from the Veterans Health Administration. *Health Affairs* 26(2):w156-w168.

LaBresh, K. A., A. G. Ellrodt, R. Gliklich, J. Liljestrand, and R. Peto. 2004. Get with the guidelines for cardiovascular secondary prevention: Pilot results. *Archives of Internal Medicine* 164(2):203-209.

Larrabee, J. H., M. A. Janney, C. L. Ostrow, M. L. Withrow, G. R. Hobbs, Jr., and C. Burant. 2003. Predicting registered nurse job satisfaction and intent to leave. *Journal of Nursing Administration* 33(5):271-283.

Leape, L. L., D. J. Cullen, M. D. Clapp, E. Burdick, H. J. Demonaco, J. I. Erickson, and D. W. Bates. 1999. Pharmacist participation on physician rounds and adverse drug events in the intensive care unit. *JAMA* 282(3):267-270.

Levin, R., M. J. Vetter, E. Fineout-Overholt, B. M. Melnyk, and M. Barnes. 2007 Advancing research and clinical practice through close collaboration (ARCC): A pilot test of an intervention to improve evidence-based care and patient outcomes in a community health setting. Paper presented at 8th Annual National/International Evidence-Based Practice Conference Translating Research into Best Practice with Vulnerable Populations, February 23, Phoenix, AZ.

Logemann, C. 2003. Patient safety initiatives: The importance of an accurate medication list. Paper presented at Faculty Seminar, College of Pharmacy, University of Iowa, Ames, April 9.

Maljanian, R., L. Caramanica, S. K. Taylor, J. B. MacRae, and D. K. Beland. 2002. Evidence-based nursing practice. Part 2. Building skills through research roundtables. *Journal of Nursing Administration* 32(2):85-90.

Marantz, P. R., W. Burton, and P. Steiner-Grossman. 2003. Using the case-discussion method to teach epidemiology and biostatistics. *Academic Medicine* 78(4):365-371.

Maviglia, S. M., R. D. Zielstorff, M. Paterno, J. M. Teich, D. W. Bates, and G. J. Kuperman. 2003. Automating complex guidelines for chronic disease: Lessons learned. *Journal of the American Medical Informatics Association* 10(2):154-165.

McGlynn, E., S. Asch, J. Adams, J. Keesey, J. Hicks, A. DeCristofaro, and E. Kerr. 2003. The quality of health care delivered to adults in the United States. *New England Journal of Medicine* 348(26):2635-2645.

McKenney, J. M., and A. J. Wasserman. 1979. Effect of advanced pharmaceutical services on the incidence of adverse drug reactions. *American Journal of Hospital Pharmacy* 36(12):1691-1697.

McMullin, S. T., J. A. Hennenfent, D. J. Ritchie, W. Y. Huey, T. P. Lonergan, R. A. Schaiff, M. E. Tonn, and T. C. Bailey. 1999. A prospective, randomized trial to assess the cost impact of pharmacist-initiated interventions. *Archives of Internal Medicine* 159(19):2306-2309.

Medical School Objective Project Writing Group. 1999. Learning objectives for medical student education—guidelines for medical schools. Report 1. *Academic Medicine* 74(1):13-18.

Melnyk, B. M., and E. Fineout-Overholt. 2002. Putting research into practice. *Reflections on Nursing Leadership* 28(2):22-25, 45.

———, 2005. Evidence-based practice in nursing and healthcare: A guide to best practice. Philadelphia, PA: Lippincott, Williams & Wilkins.

Melnyk, B. M., E. Fineout-Overholt, N. Feinstein, H. Li, L. Small, and L. Wilcox. 2003. Nurses' perceived knowledge, beliefs, skills, and needs regarding evidence-based practice: Implications for accelerating the paradigm shift. *Worldviews on Evidence-Based Nursing* 1:185-193.

Melnyk, B. M., E. Fineout-Overholt, C. Stetler, and J. Allan. 2005. Outcomes and implementation strategies from the first U.S. evidence-based practice leadership summit. *Worldviews on Evidence-Based Nursing* 2(3):113-121.

Melnyk, B. M., E. Fineout-Overholt, N. Feinstein, L. S. Sadler, C. Green-Hernandez. 2008. Nurse practitioner educators' perceived knowledge, beliefs, and teaching strategies regarding evidence-based practice: Implications for accelerating the integration of EBP in graduate programs. *Journal of Professional Nursing* 24(1):7-13.

National Association of Boards of Pharmacy. 2005. *North American Pharmacist Licensure Examination (NAPLEX) blueprint.* http://www.nabp.net/ftpfiles/NABP01/updatednaplexblueprint.pdf (accessed July 10, 2007).

National Association of Boards of Pharmacy. 2007. *Foreign Pharmacy Graduate Equivalency Examination study guide.* http://www.nabp.net/ftpfiles/bulletins/FPGEEstudyguide.pdf (accessed July 10, 2007).

National Board of Medical Examiners. 2003. *NBME subject examinations: Content outlines and sample items.* http://www.nbme.org/PDF/NBME2003SubjExams.pdf (accessed April 21, 2007).

National Institutes of Health Guide for Grants and Contracts. 2005. *Institutional clinical and translation science award (U54).* http://209.85.165.104/search?q=cache:2RDzml-fcnkJ:grants.nih.gov/grants/guide/rfa-files/rfa-rm-07-002.html (accessed July 10, 2007).

National League for Nursing. 2005. *Transforming nursing education: Position statement.* http://www.nln.org/aboutnln/PositionStatements/transforming052005.pdf (accessed May 21, 2007).

Nester, T. M., and L. S. Hale. 2002. Effectiveness of a pharmacist-acquired medication history in promoting patient safety. *American Journal of Health-System Pharmacy* 59(22):2221-2225.

Pagoto, S. L., B. Spring, E. J. Coups, S. Mulvaney, M. F. Coutu, and G. Ozakinci. 2007. Barriers and facilitators of evidence-based practice perceived by behavioral science health professionals. *Journal of Clinical Psychology* 63(7):695-705.

Pravikoff, D. S., S. T. Pierce, and A. Tanner. 2005. Evidence-based practice readiness study supported by academy nursing informatics expert panel. *Nursing Outlook* 53(1):49-50.

Ross, R., and A. Verdieck. 2003. Introducing an evidence-based medicine curriculum into a family practice residency—is it effective? *Academic Medicine* 78(4):412-417.

Rosswurm, M. A., and J. H. Larrabee. 1999. A model for change to evidence-based practice. *Image—the Journal of Nursing Scholarship* 31(4):317-322.

Rucker, L., and E. Morrison. 2000. The "EBM R_X": An initial experience with an evidence-based learning prescription. *Academic Medicine* 75(5):527-528.

Sackett, D. L., S. E. Straus, W. S. Richardson, W. Rosenberg, and R. B. Haynes. 2000. *Evidence-based medicine: How to practice and teach EBM.* 2nd ed. Oxford, United Kingdom: Churchill Livingstone.

Schultz, A. A. 2005. Clinical scholars at the bedside: An EBP mentorship model for today. *Online Journal of Excellence in Nursing Knowledge.* Indianapolis, IN: The Honor Society of Nursing, Sigma Theta Tau International.

Schumock, G. T., P. D. Meek, P. A. Ploetz, and L. C. Vermeulen. 1996. Economic evaluations of clinical pharmacy services—1988-1995. The Publications Committee of the American College of Clinical Pharmacy. *Pharmacotherapy* 16(6):1188-1208.

Stetler, C. B. 2001. Updating the Stetler model of research utilization to facilitate evidence-based practice. *Nursing Outlook* 49(6):272-279.

Strout, T. D. 2005. Curiosity and reflective thinking: Renewal of the spirit. In *Clinical scholars at the bedside: An EBP mentorship model for today,* edited by A. A. Schultz. Excellence in Nursing Knowledge. Indianapolis, IN: The Honor Society of Nursing, Sigma Theta Tau International.

Titler, M. 2002. Use of research in practice. In *Nursing research: Methods, critical appraisal and utilization.* 5th ed., edited by G. LoBiondo and J. Haber. New York: Mosby.

U.S. Department of Health and Human Services. 2000. *Report to Congress. The pharmacist workforce: A study of the supply and demand for pharmacists.* ftp://ftp.hrsa.gov//bhpr/nationalcenter/pharmacy/pharmstudy.pdf (accessed November 2007).

———. 2003. *Changing demographics: Implications for physicians, nurses and other health workers. 2003.* Bureau of Health Professions National Center for Workforce Analysis, Health Resources and Services Administration. ftp://ftp.hrsa.gov/bhpr/nationalcenter/changedemo.pdf (accessed November 2007).

———. 2004. *The national sample survey of registered nurses (NSSRN).* Bureau of Health Professions, Division of Nursing, Health Resources and Services Administration. http://bhpr.hrsa.gov/healthworkforce/reports/rnpopulation/preliminaryfindings.htm (accessed November 2007).

U.S. Department of Labor. 2006. Registered nurses. In *Occupational outlook handbook, 2006-07 edition.* Bureau of Labor Statistics. http://www.bls.gov/oco/ocos083.htm (accessed June 17, 2007).

Walsh, J. M., K. M. McDonald, K. G. Shojania, V. Sundaram, S. Nayak, R. Lewis, D. K. Owens, and M. K. Goldstein. 2006. Quality improvement strategies for hypertension management: A systematic review. *Medical Care* 44(7):646-657.

Winawer, S., R. Fletcher, D. Rex, J. Bond, R. Burt, J. Ferrucci, T. Ganiats, T. Levin, S. Woolf, D. Johnson, L. Kirk, S. Litin, and C. Simmang. 2003. Colorectal cancer screening and surveillance: Clinical guidelines and rationale-update based on new evidence. *Gastroenterology* 124(2):544-560.

Zucker, B., C. Goss, D. Williams, L. Bloodworth, M. Lynn, A. Denker, and J. D. Gibbs. 2006. Nursing retention in the era of a nursing shortage: Norton navigators. *Journal for Nurses in Staff Development* 22(6):302-306.

7

Healthcare Delivery Organizations

Coordinator

Robert M. Crane, Kaiser Permanente Institute for Health Policy

Other Contributors

Madhulika Agarwal, Veterans Health Administration; Denis Cortese, Mayo Clinic; Benjamin Druss, Emory University; Kate Meyers, Kaiser Permanente Institute for Health Policy, Jonathan Perlin, HCA, Inc.; Richard Platt, Harvard Medical School and Harvard Pilgrim Health Care; Laura Tollen, Kaiser Permanente Institute for Health Policy

SECTOR OVERVIEW

This chapter focuses on healthcare delivery organizations and is limited to two major entities: (1) integrated delivery systems (IDSs) and large physician groups and (2) hospitals. The discussion excludes physicians in solo and small group practices because such practices are too small to provide the organizational infrastructure that is the focus of this sector. However, it should be noted that physicians in solo or small group practices (2 to 10 physicians) make up fully 99 percent of office-based physician practices and that 89 percent of the physicians in the United States are in solo or small group practices (Hing and Burt, 2007).

Without major changes in clinical practice by these physicians, no amount of change by the more organized delivery sector will enable achievement of the Roundtable's goal (smaller clinical practices are addressed in Chapter 5, which describes the healthcare professional sector). Despite the number of nonorganized physicians, however, healthcare delivery organizations play a critical role because of their ability to drive practice trends, set standards, and influence smaller practices by sharing information, resources, and guidelines. A key to achieving the Roundtable's goal will be to improve the organizational infrastructure for physicians who are currently nonorganized and/or in small groups, and healthcare delivery organizations can play an important role in facilitating that improvement.

The task in this chapter is to describe how healthcare delivery organizations can enable the generation and use of evidence. "Evidence" itself is a murky concept, and there has been much debate over what type of information qualifies as evidence for the purpose of "evidence-based medicine." Most experts agree that the results of randomized controlled trials (RCTs) would qualify as evidence, but there is less agreement about the validity of other types of information, such as observational research and expert opinion and consensus. For the most part, the means of the "generation of evidence" in this chapter excludes expert opinion and refers mainly to more formal types of research and observational analysis (such as the analysis of large datasets created as part of the usual delivery of care), whether or not the findings are published in peer-reviewed journals. Also included is evidence generated by mathematical modeling techniques. When the "use of evidence" or the "dissemination of evidence" is addressed in this chapter, the origins of such information are not specified but are assumed to come from sound research rather than from accepted standards of community practice. For further discussion of the definition of "evidence," see the charter statement for the Institute of Medicine's (IOM's) Roundtable on Evidence-Based Medicine (IOM Roundtable on Evidence-Based Medicine, 2006).

To answer the question of how healthcare delivery organizations can enable the generation and use of evidence, semistructured interviews were conducted with sector members and other experts from relevant organizations.[1] Over the course of these interviews, two general themes emerged: (1) significant data aggregation is critical, and information technology is fundamental to such aggregation; and (2) healthcare organizations need to have a culture of using everyday healthcare delivery as a learning tool and a means of generating evidence.

Data Aggregation and Information Technology

Without information technology to enable the aggregation of data across settings and time, the practice of evidence-based medicine becomes nearly impossible. Data aggregation can take place at the level of a single delivery organization by using a comprehensive electronic health record (EHR), or it can take place at the level of an external third party, such as a payer, that can combine claims data from multiple providers. An example of the former is Kaiser Permanente's implementation of KP HealthConnect, a system that integrates the electronic medical record with appointments,

---

[1]For a list of interviewees see below references.

registration, and billing, linking facilities and providing physicians and patients with online access to clinical information 24 hours per day (Kaiser Permanente, 2007a). Another example is the Veterans Health Information Systems and Technology Architecture (VistA), which integrates patient records and administrative data to provide real-time data access across more than 150 healthcare facilities and 800 clinics throughout the United States and in several U.S. territories. Examples of multiorganization systems include the Cancer Research Network, sponsored by the National Cancer Institute and the HMO Research Network, and the American Medical Group Association's collaborative database of 1.5 million patient records. All of these systems have in common not just the ability to aggregate data but also the analytic capacity to organize and retrieve data in useful ways.

Culture of Continuous Learning

The interviewees agreed that there simply are not enough RCTs to keep up with the ever-advancing onslaught of new technologies, procedures, drugs, and so forth in medical care (let alone the already established technologies for which evidence to support their use may or may not be available). Such trials are costly and time intensive, and their results may not be generalizable to patient populations not included in the study, rendering RCTs unrealistic as the only acceptable standard of evidence generation for the majority of medical practices. Some experts have also noted that the peer-review process for publication of RCTs is narrow: typically, only a handful of reviewers, selected by the journal, examine a research study and its findings before it is deemed publishable. It is only after publication, when the study has already, arguably, become "evidence," that a broad array of experts can examine it and test its findings against their own experience in real-world situations. Furthermore, the amount of evidence available to support each and every medical decision will increase exponentially in the coming years and decades as massive amounts of information become available from the fields of genomics and proteomics. Organizations need to learn to make continuous use of their own observational data and, in the words of Lynn Etheredge (2007), become "rapid-learning health systems" as they face a learning curve that becomes continually steeper. Rapid-learning health systems are those that can combine the clinical experiences of their patients (and, possibly, the experiences of other organizations' patients) in a searchable database that can be used for research. Such organizations view every patient encounter as adding to the collective knowledge of the group and as a means to test a hypothesis so that others in the group can benefit from the knowledge that is generated.

Although this chapter focuses on physician group practices and hospitals separately, it is important to emphasize that both types of organizations will provide the greatest value to the field of evidence-based medicine by cooperating with other organizations within the larger delivery system. For example, data obtained from inpatient settings alone can be misleading, as patients receive care in many settings. Research into what works must take into account the fact that critical follow-up care after hospitalization takes place in the community. This follow-up care can have a huge impact on whether or not the care provided in the hospital can be considered effective. As a result, evidence about hospital-based care is not entirely separable from evidence about physician organizations. IDSs that are fully integrated and that combine inpatient and outpatient care delivery are particularly well positioned to track the delivery of care across settings.

The following sections of this chapter present an overview of the specific practices that healthcare delivery organizations use to generate and use evidence in clinical decision making. The chapter also provides a description of the challenges and a set of opportunities. At the outset, however, it is important to recognize the distance between the status quo and the goal of the IOM's Roundtable on Evidence-Based Medicine. Reaching the goal of having 90 percent of clinical decisions being evidence based by 2020 will not be easy. Healthcare delivery organizations know how to generate data; but data are not the same as usable information, and the availability of usable information does not guarantee its use. Furthermore, the generation of evidence is not without cost. Although the current practices, challenges, and recommendations are a useful start, overcoming the gaps in data, information, and the will to change must not be underestimated. Reaching the Roundtable's goal by 2020 will take more than tinkering around the edges of the healthcare delivery system. Rather, it will take fundamental restructuring and rethinking by all stakeholders, as was recommended by the IOM in its 2001 report *Crossing the Quality Chasm* (Institute of Medicine, 2001).

Current Practices

As noted above, this chapter addresses two major classes of healthcare delivery organizations: (1) IDSs and large physician groups and (2) hospitals. A simple description of each of these subsectors is warranted.

Integrated Delivery Systems and Large Physician Group Practices

As described by Enthoven and Tollen (2005), IDSs are organizations built on the core of a large, multispecialty medical group practice, often with links to hospitals, laboratories, pharmacies, and other facilities and often with a sizable amount of revenue based on per capita prepayment. Examples of IDSs include delivery organizations that also have an insurance function, such as Kaiser Permanente and Group Health Cooperative. Also included in this category, although it is not technically an insurer, is the Veterans Health Administration (VHA), which delivers extensive healthcare services and also purchases (finances) services that are not available within the organization.

This chapter also discusses large public and private physician group practices, which may or may not have links to a specific health plan. Many of the nation's largest and most well-known private multispecialty physician groups, including the Cleveland Clinic and the Mayo Clinic, are members of the Council of Accountable Physician Practices, which seeks to foster the development and recognition of accountable physician practices as a model for transforming the American healthcare system (Council of Accountable Physician Practices, 2007).[2] Other groups that represent IDSs and large physician group practices include the American Medical Group Association and the Alliance of Community Health Plans (Alliance of Community Health Plans, 2007; American Medical Group Association, 2007). Many publicly funded community clinics also function similarly to large multispecialty physician groups.

Because there is no generally agreed-upon definition of an IDS, it is difficult to provide an exact count of the number of IDSs in existence today. More readily available, however, are data on medical groups, and as noted above, the core of an IDS is a large, multispecialty medical group, whether it is public or private.

According to the U.S. Department of Health and Human Services (HHS), in 2003-2004 (the most recent year for which complete data are available), there were 311,200 office-based physicians in the United States practicing in 161,200 medical practices (Hing and Burt, 2007). As previously noted, physicians in solo or small group practices (2 to 10 physicians) make up fully 99 percent of the physicians in office-based physician practices and 89 percent of the physicians in the United States. Therefore, physicians who are the focus of this sector—those in larger groups—constitute only 1 percent of practices and 11 percent of physicians. Nearly 79 percent of physicians are in solo practice or single-specialty groups, whereas only 21 percent are in multispecialty groups. Although the percentage of physicians in large or multispecialty groups, or both, seems small, these physicians do care for a significant percentage of the U.S. population. For example, the members of the American Medical Group Association care for more than 50 million Americans (American Medical Group Association, 2007).

Hospitals

Hospitals and hospital systems comprise another important part of the healthcare delivery organizations sector. As stand-alone entities or

---

[2]For a list of Council of Accountable Physician Practices members, see www.amga.org/CAPP.

as part of healthcare systems or networks, public and private hospitals account for about 30 percent of the expenditures on health care in the United States (California HealthCare Foundation, 2006). The following data on hospitals are from the American Hospital Association (2007). There are nearly 5,800 hospitals in the United States, most of which are classified as community hospitals (nonfederal, short-term general, and other specialty hospitals, such as cancer centers or orthopedic specialty centers, including academic medical centers, fit these criteria). More than 80 percent of community hospitals are not for profit or public (state and local).

About 2,700 community hospitals are part of a "system," defined by the American Hospital Association as "a multihospital or a diversified single hospital system. A multihospital system is two or more hospitals owned, leased, sponsored, or managed under contract by a central organization. Single, freestanding hospitals may be categorized as a system by bringing into membership three or more and at least 25 percent of their owned or leased nonhospital preacute or postacute healthcare organizations." About 1,400 community hospitals are part of a "network," defined by the American Hospital Association as "a group of hospitals, physicians, other providers, insurers and/or community agencies that work together to coordinate and deliver a broad spectrum of services to their community." By these definitions, systems and networks are not mutually exclusive: an entity can be classified as both part of a system and part of a network (American Hospital Association, 2007).

As defined by the National Association of Public Hospitals and Health Systems (2006), safety net hospitals "include healthcare providers owned and operated by cities, counties, states, universities, non-profit organizations, or other entities" that have "a common . . . mission of providing health care to all, regardless of ability to pay." In addition to inpatient care, many safety net hospitals also deliver outpatient care. On average, the 100 members of the National Association of Public Hospitals and Health Systems take care of the individuals involved in more than 400,000 ambulatory care visits per year, or approximately 36 percent of outpatient visits in the safety net.

Hospitals and hospital systems are clearly not a homogeneous group, and their differences have bearing on their current and future roles in promoting the goals of the IOM's Roundtable on Evidence-Based Medicine. Although the definition is not comprehensive, use of the following definitions is one useful way to parse hospitals and hospital systems when their role in the generation and use of evidence is considered: (1) integrated hospital systems comprise hospitals that are closely integrated with multispecialty medical groups (such as the Mayo Clinic and Kaiser Permanente), (2) academic medical centers are integrated with medical schools, and

(3) nonprofit or for-profit community hospitals may or may not have affiliations with other hospitals or a network. The VHA hospitals represent a fourth category, as they combine aspects of the first two categories provided above. Another way to categorize hospitals is by the organizations that they choose to represent them at the national level, such as the American Hospital Association, the Federation of American Hospitals, and the National Association of Public Hospitals and Health Systems. Each broad category of hospitals has different types of incentives and infrastructures for the generation and use of evidence, which will be discussed in more detail in subsequent sections of this chapter.

ACTIVITY CATEGORIES

Many experts believe that healthcare delivery organizations, including hospitals, are better positioned than physicians in solo and small group practices to generate and use evidence in clinical decision making (Casalino et al., 2003a; Crosson, 2005; Enthoven and Tollen, 2005). Ultimately, they accomplish this by developing evidence-based practice guidelines and making them available to providers at the point of care. According to Berwick and Jain (2004), doing this requires a number of support systems that can "(1) find the science, (2) embed the science in sound standards of practice, (3) make the relevant knowledge available to clinicians and patients at the point of care and at the time of care, and (4) track performance and improve it continually." They also note that in creating such systems, "prepaid group practices are at the forefront." That statement can be expanded to include not just prepaid group practices but also large IDSs, large physician group practices (prepaid or not), and sophisticated hospitals.

How do healthcare delivery organizations develop the four systems described by Berwick and Jain? On the basis of the responses from the interviews, the primary mechanisms that these organizations use are described below.

Information Technology

As noted earlier, the aggregation of data across care settings and time is critical to the generation of evidence, and large delivery organizations have an advantage in this area for three reasons: (1) they have a sufficient patient base to support the meaningful (statistically relevant) aggregation of data; (2) they are more likely to have the resources required to implement and maintain the electronic data systems that are necessary for data aggregation and the provision of real-time decision support to clinicians; and (3) in the case of integrated systems, they have access to data from the many settings in which patients receive care.

According to Jha and colleagues (2006), although there is no universally accepted definition of the EHR, "consensus is emerging that electronic documentation of providers' notes, electronic viewing of laboratory and radiology results, and electronic prescribing are key components of an EHR." These tools facilitate the use of evidence-based practice because they provide clinicians with decision support (in the form of reminders, order sets, and templates) and current practice guidelines at the point of care.[3] However, it is not necessary for all of these elements to be in place for a healthcare delivery organization to benefit from electronic data capture. Disease registries can also provide an important platform for conducting research and implementing evidence-based care by providing information about every patient in a provider's population with a given condition.

Although the use of EHRs is on the rise, only about 25 percent of physicians use them, and among office-based physicians, that number is closer to 19 percent (Jha et al., 2006). Large physician group practices and IDSs have been leaders in implementing EHRs (Halvorson, 2004). In fact, the predominant factor affecting the use of information technology is practice size (Audet et al., 2004). Audet and colleagues (2004) found that 87 percent of physicians in large group practices but only 36 percent of physicians in solo practice have access to electronic test results. Other information technologies follow a similar pattern. Physicians in large group practices are more likely than solo practitioners to use EHRs, receive electronic drug alerts, and use e-mail to communicate with colleagues and patients (Audet et al., 2004).

Evidence on the use of EHRs in the inpatient setting is lacking. One systematic review of surveys on the adoption of EHRs found that the only higher-quality studies in the inpatient setting focused exclusively on computerized physician order entry (CPOE), or electronic prescribing, which is just one component of an EHR. That review concluded that just 5 percent of hospitals use CPOE and that no high-quality estimate of inpatient EHR use could be made (Jha et al., 2006). Another study that used some of the same source data on CPOE that Jha and colleagues (2006) used found that investment in this technology was more likely in government (nonfederal, in the study of Cutler [2005]) and teaching hospitals than in other types of hospitals, with for-profit hospitals being the least likely, and that larger hospitals were more likely than others to invest in CPOE (Cutler, 2005).

As with integrated systems and large physician group practices, hospital investment in information technology supports the generation and

---

[3]It should be noted, however, that if the guidelines available through the EHR are not themselves evidence based, the EHR will do little to improve practice. The EHR is only a tool to convey information; other processes must be in place to ensure that the information is evidence based.

use of evidence. Given the limited use of EHRs in hospitals at present, this potential is far from being realized. Different types of hospitals may have various incentives and capabilities to implement EHRs. Integrated hospital systems likely have the greatest capacity and incentive to invest in EHRs because of the economies of scale and the purchasing power of a larger system and because of their ability to share best practices about implementing the technology. Prepaid integrated hospital systems may have additional capacities and incentives to invest in these technologies because of global budgets. Academic medical centers may have incentives to create such systems to remain on the cutting edge and to enable better research and training, but they would typically not enjoy the same incentives as the prepaid integrated systems. Other nonprofit and for-profit community hospitals typically have less of a capability or incentive to purchase and implement large-scale information systems because of an inability to spread costs over their smaller institutions.

In a practice or hospital setting not supported by information technology, providers must rely on their memories to keep up with best practices. This is a nearly impossible task when one considers that the results of 10,000 RCTs are published each year (Chassin, 1998). According to David Eddy (1999), a leader in the field of evidence-based medicine, "The complexity of modern medicine exceeds the inherent limitations of the unaided human mind." However, having an EHR does not guarantee support for evidence-based practice. The structure—and, therein, the utility—of the data repository is important in determining how much providers can learn in real time. Issues that play a role in maximizing the usefulness of electronic data include which data are captured in the clinical information system, which data are captured as free-text notes that may not be searchable versus which data are captured as defined fields that are searchable, and whether individual data systems are connected to one another to give a comprehensive picture of a patient's clinical situation across practice settings.

Significant Research Capacity

The large patient populations that healthcare delivery organizations serve provide a foundation for conducting research to support evidence-based guidelines. According to Fink and Greenlick (2004), before the 1950s, little was known about the use of health services by noninstitutionalized populations. At about that time, the emergence of several IDSs as a source of care for large populations provided an unprecedented opportunity for research across the full spectrum of care. Some of the pioneering IDSs that established research centers include Kaiser Permanente, the HIP Health Plan of New York, and the VHA.

Today, Kaiser Permanente's eight research centers together comprise one of the largest nonacademic research institutions in the United States (Kaiser Permanente, 2007b). Similar to the Kaiser and HIP research programs, the Mayo Clinic's Department of Health Services Research also evolved out of large-scale epidemiological projects, including the Olmsted County project, the medical information (medical records, laboratory test and radiological examination results, and tissue specimens) from which the Mayo Clinic has retained for more than 50 years. This information has been the basis of many large-scale observational studies that have led to the development of new knowledge, supporting the Mayo Clinic's clinical practice, education programs, and research.

The VHA also has an expansive national research program, with studies being conducted at more than 100 medical centers on topics that include mental illness, long-term care, traumatic injury, and special populations, such as female veterans. VHA research has made direct contributions to current clinical practices for hypertension, posttraumatic stress disorder, diabetes, and other chronic diseases. The VHA has established a unique program, the Quality Enhancement Research Initiative, whose mission is to bring researchers into partnership with healthcare system leaders to ensure that the care provided is based on the most current scientific evidence, thereby bringing scientific discovery from the bedside to the bench and then back to the bedside (Francis and Perlin, 2006). In collaborating with external, academic research institutions, the VHA can serve as a model for other healthcare system-based research organizations.

In addition to these system-specific research centers, many healthcare delivery organizations have joined together in various networks to pool research data and capabilities. Examples include the HMO Research Network and the Cancer Research Network.[4] All of these research institutions can provide important insight into evidence-based practice.

Systematic Use of External Resources

In addition to generating their own research, another means by which healthcare delivery organizations gather evidence for clinical decision making is by availing themselves of external resources. Many healthcare delivery organizations have standing internal technology assessment committees or

---

[4]Members of the HMO Research Network include seven regions of Kaiser Permanente, HealthPartners Research Foundation, Group Health Cooperative, Harvard Pilgrim Health Care, Henry Ford Health System-Health Alliance Plan, Lovelace Clinic Foundation, Meyers Primary Care Institute, Fallon Community Health Plan, Fallon Foundation and the University of Massachusetts Medical School, Scott and White Health System, Geisinger Health System, and Marshfield Clinic Research Foundation. See www.hmoresearchnetwork.org. For information on the Cancer Research Network, see http://crn.cancer.gov/.

pharmacy and therapeutics committees whose purposes are to assess all available information on new procedures, devices, and drugs and determine what should be used in practice and how. These committees rely on the internal analysis both of the data and the medical literature and of information from external organizations that provide independent research and analysis, including the Blue Cross Blue Shield Association's Technology Evaluation Center, Hayes, Inc., UpToDate, ECRI Institute, the Evidence-Based Practice Centers sponsored by the Agency for Healthcare Research and Quality, the Cochrane Collaboration, and the Center for Evidence-Based Policy at the Oregon Health and Science University (Agency for Healthcare Research and Quality, 2007; BlueCross BlueShield Association, 2000; Cochrane Collaboration, 2007; ECRI Institute, 2007; Hayes, Inc., 2007; Oregon Health and Science University, 2007; UpToDate, 2007).

Quality Measurement and Reporting

Critical to the successful implementation of evidence-based practice guidelines is a system of accountability to ensure that the guidelines are being used. One of the ways that healthcare delivery organizations do this is through systematic quality measurement. Because of their size and organizational capacity, such organizations are more likely than smaller practices to have in place quality measurement systems whose capabilities go beyond those required for accreditation. Reporting on the results of the Community Tracking Study survey, Casalino and colleagues (2003b) found that the advantages of medical groups of at least moderate size are their ability to create organized processes to proactively improve care, serve as units of analysis for which statistically reliable and valid measurements of quality can be made, and monitor clinical performance and implement clinical protocols.

Hospitals, too, can implement performance measurement and reporting systems within their institutions to help physicians understand how their performance on particular evidence-based quality measures compares with that of their peers. Quality measurement can be used as an internal means of monitoring performance, or it can be tied to financial incentives, as in pay-for-performance programs. If it is done correctly, pay-for-performance can help accelerate the adoption of evidence-based medicine, but to do so, such schemes must reward adherence to evidence-based practice rather than simply reporting on processes.

Culture and Leadership

An intangible but important element of improving the use of evidence-based clinical decision making is the organizational culture and leadership.

Physicians and other clinicians must be comfortable with the notion that there is in fact a best practice that may not be their own current practice. This way of thinking can be in conflict with physicians' training, in which they are taught to be self-reliant, independent thinkers. For some, the use of guidelines may feel like "cookbook medicine" and may be viewed with suspicion. In an essay on group responsibility in medicine, Crosson and colleagues (2004) note, "It was not so long ago that physicians held a God-like sway over the healthcare universe. After all, it was a universe that consisted, for the most part, of tens of thousands of highly personalized, independent solo practices, each tending to the healthcare needs of hundreds of individual patients, one at a time. Within that intimate relationship between physician and patient, the physician held all the knowledge, all the power, all the authority."

Today, medicine has become so highly complex that individual physicians can no longer hold all the knowledge that is relevant to their practice, and they must rely on others—colleagues and organizational structures—to help them do this. This is best accomplished within an organizational culture and with strong leadership that emphasize the use of evidence-based medicine, collaboration, and group responsibility for a population of patients rather than the outmoded model of one patient and one provider.

Human Factors Principles

Organizations that provide a physical space for the delivery of care can establish systems within their institutions that support medical staff in doing the right thing for the right patient at the right time. Systems that address human factors build evidence-based and safety principles into the design of buildings, technology, and the workflow. Examples include medication management tools (to avoid the prescription of incorrect doses or the contraindicated use of medications) and establishing standard codes among different hospitals in the same area to reduce errors when staff work in more than one facility. Hospitals can also identify what processes are needed to address quality gaps and to bundle those processes, making it the standard of care for patients with given circumstances to receive that bundle of interventions, which are supported by tools such as standing orders, protocols, and care team training. The VHA Center for Patient Safety offers an outstanding example of a systemwide safety program that is predominantly electronic in nature and that produces aggregate data for performance improvement activities and incident avoidance.

Case Studies

The following case studies illustrate the ways in which healthcare delivery organizations have incorporated the practices described above to support the use of evidence-based medicine. Each organization uses a combination of the techniques described, as no single practice is sufficient to achieve the type of culture change needed to reorient an organization toward evidence-based decision making.

Kaiser Permanente Care Management Institute

As the nation's largest nonprofit health plan and largest nonfederal integrated healthcare delivery system, Kaiser Permanente cares for 8.7 million members in eight geographic regions. One of Kaiser Permanente's assets in improving the generation and use of evidence is the Care Management Institute (CMI), which works to improve health outcomes through the identification, implementation, and evaluation of nationally consistent evidence-based population care management programs. Focusing on some of the most common and costly chronic diseases (e.g., diabetes, asthma, depression, hypertension, and chronic pain) as well as on the unique needs of specific populations, such as older adults, CMI acts as a central hub for the development of evidence-based guidelines, models of care, and common measurement systems for use across Kaiser Permanente.

CMI's guiding philosophy is "making the right thing easier to do." With collaboration among 55 staff members, work groups of clinicians, and other experts and with the use of regional implementation and measurement counterparts, its specific streams of work include creating and sharing knowledge about successful clinical approaches, designing and collecting empirical measurement and modeling projections to inform decision making, identifying and diffusing successful practices and innovations, and creating and supporting systems that enhance health care.

One example of CMI's work focuses on decreasing the risk of cardiovascular events among people with diabetes and coronary artery disease. There is compelling clinical evidence that a combination of three medications, aspirin, lisinopril, and lovastatin (ALL), can reduce the risk of heart attack, stroke, and death in patients over 55 year of age with diabetes and in patients with coronary artery disease by more than 70 percent. CMI's ALL initiative tracks regional performance on ALL use and facilitates the sharing of successful practices to increase the rate of use of this combination of medications in the target population. These practices include programs for mailed prescriptions, group visits, phone consultations with pharmacists, electronic reminders for physicians, tools for panel management support, patient coaching outside of the office, and the involvement of the entire healthcare team. From 2002 to 2005, the proportions of members with coronary artery disease and those over age 55 years with diabetes who took the ALL medications increased from 49 to 67 percent (personal communication, Michelle Wong, Kaiser Permanente Care Management Institute, 2007).

Safety Net Clinics

Community clinics are an integral part of the safety net, with more than 1,000 health centers serving an estimated 14.8 million patients in 2006 (personal communication, D. Geolot, Center of Quality, and colleagues, Health Resources and Services Administration, U.S. Department of Health and Human Services, 2007). Driven by a mission of serving the underserved, safety net clinics engage in a number of practices aimed at improving the quality of care on the basis of a general evidence-based approach. These safety net clinics and health centers use a range of technologies to help support evidence-based practice, including practice management tools, registries, care management systems, and EHRs that integrate these different functions and more. At present, only about 8 percent of health centers have full EHRs, but the majority of those that do not are actively considering investing in EHR systems and doing research to make informed choices so that they may select the system that best meets their needs.

Safety net clinics were early adopters of the notion of evidence-based practice and quality improvement processes, as demonstrated by a partnership with the Institute for Healthcare Improvement to form Health Disparities Collaboratives, which began in 1998. This evidence-based systems change initiative is, at its core, a quality improvement effort based on known quality deficiencies in the treatment of chronic diseases and cancer and in the prevention of these diseases. It focuses on the translation of evidence into practice by identifying the optimal ways to deliver the right care and applies evidence-based criteria to clinical, operational, and fiscal components. It is explicitly an evidence-based practice framework applied to all components of delivery of care, using national clinical experts, national management experts, and national experts in systems change. More than 90 percent of health centers participated in the collaboratives in 2007. Through this process, health centers have adopted the use of the same terminology and models for quality improvement, enabling the more rapid communication and dissemination of successful practices.

The collaboratives focused on improving processes of care and succeeded in this regard. One evaluation found that the centers participating in the collaboratives had significantly greater improvement than external and internal control centers in certain measures of prevention, screening, disease treatment, and monitoring, including "a 21 percent increase in foot examinations for patients with diabetes, . . . a 14 percent increase in the use of anti-inflammatory medication for asthma, and a 16 percent increase in the assessment of glycated hemoglobin" (Landon et al., 2007). However, the same evaluation showed no improvement in any of the intermediate clinical outcomes assessed to date. Given that finding, safety net clinics are now looking at ways to integrate more monitoring of outcomes through the development of core measures. Although the collaboratives have mainly focused on ways of "pushing" evidence to clinicians and translating evidence into practice, plans for future work emphasize the "pull" for evidence-based care by the use of more standardized quality measures across the program in areas where the evidence is strong. This measurement will enable the identification of model programs that can be disseminated elsewhere and can provide centers with information on comparable patient populations.

Veterans Health Administration

As the largest public IDS in the United States, the VHA annually serves 5.3 million patients at nearly 1,400 sites of care (Kupersmith et al., 2007). Although its patients are older, sicker, and poorer than the general U.S. population, the VHA's performance surpasses that of other health systems on standardized quality measures (Asch et al., 2004). The transformation of the VHA was enabled by the adoption of evidence-based practice guidelines and quality measures; a renewed focus on the safety of vulnerable groups of people, such as individuals with mental or chronic illnesses; and the development of a performance management system that held senior managers accountable for evidence-based quality measures (Jha et al., 2003).

All of this work was supported by the creation of a comprehensive EHR, now known as VistA, which includes a suite of more than 100 applications supporting clinical, financial, and administrative functions. Access to VistA was made possible through a user interface known as the computerized patient record system (CPRS). With VistA/CPRS, providers can securely access patient information at the point of care, update a patient's medical history, place orders, and review test results and drug prescriptions. Because VistA also stores medical images such as x-rays and photographs directly in the patient record, clinicians have access to all of the information that they need for diagnosis and treatment. As of December 2005, VistA systems contained 779 million clinical documents, more than 1.5 billion orders, and 425 million images.

Many clinicians initially resisted the use of the EHR. Convincing them otherwise took several approaches. The most important approach was involving clinicians at the onset. This meant working to ensure the usability and integration of the EHR system with clinical processes. Local and national supports were created. Local "superusers" were designated to champion the project; and a national Veterans Electronic Health University facilitated collaboration among the local, regional, and national sponsors of the EHR rollout. National performance measures and the gradual withdrawal of paper records made the use of EHR an inescapable reality. Finally, the economic costs to clinicians were blunted by a salaried environment, and other benefits (such as reductions in time wasted searching for paper records) also emerged. Over time, staff came to view VistA/CPRS as indispensable for good clinical care (Brown et al., 2003).

VistA/CPRS allows clinicians to access and generate clinical information about their individual patients, but additional steps are needed to yield insights into population health. Structured clinical data in the EHR can be aggregated within specialized databases, providing a rich source of data for VHA administrators and health services researchers. Additionally, unstructured text data, such as clinicians' notes, can be reviewed and abstracted electronically from a central location. This is of particular benefit to researchers: VHA multisite clinical trials and observational studies are facilitated by immediate 100 percent chart availability.

The greatest advantage of EHRs in the VHA is their ability to influence the behavior of patients, clinicians, and the system itself. For instance, the VHA's diabetes registry has been used to construct performance profiles for administrators, clinical managers, and clinicians. These profiles included comparisons of facilities and identified the proportion of veterans with substantial elevations in their hemoglobin HbA1c and cholesterol levels and blood pressure. Patient lists also facilitated follow-up with high-risk patients. The EHR system also allows the consideration of options that can be used to intensify therapy in response to that risk level (such as starting or increasing the dose of a cholesterol-lowering medication when the patient's low-density lipid cholesterol level is elevated). This approach credits clinicians with providing optimal treatment and informs them about what might be required to improve care (Kerr et al., 2003).

The VHA has been an EHR innovator, developing from the ground up a clinically rich system that has become so integrated into the delivery of care and the conduct of research that one cannot imagine a veterans' health system without it. However, many factors in addition to the EHR contributed to the VHA's quality transformation, including a culture with academicians-clinicians who value quality, scientific evidence, and accountability; the presence of embedded researchers who are active clinicians, managers, policy makers, and the developers of VistA/CPRS; and a research infrastructure that can be applied to this topic (Greenfield and Kaplan, 2004; Perlin, 2006).

Mayo Clinic

The Mayo Clinic has a long and distinguished history as a leader in the provision of high-quality health care and as a learning organization through its use of core strategies of integrated medical practice, education, and research, all underpinned by the provision of information in an accurate, timely, and reliable manner. The Mayo Clinic's culture is centered on the notions of systems engineering. The organization has included a formal focus on systems engineering through its Department of Systems and Procedures since 1947. Several specific actions taken in recent years demonstrate the Mayo Clinic's efforts to provide quality and high-value care using evidence-based decisions and distributing evidence at the point of care. Building on their existing EHR, Mayo Clinic staff members are developing the Enterprise Learning System (ELS), which distributes clinical knowledge and patient-specific triggers to physicians in a timely way. Future plans for the ELS include the ability to provide continuing medical education as just-in-time learning when an individual accesses specific information in the ELS. In addition, the Mayo Clinic is building an Enterprise Information Technology Data Trust for all patient-related data that will improve its efforts to modify old information and to generate new knowledge. Several components of the Mayo Clinic's organizational structure also support the generation and use of evidence. For example, the Mayo Clinic has an enterprise-wide Quality Academy, through which the organization is taking significant steps to improve transparency, both internally and externally. In addition, it has a Department of Health Sciences Research that supports quality efforts and generates knowledge about clinically related questions.

Institute for Clinical Systems Improvement

In an impressive example of a virtual system working to improve the use of evidence-based medicine, 11 competing hospital systems (operating a combined total of 26 hospitals in southeastern Minnesota) created the Safest in America program. Members of the group work toward the ideal of being the safest in America by sharing data, exchanging information, implementing best practices, and implementing community standardization where appropriate. Safest in America is facilitated by the Institute for Clinical Systems Improvement, an independent, nonprofit organization that facilitates collaboration on healthcare quality improvement by medical groups, hospitals, and health plans in the state of Minnesota and in adjacent areas of surrounding states. Founded in 1993 by HealthPartners Medical Group, the Mayo Clinic, and Park Nicollet Health Services, the Institute for Clinical Systems Improvement today has 62 members and is funded by all six health plans in Minnesota. The medical groups and hospital systems combined represent more than 7,600 physicians (Institute for Clinical Systems Improvement, 2007).

Safest in America hospitals have put competition aside to collectively set goals for the prevention of ventilator-associated pneumonia, the implementation of rapid response teams, reductions in the incidence of hyper- and hypoglycemia, and other patient safety issues. A key value of Safest in America has been its ability to facilitate community-wide standardization, when appropriate. For example, one of Safest in America's first projects in 2000 was a community-wide ban on the use of nine unsafe prescription abbreviations. In recent years, hospitals implemented a standard safe-site surgery protocol to verify the surgical site, patient, and procedure. This year, Safest in America hospitals will implement a standard protocol to prevent the retention of unintended foreign objects in the patient's body during surgical procedures.

Archimedes

Evidence-based medicine is often thought of as syntheses of data points from clinical trials or other sources that can be used to determine the best course of action for a particular patient population. Mathematical modeling goes beyond this paradigm to include projections about what would likely happen (as opposed to what has happened in past studies) to certain types of patients in certain scenarios on the basis of what is already known from existing clinical trials or other data. The Archimedes model, developed by David Eddy and Len Schlessinger, creates a virtual reality that is able to simulate a series of events for specific patient populations. In the model, "all the important objects and events in the real world have corresponding objects and events in the model's world. When a simulation is run, the objects interact and events occur as they would in the real world. [The model] has virtual people with virtual physiologies who get virtual diseases, go to virtual doctors, get virtual tests and treatments and have virtual outcomes" (Archimedes-Kaiser Permanente, 2007). The model can focus on simulated patients, doctors, offices, tests, equipment, or treatments in the areas of diabetes, coronary artery disease, congestive heart failure, asthma, stroke, hypertension, dyslipidemia, and obesity, with the potential for other conditions to be added in the future. The model has been validated against existing real-world clinical trials by simulating the different components of those trials and comparing the results of the simulation to the results of the actual trial itself (Archimedes-Kaiser Permanente, 2007). The model enables experimentation with different interventions or different assumptions about patient characteristics or care processes and has the ability to explore the impacts of these variations on outcomes of interest.

The Archimedes model can use existing clinical evidence to support care protocols, and it can also generate new evidence. The model uses existing evidence and data from clinical trials, large-scale surveys and datasets, health risk appraisals, and, once they are available, EHRs to represent real populations in its virtual world. It generates evidence by testing a variety of interventions or alternatives. For example, as described by Eddy (Eddy, 2007), the objective of a model like Archimedes is to create a virtual world that can be used to help analyze physiological processes; design guidelines, performance measures, and the "what-to-do" parts of disease management programs; design the "how-to-do-it" parts of disease management programs, case management protocols, and continuous quality improvement (CQI) projects; forecast logistics, utilization, costs, and cost-effectiveness; set clinical priorities and design strategic goals; prioritize or combine performance measures; analyze the effects of multiple diseases (co-morbidities), syndromes that affect multiple organ systems, drugs that have multiple effects, and combinations of drugs; address questions of timing, such as screening, frequency of follow-up visits, or how long a medication should be tried before the dose is changed; and help design and predict clinical trials.

Eddy and Schlessinger developed the Archimedes model with major support from Kaiser Permanente, and the model is now available to all researchers and healthcare delivery organizations. For example, the American Diabetes Association has partnered with Archimedes to create a World Wide Web–based consumer-focused tool called Diabetes PhD (American Diabetes Association, 2007). The tool allows consumers to enter personal information about their health history and to explore the effects of a variety of interventions, including losing weight, stopping smoking, and taking certain medications. Diabetes PhD creates a personalized results overview for each patient that shows the patient's current risk for diabetes, heart attack, stroke, kidney failure, and foot and eye complications. By changing the variables in the profile, such as smoking cessation or weight loss, patients can see how these changes will affect their future health.

Challenges

Although healthcare delivery organizations have made strides in improving the development and use of evidence in clinical decision making, there are many challenges to reaching the Roundtable's goal of having 90 percent of clinical decisions being evidence based by 2020. Among healthcare delivery organizations, hospitals may face special constraints as institutions with various levels of control or influence over the practices of the physicians who care for patients in their facilities. Ultimately, hospitals will be most successful at achieving improvement in the evidence-based delivery of care when they are able to collaborate with their physicians to identify gaps and potential solutions.

The interviewees identified the primary challenges for organizations in implementing evidence-based decision making. The following sections describe these challenges.

The Information Technology Gap

Information technology generally and EHRs specifically are critical to the improved use of evidence in clinical decision making. Although many healthcare delivery organizations are ahead of the curve in implementing this technology, the majority of providers lag far behind. Only one-fourth of the physicians in the United States use an EHR, and only 5 percent of the hospitals use electronic prescribing tools (Jha et al., 2006). The likelihood that these tools will be used increases with practice size (Audet et al., 2004; Burt and Sisk, 2005). Significant expansions in the availability and use of information technology will be necessary to bridge this digital divide and to reach the Roundtable's goal of having 90 percent of clinical decisions be evidence based by 2020. It is also critical that expansions in the use of information technology be strongly rooted in the concept of interoperability so that various systems can "talk" to one another. Interoperability will ensure that all providers have systems that meet their needs and will also allow patients to travel from one delivery system to another without a loss of their medical information.

Restrictions on Support of Technology

Given the important role that information technology plays in the generation and use of evidence, hospitals would be better equipped to improve the quality of care that they provide if their affiliated physicians had access to EHRs. However, hospitals are challenged in their ability to support affiliated physicians' purchase of information technology by the federal Stark laws. These rules originally banned hospitals from funding such technology, and although the Centers for Medicare and Medicaid Services established "safe harbors" in August 2006, many hospitals are proceeding cautiously, as unresolved issues remain (Serb, 2007). For many hospitals, these safe harbors do not appear to be safe enough, so the investment in and the adoption of information technology by affiliated physician groups is progressing slowly. However, a recent Internal Revenue Service determination clarified that hospital subsidies for physicians' costs for HHS-approved information technology will not jeopardize the tax-exempt status of nonprofit hospitals (Lerner, 2007). This determination may remove one of the barriers to hospital subsidization of information technology for physicians, at least in the nonprofit sector.

The Inferential Gap

Much of the clinical evidence available today (which largely comes from RCTs) fails to meet the needs of its end users. Research on strictly defined populations may not be directly applicable to the populations of aging individuals and individuals with comorbid conditions who clinicians see in their offices every day. Walter Stewart and colleagues from the Geisinger Health System have referred to this problem as the "inferential gap" or "the gap between the paucity of what is proved to be effective for selected groups of patients versus the infinitely complex clinical decisions required for individual patients" (Stewart et al., 2007). Stewart and colleagues believe that EHRs will help narrow this large gap by accelerating the creation of evidence relevant to everyday practice needs and facilitating the real-time use of knowledge in practice. They envision a future state similar to that which was described earlier as a rapid-learning healthcare system (Etheredge, 2007).

The Science of Behavior Change

Experts in the field of evidence-based medicine have put a great deal of effort into understanding and improving the generation of evidence and making it available to clinicians. Equally important is the issue of changing clinicians' and patients' behavior when they are provided with sound, convenient, and relevant information. With respect to physicians, a landmark study by the RAND Corporation starkly illustrated this problem, finding that patients receive the recommended care only about 50 percent of the time (McGlynn et al., 2003). How can the use of the available recommendations and information be ensured?

The best methods of changing physician behavior are not yet known. Research has shown that the provision of didactic continuing medical education courses is not effective in changing behavior, and more participatory forms of continuing medical education (e.g., rounds) are only slightly more effective. Other possible means of changing physician behavior include pay-for-performance programs and the use of information technology, academic detailing, and even peer pressure in the form of quality measurement and internal reporting at the individual physician level. More research is required to determine which methods are the most effective. There are similar issues with respect to patients. Although some evidence provides information about the tools and shared decision-making practices that are most effective in motivating patients to adopt healthy behaviors, physicians do not necessarily know that these tools are available, nor do they know how to use them.

Financial Incentives

One of the most important potential barriers to the use of evidence-based practice is the predominant fee-for-service (FFS) payment system.

Under the FFS system, providers and hospitals are rewarded for taking actions: doing procedures, prescribing drugs, performing tests, and so forth. This type of payment system may encourage the application of evidence in determining a course of care when the evidence calls for doing more. However, the best evidence sometimes calls for not doing something or for taking a more conservative course of action. In such cases, the payment system can discourage the use of best practices. In addition, the FFS payment system causes physicians to ask the wrong questions in evaluating adherence to best practices. Physicians ask, "Did the patient survive the bypass surgery?" rather than, "Could the patient's bypass surgery have been avoided?" FFS system incentives to do more may stand in the way of evidence-based practices that call for more streamlined or less invasive care paths or the use of low-tech interventions to improve quality (such as the use of better hygiene practices in clinical encounters).

Leadership Practices

As noted earlier, the key to the improved use of evidence in decision making is a culture of group responsibility and an appreciation for the fact that no single physician can keep track of all relevant best practices in his or her head. These intangibles require strong physician leadership, which is often lacking in organizations compelled to respond to financial imperatives. The critical importance of evidence-based decision making does not yet seem to be on the radar screen of the majority of physician and hospital leaders, although the tipping point may be near.

Followership Practices

Although greater leadership is needed to advance the practice of evidence-based medicine, rank-and-file practitioners also need a more thorough understanding of the concept. Many experts interviewed for this statement believe that outside of highly academic and elite health and medical policy circles, there is little discussion of the implications of evidence for clinical decision making or understanding that much of current practice is not, in fact, evidence based. Healthcare providers need to become much more acculturated to this concept and willing to recast professional norms so that they align more with evidence than with autonomy.

Privacy Rules

Current privacy expectations, mores, and fears of misuse can lead to the zealous protection of medical information. To a certain extent, laws that do not go far enough in terms of prohibiting the misuse of personal health information (e.g., for insurance rating and employability) can have a chilling effect on the use of deidentified health information as a public utility for understanding and improving healthcare services and delivery. In addition, deidentified data often lack sufficient detail to allow the tracking of outcomes and the establishment of linkages across data systems (for example, without a date of birth or social security number, it is not possible to check the National Death Index to determine mortality for a specific patient). The Health Insurance Portability and Accountability Act (HIPAA) was developed more than a decade ago, before the establishment of the current notions of learning healthcare organizations. It may be time to revisit the HIPAA privacy requirements to allow the improved and more rapid use of patient information to support research and quality improvement.

Multiple Payers and Reporting Requirements

As noted above, quality measurement and reporting are means by which large healthcare delivery organizations can improve their use of evidence-based decision making. However, large providers are often subject to multiple and conflicting reporting demands from different payers. Each payer's reporting requirements divert resources and attention from another's, creating barriers to organizations' ability to focus on a critical (and manageable) set of evidence-based practices.

Physician Supply and Resources

The practice of evidence-based medicine can be time intensive for physicians. Some experts argue that it will require much more than the usual 15-minute office visit to ensure that 90 percent of clinical decisions are evidence based. Anecdotal evidence suggests that physicians in primary care are already overwhelmed with the number of protocols and best practices that they must fit into brief office visits, and the field is not even close to having 90 percent of clinical practice being supported by evidence. If office visit times (or inpatient visits) need to be lengthened to accommodate a greater reliance on evidence for decision making, will the country need more physicians and more beds? Can non-visit-based types of care (phone, e-mail, etc.) or care in nontraditional settings help offset any additional time that physicians may wish to spend with patients in their offices or in the hospital?

Special Challenges for the Safety Net

In addition to the challenges described above, safety net providers may face other difficulties in improving the use of evidence-based decision making because of resource constraints. Many safety net organizations are highly committed to the principles of evidence-based quality improvement. More than 80 percent of the health centers that receive funding from the Bureau of Primary Health Care participate in a Health Disparities Collaborative for quality improvement in chronic diseases, cancer, and prevention. Many public hospitals are closely affiliated with academic medical centers and partner with them on the development of evidence through clinical research and the use of evidence through care protocols. Some clinic practices are also large and multispecialty, but a lack of resources can make it difficult to devote staff and expertise to seeking out the available evidence and embedding it into best practices. A lack of resources can also make referrals to specialists difficult, even when the best evidence clearly calls for it. In addition, the multiple comorbidities and poor socioeconomic condition of many individuals who comprise the safety net patient population add to the problem of the inferential gap described earlier.

Special Challenges for Hospitals

As noted above, hospitals will be most effective in increasing the use of evidence-based decision making when they can influence the behavior of physicians who practice within their walls. The interviewees identified two major challenges to this.

Adversarial hospital-physician relationships   Relationships between hospitals and medical staff have evolved over the last few decades. According to Berenson and colleagues (2007), traditionally, physicians "have been relatively independent of hospitals and have used them as 'workshops' in which to carry out their professional services." Since the 1990s, greater competition between physicians and hospitals has emerged in some areas of the country, with reports of greater strain in hospital-physician relations in 2005 than in 2000-2001 (Berenson et al., 2007). This tension limits the amount of leverage that hospitals have to compel physicians to generate and use evidence in their delivery of care. There may be differences in this potential leverage among different types of physicians and hospitals. For example, hospitals may hold more sway with specialist physicians who are directly employed by or contracted as a group with the hospital, such as hospitalists, intensivists, radiologists, anesthesiologists, and emergency physicians, due to their more explicit employer-employee relationships. Integrated hospital systems have the most potential to influence medical staff, as they can provide direct financial incentives to physicians to adhere to evidence-based practices and protocols and are better able to measure the rate of adherence and to compare the performance of physicians with those of other physicians within the system. Some academic medical centers are moving toward establishing participation in evidence-based medicine activities as part of their contracts with new physicians but may have less of an opportunity to influence their more senior physicians. In many community hospitals, relationships with physicians are more adversarial, and hospitals have less leverage.

Difficulty of sanctions   Even when evidence-based practices and protocols can be instituted within hospitals, the financial interdependence between hospitals and physicians, as well as their intertwined professional networks, may make it difficult for hospitals to enforce guidelines and issue sanctions against noncompliant physicians. Furthermore, few options for managing noncompliance exist. The use of blunt instruments, such as revoking hospital privileges or malpractice insurance coverage, are drastic approaches to punishing undesired behavior and can be used only in rare circumstances in which there is absolutely no doubt about the right care. Otherwise, further deterioration in relationships between hospitals and physicians will occur.

LEADERSHIP COMMITMENTS AND INITIATIVES

The experts interviewed for this chapter described the following opportunities for improved evidence-based decision making.

Create a Focal Point for the Development and Dissemination of Evidence

There is a need for national agenda setting and coordination of the generation and communication of evidence. As noted earlier, there is a gap between the evidence available and the evidence needed for everyday decision making. Currently, no single entity in the healthcare system serves as a focal point for determining where the most urgent evidence gaps lie and deciding how limited research dollars should be spent to fill those gaps. Such a focal point, presumably, an entity publicly charged with coordinating the generation and communication of evidence, would determine where the most urgent evidence gaps lie, support comparative effectiveness analysis of treatments, and provide information to physicians and patients. To maximize its effectiveness, the entity should be inclusive of a broad range of stakeholders; have adequate resources to accomplish the goal of the IOM's Roundtable on Evidenced-Based Medicine; and be transparent about the methods, the processes, and the priorities for study.

Support Information Technology and Identify Strategies to Eliminate the Digital Divide

To improve the generation and use of evidence, more healthcare delivery organizations must implement fully operational EHRs with decision support capabilities. Structured correctly, such systems can provide useful information based on real-time clinical care, enabling organizations to be rapid-learning systems that use observable data to create evidence on what works (Etheredge, 2007). Too few physicians currently have access to this technology, and the digital divide is even greater for hospitals. Policies that support provider adoption of EHRs should be encouraged.

Improve Leadership Training

Tomorrow's leaders of complex healthcare organizations must become conversant in the concepts of evidence-based medicine and committed to establishing a culture of continuous learning. According to the IOM (Institute of Medicine, 2005), the healthcare industry has neglected to use engineering strategies and technologies that have revolutionized quality, productivity, and performance in many other industries. Remedying this problem, essentially undoing the learning that health care is delivered one patient at a time, will require the training of clinician leaders in new fields, such as systems and industrial engineering and the management of organizational change. Leaders need to be reoriented to view healthcare organizations as having a collective responsibility for groups of patients. Today, most leaders of healthcare organizations come from a medical or business background. Neither of these disciplines yet consistently incorporates the concepts of systems engineering and group responsibility that are foundational to the use of evidence-based medicine.

Improve Clinician Training

Leaders are not the only actors in healthcare organizations who need to become more familiar with the concepts of evidence-based medicine. Frontline clinicians (both physicians and other healthcare professionals) delivering care on a daily basis need to have ongoing training in the use of evidence in decision making. The continuing medical education system is one mechanism for bringing this content to clinicians, although its effectiveness is questionable, as noted above. Another idea is to incorporate training in evidence-based medicine into requirements for board certification in the medical specialties. By incorporating evidence-based medicine concepts into medical training, a demand for this style of practice is created among clinicians, so that when they leave school and practice in the community, they will expect to have the organizational support that they need to practice in this way.

Engage and Leverage Boards of Directors

To ensure that evidence-based practice is a priority for healthcare delivery organizations, boards of directors should be educated about the principles of evidence and make evidence-based practice a stated goal of the organization. Two levers for influencing boards include framing evidence-based care as a mechanism for fulfilling the organization's mission or "contract with the community" and as part of their fiduciary duty to deliver effective, efficient care. A more limited role for hospital boards could be to make participation in evidence-based practice a condition of hospital privileges, but this is complicated, as discussed above.

Increase Patient Demand for Evidence-Based Medicine

Although increasing physician demand for evidence-based practice is important, so, too, is creating consumer or patient demand. If patients know what evidence-based medicine is and understand the organizational structures that must support it, they may be more likely to demand this style of practice from their clinicians. Today, it would most likely come as a surprise to the majority of patients that some of their care is not evidence based. One means of improving consumers' understanding is to incorporate basic concepts of health literacy into the health education that students receive in middle and high school. Such training would need to be reinforced for adults through media outreach and public information campaigns. Another means of creating consumer demand for evidence-based medicine is to design insurance benefit packages that require smaller amounts of cost-sharing for evidence-based care than for other types of care.[5] The science of evidence-based medicine may not yet allow this to happen on a broad scale, but as the science develops, so, too, can consumer incentives.

Link Performance Standards to Use of Evidence

Healthcare delivery organizations can and must identify standards of care and measure individual physicians' performance against them. Such standards can be used internally for quality improvement, or they can be reported to external entities, where they may become the basis for payment differentials (see "Restructure Financial Incentives" below). Organizations can identify standards of care, measure an individual physician's performance, and report back to enable physicians to compare their performance

---

[5]For more on the concept of evidence-based benefit design, see the work of the Employers-Employees Sector of the IOM Roundtable on Evidence-Based Medicine in Chapter 12.

with that of their peers. The use of peer pressure as an incentive can be even more effective than the use of financial incentives. When financial incentives are used, they should focus on paying for value and outcomes and not just for performance on process measures. Work by organizations such as the National Committee for Quality Assurance and the Leapfrog Group to standardize performance measures should incorporate concepts of evidence-based decision making.

Restructure Financial Incentives

The FFS payment system creates incentives to provide care and services which may or may not be based on evidence-based care. Value-based purchasing initiatives built on foundations of comparative effectiveness research have the potential to correct this problem. As discussed above, pay-for-performance and capitation, types of value-based purchasing, can be important tools if they are structured correctly. However, capitation alone does not encourage the use of evidence-based medicine when the evidence calls for doing more (or more expensive) treatments.

Enable Passive Generation of Evidence

Even without EHRs, healthcare delivery organizations routinely collect a variety of patient care data that could be aggregated by a common entity, such as a payer (e.g., the Centers for Medicare and Medicaid Services, which has claims data from the vast majority of hospitals and physicians). This would add to the ability to use real-time data to learn about best care and would help to bridge the inferential gap that occurs when published research findings are based on data for very narrowly defined populations.

Encourage "Systemness"

Hospitals and physicians that are parts of systems have a greater ability and more incentives to invest in information technology and to share information on evidence-based care guidelines. Improved collaboration among hospitals and medical staffs, in a variety of organizational forms, will allow the more effective capture and use of evidence. In different geographic areas, different models of hospital-physician collaboration or integration will work better than others, and "systemness" can be either real or virtual. For example, regional health information organizations, which share patient data among the providers in a community, are types of virtual organizations that may prove to be a bridge to improved systemness without full organizational integration.

Invest in Understanding the Drivers of Behavior Change

Further research is needed to determine which methods work best in changing clinicians' and patients' behavior. A large body of literature in the disciplines of sociology and psychology, as well as health services research, has explored this question. Ideas and experts from these fields must be integrated more fully into discussions of evidence-based medicine to ensure the use of the most effective means of translating evidence into practice.

Advocate for Changes to HIPAA

As noted above, the patient privacy provisions of HIPAA have had a chilling effect on the use of large datasets of patient information, even when that information is deidentified. Greater flexibility in the use of patient information for research and quality improvement is needed, provided that the patients' information is not put at risk of being revealed for other purposes. The IOM is conducting a study, entitled Health Research and the Privacy of Health Information—The HIPAA Privacy Rule, that can serve as a foundation for revisiting HIPAA in light of the need for the improved generation and use of evidence in the everyday delivery of care (Institute of Medicine, 2007). In addition, the high visibility of consumer messages about the right to privacy may have inadvertently created a culture in which consumers do not expect and are not willing to permit data about themselves to be used for any purpose. More accurate and nuanced messages need to be created for consumers.

Improve Collaboration Among End Users

As described above in the case studies, many healthcare delivery organizations have processes in place to review internal and external evidence, create clinical guidelines, and translate them into practice. This effort is essential to provide safe, high-quality care but requires significant resources. Today, a sufficient cadre of highly capable entities perform evidence translation, and it may be unnecessary to internally and individually create the capacity. Rather, evidence-based knowledge products (reviews and practice guidelines) can be created jointly by use of a cooperative mechanism.

Optimize Human Resources

Hospitals and large physician group practices can create infrastructures that fully utilize the expertise that they have within the medical staff. By supporting information exchange and consultation among physicians around emergent or complex medical needs, such as rapid response teams that bring critical care experts to a patient's bedside within minutes of being called, hospitals can increase best practices and improve outcomes. Similarly, physician organizations, such as the Mayo Clinic, have improved diabetes care by providing the primary care physicians at the clinic in Rochester, Minnesota, virtual consultations with endocrinologists through e-mail. The endocrinologists review an abstract of the EHR and provide performance-triggered suggestions with supporting evidence to the clinicians and their families.

NEXT STEPS

Although all of the opportunities described above are important for improving evidence-based decision making, several key initiatives that have the potential to transform the way in which the healthcare delivery organization sector generates and uses evidence have been identified.

Create a National Entity to Develop and Disseminate Evidence

As noted earlier, there is a need for national agenda setting and coordination of the generation and communication of evidence. An increased and focused investment is also needed. Many large healthcare delivery organizations already do this work independently. National coordination and prioritization would allow the sector as a whole to eliminate redundancy and make better use of the resources devoted to evidence generation.

First Step

The most important first step for healthcare delivery organizations in creating a national entity for the development and dissemination of evidence is to advocate for this change with policy makers and other stakeholders. Policy makers must be educated about the need for such an entity and encouraged to authorize and establish funding for it. Because of their high visibility and significant clinical expertise, sector members must play a central role in efforts to design and advocate for the agenda-setting entity. Such work may include active communication of the work of the IOM's Roundtable on Evidence-Based Medicine.

Cross-Sector Collaboration

A number of other healthcare sectors are advocating for the entity described here. Rather than working alone or at cross-purposes with these sectors, healthcare delivery organizations should work with the organizations already active in this area as they develop a vision and legislation to authorize the entity. Some of the organizations taking a lead in this area include America's Health Insurance Plans, the BlueCross BlueShield Association, the Health Industry Forum, and AcademyHealth. These existing efforts could benefit from the clinical and research expertise of the large healthcare delivery organizations.

Support the Adoption and Use of Information Technology

The broader implementation of EHRs across the entire healthcare delivery organization sector will both support the delivery of care and create rapid-learning organizations. The digitization of healthcare delivery through the use of the EHR is one of the most important changes that can be made to improve care and support learning. Large delivery organizations, in addition to leading this change, can also help smaller physician groups learn about EHRs by providing technical assistance and sharing their expertise through the establishment of learning networks. Unless all (or nearly all) healthcare providers can connect and share information electronically, there will continue to be a significant amount of information lost and missed opportunities for learning. It is therefore critical that the digital divide be closed. Healthcare delivery organizations can play a leadership role in making this happen.

First Steps

One of the major barriers to the widespread adoption of EHRs is a lack of standardization of the data produced by clinical information systems. The federal government is in the best position to convene stakeholders to establish these needed standards and to enforce adherence to the standards, once they are established. However, as noted above, healthcare delivery organizations are leaders in the implementation of EHRs and therefore have a wealth of expertise that can and should be brought to bear on efforts to create interoperability and other information technology standards. This sector can also be a leader in establishing learning networks of organizations that have implemented EHRs to disseminate knowledge to all providers, both organized and nonorganized.

Cross-Sector Collaboration

The federal government is leading the way in standard setting for health information technology interoperability. In 2005, HHS announced the formation of the American Health Information Community (AHIC), which will provide input and recommendations to HHS on how to make health records digital and interoperable and ensure that the privacy and security of those records are protected (U.S. Department of Health and Human Services, 2007). Initially, HHS appointed 16 members, including a few representing healthcare delivery organizations, to the AHIC commission. Plans are now being made to transition AHIC to an independent and sustainable public–private partnership by fall 2008. Because of their expertise with these systems and their significant financial investments in them, healthcare delivery organizations should take every opportunity to participate in this and other processes that support standardization. Healthcare delivery organizations should also continue to collaborate with the federal government in this area by participating in various Medicare demonstration projects to test and measure the effect of program changes on the adoption and use of healthcare information technology (primarily in the FFS delivery system).

Improve Understanding of and Support for Evidence-Based Care

The concept of evidence-based medicine and its potential to drastically improve quality need to be communicated broadly to the public in much the same way as the concept of medical errors and the opportunities to make health care safer were communicated when the IOM published *To Err Is Human* in 1999 (Institute of Medicine, 1999). Many of the opportunities identified above call for educating key stakeholders (clinical leaders, rank-and-file clinicians, boards of directors of healthcare delivery organizations, and patients-consumers) about the need for the improved use of evidence-based decision making and outlining some potential strategies for doing so. As these strategies make clear, there is no single way to reach all of these audiences with messages about evidence-based care; multiple channels will need to be used. As entities with many opportunities to reach both patients and providers, healthcare delivery organizations have a unique opportunity to develop and deliver messages about the importance of evidence-based care to these audiences.

First Steps

Although the strategies for reaching the main stakeholders differ, the healthcare delivery organizations sector has unique access to all of these groups and therefore a unique potential to influence them. As a first step toward improving the understanding of and support for evidence-based care, healthcare delivery organizations should work collaboratively to develop the messages, materials, or curricula to be used with key audiences and then work independently to influence their own boards, clinical leaders, clinicians, and patients. To make such an education part of the culture of medicine and the delivery of care and to influence the public in a more meaningful way, longer-term strategies involving the efforts and resources of multiple sectors (including the media) will be necessary.

Cross-Sector Collaboration

Collaboration across healthcare sectors and beyond will be critical to improving the understanding of and support for evidence-based care. For example, the healthcare professions education sector and professional societies and associations will need to play active roles in efforts to change the training of clinicians (and clinician leaders). The consumer sector will need to collaborate with healthcare delivery organizations, insurers, and others outside of traditional healthcare circles (including the broader public education sector) to include information on evidence-based care in health education, in public awareness campaigns, and through health insurance benefit design. There may be a role for an entity such as the IOM to organize and facilitate this work, given the cross-sector collaboration required.

Link Measures of Evidence-Based Care to Performance Standards and Incentives

Performance measurements and incentives need to be structured to encourage the use of evidence-based care. Healthcare delivery organizations can play an important role in this work by identifying care standards based on the evidence and structuring incentives (such as payment differentials) to reward value and outcomes. This can help place a focus on the most important standards and narrow the range of different requirements from different payers. A lack of consistent pay-for-performance expectations has been shown to reduce the impacts of these programs.

First Steps

Healthcare delivery organizations should review their existing performance measures and care standards to assess the extent to which they are already evidence based. Measures and standards that are evidence based should be prioritized, and those that are not should be considered for adaptation or elimination. In addition, healthcare delivery organizations should examine their existing internal payment incentives (such as provider bonuses) to ensure that they are paying for evidence-based care.

Cross-Sector Collaboration

A number of sectors will need to be involved in efforts to align performance measurement and incentives with evidence-based care. For example, as noted earlier, organizations such as the National Committee for Quality Assurance and the Leapfrog Group can set the standard for creating performance measures based on evidence, and purchasers can adopt more consistent evidence-based standards. The Agency for Healthcare Research and Quality should also play a role in this work. Although healthcare delivery organizations can serve as subject matter experts and learning laboratories for testing measurement and incentive approaches, the national entities described above are in a better position to standardize measures and approaches to providing incentives across organizations. In addition, employers and large public purchasers should play a central role in creating value-based purchasing initiatives (such as pay for performance) that align incentives for medical care to adhere to the evidence.

Conclusion

The healthcare delivery organizations sector plays a central role in efforts to improve the use of evidence-based care. As entities that organize and employ physicians and other clinicians, deliver care to patients, and, in some cases, conduct research, sector members have opportunities to influence the generation and use of evidence through many channels. Because sector members are organized and can act purposefully as goal-setting institutions, they may have a greater ability than nonorganized providers to influence the transformational initiatives outlined above.

Momentum is building nationally to improve the use of evidence-based care, and now is the time for healthcare delivery organizations to take action to assist in this effort. Change will not come overnight, nor will it come from only one sector. Reasonable goals for the healthcare delivery organizations sector in the next 3 to 5 years include working with others to accomplish the following: enact authorizing legislation for a national entity to develop and disseminate evidence, develop widely accepted standards for information technology interoperability, begin a public outreach and awareness campaign about evidence-based medicine, and standardize and streamline quality measurement and incentive programs to focus resources on a defined set of evidence-based practices.

Sector members can also provide leadership in efforts to improve the use of evidence-based care by modeling what works for nonorganized providers. To date, as examined in the case studies presented earlier in this chapter, many healthcare delivery organizations are already active in this arena. By providing models of effective generation and use of the evidence, healthcare delivery organizations can help nonorganized providers better understand the quality benefits of integration and organization, which could ultimately encourage the spread of evidence-based care.

REFERENCES

Agency for Healthcare Research and Quality. 2007. *Evidence-based practice centers.* http://www.ahrq.gov/clinic/epc/ (accessed August 31, 2007).

Alliance of Community Health Plans. 2007. *Alliance of Community Health Plans website.* http://www.achp.org/ (accessed April 30, 2008).

American Diabetes Association. 2007. *Diabetes personal health decisions (PHD).* http://www.diabetes.org/diabetesphd/default.jsp (accessed April 30, 2008).

American Hospital Association. 2007. *Fast facts on U.S. hospitals.* http://www.aha.org/aha/resource-center/Statistics-and-Studies/fast-facts.html (accessed March 22, 2007).

American Medical Group Association. 2007. *American Medical Group Association website.* http://www.amga.org/ (accessed April 30, 2008).

Archimedes-Kaiser Permanente. 2007. *The Archimedes model.* http://archimedesmodel.com/archimedes.htm (accessed April 30, 2008).

Asch, S., E. McGlynn, M. Hogan, R. Hayward, P. Shekelle, L. Rubenstein, J. Keesey, J. Adams, and E. Kerr. 2004. Comparison of quality of care for patients in the Veterans Health Administration and patients in a national sample. *Annals of Internal Medicine* 141(12):938-945.

Audet, A. M., M. M. Doty, J. Peugh, J. Shamasdin, K. Zapert, and S. Schoenbaum. 2004. Information technologies: when will they make it into physicians' black bags? *MedGenMed: Medscape General Medicine* 6(4):2.

Berenson, R. A., P. B. Ginsburg, and J. H. May. 2007. Hospital-physicians relations: Cooperation, competition, or separation? *Health Affairs* 26(1):w31-w43.

Berwick, D. M., and S. H. Jain. 2004. Systems and results: The basis for quality care in prepaid group practice. In *Toward a 21st century health system: The contributions and promise of prepaid group practice*, edited by A. Enthoven and L. Tollen. San Francisco, CA: Jossey-Bass.

BlueCross BlueShield Association. 2000. *Technology evaluation center.* http://www.bcbs.com/betterknowledge/tec/ (accessed April 30, 2008).

Brown, S. H., M. J. Lincoln, P. J. Groen, and R. M. Kolodner. 2003. Vista—U.S. Department of Veterans Affairs national-scale HIS. *International Journal of Medical Informatics* 69(2-3):135-156.

Burt, C. W., and J. E. Sisk. 2005. Which physicians and practices are using electronic medical records? *Health Affairs* 24(5):1334-1343.

California HealthCare Foundation. 2006. *Snapshot: Health care costs 101.* http://www.chcf.org/documents/insurance/HealthCareCosts06.pdf (accessed March 22, 2007).

Casalino, L., R. R. Gillies, S. M. Shortell, J. A. Schmittdiel, T. Bodenheimer, J. C. Robinson, T. Rundall, N. Oswald, H. Schauffler, and M. C. Wang. 2003a. External incentives, information technology, and organized processes to improve health care quality for patients with chronic diseases. *JAMA* 289(4):434-441.

Casalino, L. P., K. J. Devers, T. K. Lake, M. Reed, and J. J. Stoddard. 2003b. Benefits of and barriers to large medical group practice in the United States. *Archives of Internal Medicine* 163(16):1958-1964.

Chassin, M. R. 1998. Is health care ready for six sigma quality? *Milbank Quarterly* 76(4):510, 565-591.

Cochrane Collaboration. 2007. *The Cochrane Collaboration website.* http://www.cochrane.org/ (accessed April 30, 2008).

Council of Accountable Physician Practices. 2007. *Better together.* http://www.amga.org/CAPP (accessed April 30, 2008).

Crosson, F. J. 2005. The delivery system matters. *Health Affairs* 24(6):1543-1548.

Crosson, F., A. Weiland, and B. Berenson. 2004. Physician leadership: "group responsibility" as key to accountability in medicine. In *Toward a 21st century health system: The contributions and promise of prepaid group practice*, edited by A. Enthoven and L. Tollen, San Francisco, CA: Jossey-Bass.

Cutler, D. M., N. E. Feldman, and J. R. Horwitz. 2005. U.S. adoption of computerized physician order entry systems. *Health Affairs (Millwood)* 24(6):1654-1663.

ECRI Institute. 2007. *ECRI Institute website.* http://www.ecri.org/Pages/default.aspx (accessed November 2007).

Eddy, D. M. 1999. *Issues in Permanente medicine: Evidence-based medicine.* San Francisco, CA: Permanente Federation.

———. 2007. Linking electronic medical records to large-scale simulation models: Can we put rapid learning on turbo? *Health Affairs* 26(2):w125-w136.

Enthoven, A. C., and L. A. Tollen. 2005. Competition in health care: It takes systems to pursue quality and efficiency. *Health Affairs* Suppl. Web Exclusives:W5-420–W5-433.

Etheredge, L. M. 2007. A rapid-learning health system. *Health Affairs* 26(2):w107-w118.

Fink, R., and M. Greenlick. 2004. Prepaid group practice and health care research. In *Toward a 21st century health system: The contributions and promise of prepaid group practice*, edited by A. Enthoven and L. Tollen. San Francisco, CA: Jossey-Bass.

Francis, J., and J. B. Perlin. 2006. Improving performance through knowledge translation in the veterans health administration. *Journal of Continuing Education in the Health Professions* 26(1):63-71.

Greenfield, S., and S. H. Kaplan. 2004. Creating a culture of quality: The remarkable transformation of the Department of Veterans Affairs health care system. *Annals of Internal Medicine* 141(4):316-318.

Halvorson, G. 2004. Prepaid group practice and computerized caregiver support tools. In *Toward a 21st century health system: The contributions and promise of prepaid group practice*, edited by A. Enthoven and L. Tollen. San Francisco, CA: Jossey-Bass.

Hayes, Inc. 2007. *Hayes, Inc. website.* http://www.hayesinc.com/hayes/ (accessed April 30, 2008).

Hing, E., and C. W. Burt. 2007. Office-based medical practices: Methods and estimates from the national ambulatory medical care survey. *Advance Data* (383):1-15.

Institute for Clinical Systems Improvement. 2007. *Institute for Clinical Systems Improvement website.* http://www.icsi.org/ (accessed November 2007).

Institute of Medicine. 1999. *To err is human.* Washington, DC: National Academy Press.

———. 2001. *Crossing the quality chasm: A new health system for the 21st century.* Washington, DC: National Academy Press.

———. 2005. *Building a better delivery system: A new engineering/health care partnership.* Washington, DC: The National Academies Press.

———. 2007. *Health research and the privacy of health information—The HIPAA privacy rule.* http://www.iom.edu/CMS/3740/43729.aspx (accessed November 2007).

IOM Roundtable on Evidence-Based Medicine. 2006. *Charter and vision statement: Roundtable on Evidence-Based Medicine.* Washington, DC.

Jha, A. K., J. B. Perlin, K. W. Kizer, and R. A. Dudley. 2003. Effect of the transformation of the Veterans Affairs health care system on the quality of care. *New England Journal of Medicine* 348(22):2218-2227.

Jha, A. K., T. G. Ferris, K. Donelan, C. DesRoches, A. Shields, S. Rosenbaum, and D. Blumenthal. 2006. How common are electronic health records in the United States? A summary of the evidence. *Health Affairs* 25(6):w496-w507.

Kaiser Permanente. 2007a. *KP healthconnect.* http://www.kphealthconnectq4update.org/index.html (accessed November 2007).

— . 2007b. *Medical research at Kaiser Permanente.* http://newsmedia.kaiserpermanente. org/kpweb/ourmedicalres/entrypage.do (accessed November 2007).

Kerr, E. A., D. M. Smith, M. M. Hogan, T. P. Hofer, S. L. Krein, M. Bermann, and R. A. Hayward. 2003. Building a better quality measure: Are some patients with "poor quality" actually getting good care? *Medical Care* 41(10):1173-1182.

Kupersmith, J., J. Francis, E. Kerr, S. Krein, L. Pogach, R. M. Kolodner, and J. B. Perlin. 2007. Advancing evidence-based care for diabetes: Lessons from the Veterans Health Administration. *Health Affairs* 26(2):w156-w168.

Landon, B., L. Hicks, A. O'Malley, T. Lieu, T. Keegan, B. McNeil, and E. Guadagnoli. 2007. Improving the management of chronic disease at community health centers. *New England Journal of Medicine* 356(9):921-934.

Lerner, L. 2007. *Hospitals providing financial assistance to staff physicians involving electronic health records.* Internal Revenue Service memorandum. Washington, DC: Internal Revenue Service.

McGlynn, E., S. Asch, J. Adams, J. Keesey, J. Hicks, A. DeCristofaro, and E. Kerr. 2003. The quality of health care delivered to adults in the United States. *New England Journal of Medicine* 348(26):2635-2645.

National Association of Public Hospitals and Health Systems. 2004. *America's public hospitals and health systems, 2004: Results of the NAPH annual hospital characteristics survey.* http://www.naph.org/Content/ContentGroups/Publications1/Characteristics2004. pdf (accessed March 22, 2007).

Oregon Health and Science University. 2007. *Center for evidence-based policy.* http://www. ohsu.edu/policycenter/ (accessed April 30, 2008).

Perlin, J. 2006. Transformation of the U.S. Veterans Health Administration. *Health Economics, Policy, and Law* 1(2):99-105.

Serb, C. 2007. Stark redo. Hospitals hesitate to help digitize doctors' offices until the "relaxed" rules are further clarified. *Hospitals and Health Networks* 81(2):32, 34-36, 38.

Stewart, W. F., N. R. Shah, M. J. Selna, R. A. Paulus, and J. M. Walker. 2007. Bridging the inferential gap: The electronic health record and clinical evidence. *Health Affairs* 26(2): w181-w191.

UpToDate. 2007. *UpToDate website.* http://www.uptodate.com/ (accessed April 30, 2008).

U.S. Department of Health and Human Services. 2007. *American health information community.* http://www.hhs.gov/healthit/community/background/ (accessed April 30, 2008).

INTERVIEWEES

The interviewees included Madhulika Agarwal, Chief Patient Care Services Officer, Veterans Health Administration; Ahmed Calvo, Medical Advisor, Center for Quality, Health Resources and Services Administration; Denis Cortese, President and Chief Executive Officer, Mayo Clinic; Roscoe Dandy, Office of Minority Health and Health Disparities, Health Resources and Services Administration; Carolyn Days-Mustille, Codirector, Kaiser Permanente Care Management Institute; Benjamin Druss, Rosalynn Carter Chair in Mental Health and Associate Professor of Health Policy and Management, Rollins School of Public Health, Emory University; Kay Felix-Aaron, Director, Office of Quality Data, Center for Quality, Health Resources and Services Administration; Nancy Foster, Vice President for Quality and Patient Safety, American Hospital Association; Denise Geolot,

Director, Center for Quality, Health Resources and Services Administration; Steve Mayfield, Director, American Hospital Association Quality Center; Gregg Meyer, Medical Director, Massachusetts General Physician Organization (MGPO) and Senior Vice President for Quality and Patient Safety, Massachusetts General Hospital and MGPO; Lynnette Nilan, Office of Patient Care Services, U.S. Department of Veterans Affairs; Jonathan Perlin, Chief Medical Officer and President, Clinical Services, HCA, Inc.; Richard Platt, Professor and Chair, Department of Ambulatory Care and Prevention, Harvard Medical School and Harvard Pilgrim Health Care; Paul Wallace, Medical Director for Health and Productivity Management Programs, The Permanente Federation; Deborah Willis-Fillinger, Senior Medical Advisor, Center for Quality, Health Resources and Services Administration; and Scott Young, Codirector, Kaiser Permanente Care Management Institute.

8

Healthcare Product Developers

Coordinator

Peter Juhn, Johnson & Johnson

Other Contributors

Patricia Adams, National Pharmaceutical Council; Pat Anderson, Stryker; Marc Berger, Lilly; Catherine Bonuccelli, AstraZeneca; Spencer Borden, Health Care Systems, Johnson & Johnson; Linda Carter, Global Regulatory Affairs, Johnson & Johnson; Christopher M. Dezii, Bristol-Myers Squibb; Dave Domann, Ortho McNeil Janssen, Johnson & Johnson; Mary Erslon, Covidien (formerly Tyco Healthcare); Barry Gershon, Wyeth; Kathryn Gleason, National Pharmaceutical Council; Page Kranbuhl, Stryker; Jerry McAteer, Siemens Medical Solutions Diagnostics; Newell McElwee, Pfizer; Scott McKenzie, Ortho Biotech, Johnson & Johnson; Gary Persinger, National Pharmaceutical Council; Wayne Rosenkrans, AstraZeneca; Lisa Saake, Covidien (formerly Tyco Healthcare); Phil Sarocco, Boston Scientific; Hemal Shah, Boehringer-Ingelheim; David Sugano, Schering-Plough; Steve Teutsch, Merck; Karen Williams, National Pharmaceutical Council

SECTOR OVERVIEW

The companies in the healthcare products industry represent a unique sector of health care focused on the development and implementation of innovative medical products. The pharmaceutical, medical device, and diagnostic industries have contributed technologies that increase survival and decrease disease-associated morbidities and mortalities. The greater life expectancies and improved quality of life that patients with, for example, cardiac disease, diabetes, and cancer experience can in many ways be credited to improved medical diagnostic technologies and improved therapies: from the improved ability to detect tumors by the use of new imaging procedures to the increased use of cholesterol drugs, blood thinners, and new cancer medicines; new home-based therapeutic devices, such as diabetes monitors and home oxygen therapy; and the improvements in quality of life achieved with orthopedic implants.

The medical device and diagnostic portion of the industry includes more than 20,000 companies worldwide, most with an average of 50 employees or fewer, and produce more than 80,000 brands and models of medical devices for the U.S. market. Medical technology innovation typically consists of incremental improvements to existing technologies; therefore, the product life cycles in this sector range from about 18 months to 2 years (Advanced Medical Technology Association, 2007). Other medical technology products, including those requiring large capital investments, long-term clinical data, or physician adoption for market penetration, have longer life cycles. Consequently, follower competitors typically capture the benefits from the innovator in the medical device and diagnostic market.

In contrast, the biopharmaceutical portion of the industry is much more consolidated, with some 200 pharmaceutical companies, 400 publicly traded biotechnology companies, and 1,400 privately held biotechnology companies in existence worldwide. The pharmaceutical industry introduces 25 to 30 new innovative products each year, on average, and has some 2,000 products in development that may be useful in all areas of therapy. Biotechnology has created more than 200 new therapies and vaccines and has some 400 products in active development, including products for the treatment of cancer, diabetes, human immunodeficiency virus infection/AIDS, and autoimmune disorders. The discovery and development process for biopharmaceuticals takes an average of 15 years and involves sequential steps, from discovery to preclinical animal tests and human studies. Over the course of drug development, the product attrition rate is high, and the cost of bringing an individual drug to market has been estimated to be more than $800 million (Pharmaceutical Research and Manufacturers of America, 2005a), with new data from the Tufts Center for Drug Development suggesting that the cost for the development of a new biopharmaceutical may top $1.2 billion.

Although these manufacturers produce a heterogeneous assortment of products, each has core capabilities in the design and implementation of programs that produce and disseminate evidence about the safety and efficacy of their products to patients and healthcare providers. Given the considerable requirements for regulatory and market information from this sector, it is likely that it collectively has more experience in evidence development and dissemination than any other healthcare sector.

The financial and resource investments of pharmaceutical and device manufacturers in evidence development and dissemination are substantial. In 2005, the biopharmaceutical industry spent more than $51 billion on new product development (research and development [R&D]); it spent

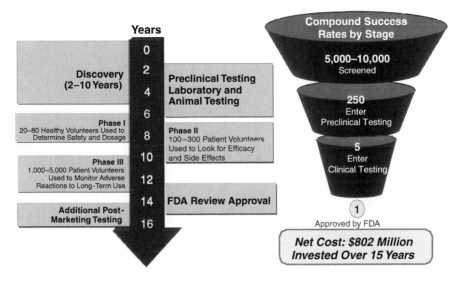

FIGURE 8-1 Financial and resource investments of pharmaceutical and device manufacturers for the development of new therapies.
SOURCES: DiMasi et al. (2003); Pharmaceutical Research and Manufacturers of America (2005b,c).

about 40 percent of that amount on preapproval clinical trials and considerably less for postmarketing assessment (Pharmaceutical Research and Manufacturers of America, 2005b). The financial and resource investments required for pharmaceutical development are shown in Figure 8-1.

Regulatory Approval Requirements

The development of evidence required for regulatory approval varies by the type of product and the disease. Medical device and diagnostic manufacturers supply data to the Food and Drug Administration (FDA) for premarketing approval applications (PMAs) or 510(k) premarketing notifications (as required by section 510(k) of the Federal Food, Drug, and Cosmetic Act), depending on the specific product under evaluation. Pharmaceutical and biotechnology manufacturers provide data in new drug applications or biologics license applications.

The diversity of medical devices and diagnostics has led to a risk-based classification system, and that system uses established standards to evaluate device safety and effectiveness distinct from those that FDA uses to evaluate drug safety and effectiveness. The system calibrates regulatory controls to the risk that specific devices pose, and only a small percentage of devices—those that pose the greatest risk—require clinical studies for PMAs. Between 50 and 80 high-risk (i.e., Class III) devices receive approval under the PMA review process annually. Most manufacturers of medical devices follow the 510(k) premarketing notification process for substantially equivalent technologies. According to FDA, more than 4,000 new, low-risk (i.e., Class I) devices that are exempt from FDA premarketing review are marketed each year; about 3,500 medium-risk (i.e., Class II) products are reviewed and approved for marketing by FDA under the 510(k) premarketing notification process, with about 8 percent of those products subject to special controls that require clinical data. Postmarketing surveillance studies are an example of special controls. Finally, investigational device exemption allows an investigational device or investigational diagnostic to be used in a clinical study to support a PMA or 510(k) premarketing notification process.

The evidentiary standard for devices is less burdensome than that for drugs because of the medical technology innovation process and its shorter cycle time. Consequently, the amount of evidence required for device evaluation is inherently different from that required for marketing applications for drugs. Also, the type of evidence permitted to substantiate the efficacy of a device is much broader than the type of evidence permitted to substantiate the efficacy of a drug. The evidentiary standard for the approval of biopharmaceuticals, however, is significant. Marketing approval requires randomized controlled trials, starting with dosing and safety studies, typically conducted with healthy volunteers (Phase I studies), and progressing to increasingly larger and logistically more complex studies with patients with the disease to demonstrate safety and efficacy (Phase II and Phase III studies). Biopharmaceutical companies must routinely make go–no go investment decisions throughout the average 15-year development cycle on the basis of the estimated clinical effectiveness and safety of the product, expected regulatory and coverage and reimbursement requirements at launch, the probability of technical and commercial success, the place of the product in expected medical practice, and the net present value of the product.

Complex Requirements for Real-World Effectiveness

The growing need for patients, providers, and payers to evaluate treatment options and the financial implications of these evaluations are resulting in increasing demands for evidence of real-world comparative effectiveness and safety for treatment- and coverage-related decision making. However, these new research questions are fundamentally different from the research questions that regulatory agencies ask when they make marketing approval decisions (Lomas et al., 2005) and add incremental costs to the existing expense of development that the manufacturers have already incurred. In addition to these different types of questions, the larger populations required to power comparative studies adequately also add to the cost. All of these costs serve to lower the net present value of products in development. This lower net present value, in turn, can result in more no go decisions in the development process and higher product attrition rates because of reduced commercial viability.

If the responsibility for the conduct and payment for the development of real-world evidence lies with the industry, then industry will need to develop a process to incorporate the costs and benefits of conducting these studies into early-phase development decisions. That process will, by definition, be inexact. It is impossible to completely anticipate future research needs, because so many research decisions are based on the results of interim research and an evolving understanding of the underlying science, which may not be known for some years. Nevertheless, much of the uncertainty could be reduced if standards for the types of studies that represent appropriate evidence and the types of findings that would allow appropriate third-party coverage were created through broad stakeholder consensus. Such standards will ensure the development of the best-quality evidence, lower the uncertainty for that element in drug development, and increase the ability of manufacturers to continue to develop new products.

Even with the increased predictability that coverage-related decision-making standards foster and the considerable effort being expended on increasing R&D productivity, these incremental costs can become unsustainable and can significantly hinder innovation. A lack of market valuation of products that show incremental improvements or the valuation of only breakthrough innovations can create a greater perceived financial risk in product development when the considerable costs are taken into account and may result in the introduction of fewer products. The introduction of fewer products also reduces the therapeutic choice options that providers have to overcome patient variability in response to therapy and reduces price competition.

For medical devices and diagnostics, the granularity of the evidence that payers need is getting tougher to obtain; that is, meeting the demand for answers from studies with smaller subpopulations or population segments requires more time and more resources. There remains a lack of clarity of how payers' reimbursement decision-making processes integrate the evidence that healthcare manufacturers generate. Finally, use of the "gold standard" type of clinical study, randomized clinical trials, is not always feasible for medical devices and diagnostics, for multiple inherent reasons. Thus, it is essential that the evolution of a consensus on the value and limitations of studies be explored by using current methodological standards.

These unintended consequences of the development and use of additional evidence for coverage-related decision making should be considered as the evidence requirements for real-world effectiveness and safety develop, as this may limit the ability to fully deliver on the promise of innovation. Members of the healthcare product sector recommend that informed members of the academic economic community evaluate the potential impact of these new evidentiary standards on the economics of innovation and consequent patient care to help guide payers and the government as they make policy decisions.

Evidence Synthesis and Development

Manufacturers generate evidence both to inform internal investment decisions regarding the market viability of emerging products and to inform stakeholders (e.g., regulatory agencies, payers, healthcare professionals, patients, and employers) about the benefits and risks of new and existing treatments. The priority given to the collection of various types of data for each product varies over time. For example, preapproval studies generally focus on dose finding, identification of the target population, and the demonstration of safety and efficacy, whereas postapproval studies may be directed toward the evaluation of comparative effectiveness, cost-effectiveness, patient preference, long-term safety, and patient adherence and may include observational studies. The unique perspectives of various stakeholders can result in a potentially broad range of questions to be addressed about the specific product or disease state. Furthermore, the type of evidence required will vary by desired treatment outcome (e.g., whether curative, preventative, or palliative treatment is needed), the time course of the underlying disease (e.g., whether an acute or a chronic intervention is needed), and whether the treatment alternatives for a given condition already exist or are in development. In the past few decades, the development of evidence in support of the first launch of a product has extended beyond traditional placebo-controlled efficacy and safety trials to include information from studies with certain subpopulations and information on comparative efficacy, quality of life, outcomes, and cost-effectiveness.

After FDA approval, manufacturers provide evidence and generate additional evidence to help providers and patients make appropriate treatment choices and to help payers facilitate their coverage-related decision making through the coverage and payment processes. This may involve the need for studies focused on real-world utilization and outcomes to supplement the findings of clinical trials that have established the defined populations, dosing, and treatment durations. Most recently, stakeholders have expressed a strong interest in information on real-world comparative effectiveness, resulting in requests for additional evidence, including the systematic collection of data from and analysis of the scientific literature, analyses of the data in clinical and claims databases, and the collection of results from studies of specific technologies. Many manufacturers have devoted significant resources to this type of evidence development for internal purposes, scientific meeting presentations, and informing or partnering with various groups developing similar types of evidence, as discussed below. Thus, healthcare manufacturers play a key role in the development of evidence. Their investments in evidence development for pre- and postmarketing approval are substantial, with significant risk, and require long-term investments for the development of pharmaceuticals.

The industry also recognizes that in addition to the sector's role in evidence development, several other public and private organizations also contribute to the development and synthesis of evidence about the products that the industry produces. These include the Cochrane Collaboration (Cochrane Collaboration, 2007); the Oregon Drug Effectiveness Review Project process (Oregon Health and Science University, 2007); the Agency for Healthcare Research and Quality (AHRQ) Comparative Effectiveness Program Centers (Agency for Healthcare Research and Quality, 2007b); and various private health technology assessment groups, including the Blue Cross Blue Shield Technology Center (BlueCross BlueShield Association, 2007) and the ECRI Institute (formerly Emergency Care Research Institute) (ECRI Institute, 2007). These organizations use a number of methodologies from evidence-based medicine, including systematic reviews; large observational studies with administrative data (e.g., data from commercial data vendors, like Ingenix and Premier, and health plans, like Kaiser, Partners, Aetna, and others); and increasingly, studies done with data from systems containing integrated health information, such as the systems of regional health information organizations and large electronic health record systems (e.g., the Cleveland Clinic, the Mayo Clinic, and Harvard Pilgrim).

It is important to recognize the dynamic aspect of product development and the associated development of evidence. There is uncertainty at every stage of product development, with significant but decreasing rates of attrition of compounds from Phase I through Phase III. At each stage, evidence development, both pre- and postapproval, builds on previous results and new understanding of the underlying science. It can therefore be impossible to anticipate the total research required during the life of a product because it is impossible to anticipate the results of research conducted at each step of the product's life. Although healthcare payers prefer data from comparative trials (i.e., trials that compare active products) because of the type of evidence that they provide, comparative trials introduce substantial additional costs as well as risks, especially when they are carried out before approval. In addition, without a consensus on the value and limitations of studies conducted by using current methods, data from these studies become difficult to interpret for coverage decisions. As such, the involvement of all stakeholders in choosing priority questions and conducting research into new methods is needed.

After the introduction of a new medicine into the market, providers go through a learning curve on appropriate product use. Appropriate product use is informed by the data that have been generated before the launch of the product, the information on the product label, data from supplemental research and case report studies, information obtained through informal and formal medical education, and most importantly, the personal experiences of the providers themselves. The use of the product beyond the product indication can be common and sometimes evolves into a recommended or best practice determined on the basis of that fact that use of the product as treatment for a reason other than its original indication has become well established within the medical community, even in the absence of a formal labeled indication (i.e., off-label use).

The learning curve associated with provider use of medical device and diagnostic technologies may be longer than that associated with provider use of drugs. Furthermore, the iterative improvements that mark device and diagnostic technology innovation tend to parallel increases in the skill levels of providers, so that outcomes depend on both product performance and practitioner expertise. Innovations in medical device and diagnostic technologies are not restricted to the premarketing phase of their development. Instead, actual practitioner use of devices in clinical practice typically spurs additional refinements and improvements. Clinical adoption thus serves as the beginning of an iterative process of feedback from medical practitioners, device redesign, use, and more feedback. Furthermore, in addition to technological refinements, these medical practitioners may use medical devices for reasons other than their original intended uses.

Evidence Interpretation

The proper synthesis and interpretation of a body of clinical evidence requires two critical but very different skill sets. Ideally, teams with collective expertise in the specific domain area, in methods of synthesis, and in the analysis of many types of clinical evidence should carry out this exercise; and they should use structured and reproducible techniques to carry out the exercise. The use of such a multidisciplinary team approach avoids the performance of evaluations by a clinical expert who tends to review and interpret the clinical literature from his or her personal perspective or by a nonclinical technical expert who might use structured methods to essentially filter out all evidence that does not conform to a predefined set of strict criteria that do not require clinical judgment. Both extremes are, of course, wrong, but in different settings they are both called "evidence-based medicine."

The challenge of this new age of health technology assessment is to find processes that are not specific either to clinical experts, who focus on evidence that supports their personal experience and views, or to methodological technicians, who focus only on the evidence that supports their preferences for the types of studies and data reporting that they are most comfortable in reviewing. Even the National Institute for Health and Clinical Excellence (2007), which probably considers the broadest scope of clinical evidence in its reviews, tends to depend more on nonclinical reviewers than on domain experts in its interpretation of clinical effectiveness. New evidence-based medicine and health technology assessment procedures must, from the beginning of the process, create teams of clinical experts and methodological experts who work hand in hand on the challenging task of assessing all potentially useful evidence for the comparison of technologies and then structuring the analysis to ensure that other groups may reproduce the synthesis and interpretation of the evidence. Ultimately, because of the various approaches used to interpret evidence, it is critical that this decision-making process be open to appeal through an independent, transparent, and facile process.

Evidence Dissemination

Healthcare product manufacturers disseminate evidence about their products strictly within a clearly defined regulatory framework that aligns with the approved product labeling. Labeled product information is proactively disseminated by multiple routes, including scientific presentations and publications, personal selling, prescriber advertising, product labels, speaker programs, product exhibits at conferences and events, and more recently, tightly controlled direct-to-consumer marketing. It is noteworthy that when new evidence outside the approved labeling information becomes available, product manufacturers cannot, because of regulatory restrictions, proactively disseminate or initiate discussions about these new data. They can, however, use these data in response to specific inquiries by providers and payers and can publish the findings of industry-sponsored clinical trials at scientific meetings and in peer-reviewed journals. Information dissemination from sources other than the industry are not subject to these regulatory restrictions, and evidence can therefore be disseminated through the broadest possible means, including continuing medical education classes, academic forums, the development of guidelines, published case studies, Internet chat rooms and blogs, pharmacist brochures, and health information websites.

Evidence Application

The translation of new evidence into improved healthcare outcomes continues to be a primary goal for healthcare stakeholders. Manufacturers rely on the routes of evidence dissemination outlined above to drive the application of evidence for their products. However, an awareness of new evidence does not automatically translate into new behaviors for patients or physicians. There are a myriad of reasons for this disconnect between knowledge and action, including the nearly overwhelming volume of new evidence available to physicians, patient nonadherence, gaps in the process of care, and a lack of decision support tools. The application of scientific evidence to medical decisions (evidence-based decision making) is complex. Factors such as baseline risk, variations in treatment response, susceptibility to adverse events, and patient preferences should be taken into consideration; but often they are not (Kravitz et al., 2004). Patient and healthcare system understanding of the applicable and actionable evidence could greatly enhance optimal product use and patient outcomes. In addition, the incorporation of this actionable evidence into direct patient care can be facilitated through systems that enable the use of health information technology, including electronic prescribing and decision support tools in electronic medical records. Accelerating the use of health information technology in healthcare will provide unparalleled opportunities to bring evidence-based information to the point of patient care and decision making.

A major underlying problem in the healthcare system continues to be that much of the important evidence about the most effective ways to treat patients that already exists is not embedded into clinical practice. In other words, healthcare providers are not using the best evidence available to make patient treatment decisions. Recent studies show that only a little more than one-half (about 55 percent) of adult patients receive the recommended care during a given encounter with the healthcare system (McGlynn et al., 2003). National medical societies are responsible for the creation of clinical practice guidelines and establishing these standards of care. Guidelines are created through the use of the evidence available from randomized controlled trials (much of it from the industry) and other forms of evidence, including medical consensus, when more rigorous evidence is not available. The best evidence available from clinical practice guidelines is disseminated to healthcare professionals by publication in medical journals and through continuing medical education and other postgraduate coursework, including relicensure and specialty recertification examinations. The evidence base for effectively treating patients, however, is constantly evolving, and best practices change over time. There are multiple opportunities for physicians and other healthcare professionals to keep abreast of new and revised guidelines and other advances and for their integration into clinical care; but there are also considerable barriers, and the diffusion of new evidence into medical practice appears to be slow and incomplete.

The balance between population-based evidence and the evidence needs for an episode of care, that is, the interaction between the individual patient and the physician, is critical. Evaluations should consider the evidence on variations in individual responses to a particular treatment to ensure that an adequate variety of treatment choices is available to meet the needs of individual patients.

The application of evidence has been supported in recent years through healthcare quality improvement initiatives in which evidence-based care is evaluated and promoted through quality indicator measurement and pay-for-performance programs. These programs are designed to improve the practice of evidence-based care through transparent quality measurement and reporting. Programs such as the Health Plan Employer Data and Information Set offered through the National Committee for Quality Assurance,[1] Ambulatory Quality Alliance,[2] and Hospital Quality Alliance[3] have created evidence-based quality measures that are increasingly applied in the institutional and ambulatory environments aligned with pay-for-performance programs directed by the organizations LeapFrog[4] and Bridges to Excellence.[5] It will be important to provide feedback to healthcare providers and payers on the quality of care that they provide and to provide incentives to practice evidence-based care. Additionally, those stakeholders responsible for generating evidence for medical practice and the use of medications must receive feedback on the types of evidence to be generated for future practice and the safe and appropriate use of medications.

Although the dissemination of evidence to health policy decision makers and healthcare providers for patient care decisions is critical, the availability of evidence for consumers is also necessary to support consumers' increasing role in making decisions about their health management. Various organizations, including WebMD,[6] Harvard Medical School,[7] the Mayo Clinic,[8] and others, have created consumer medical knowledge services available through the Internet, public health campaigns, the popular press, and broadcast consumer advertising.

Finally, the promotion of a learning environment in healthcare practice in which the best available evidence is applied and quality and outcomes are measured will be critical to advancing evidence-based care. However, until effective mechanisms to ensure the appropriate application of evidence to health care are defined, the development of new evidence will not result in meaningful improvements in patient care. General principles for apply-

---

[1] See http://web.ncqa.org/tabid/59/Default.aspx.
[2] See http://www.aqaalliance.org.
[3] See http://www.cms.hhs.gov/HospitalQualityInits/15_HospitalQualityAlliance.asp.
[4] See http://www.leapfroggroup.org/leapfrog_compendium.
[5] See http://www.bridgestoexcellence.org/.
[6] See http://www.webmd.com.
[7] See http://http://hms.harvard.edu/public/consumer/consumer.html.
[8] See http://www.mayoclinic.com/.

ing evidence are lacking. The industry needs stable processes that lead to predictable outcomes, especially in the area of coverage and reimbursement decisions, to ensure its ability to deliver innovative products.

Considerations for Developing, Disseminating, and Applying Evidence

Several factors continue to influence the healthcare product industry's ability to ensure the appropriate and safe use of their products to improve overall patient outcomes:

- With the availability of a range of new technologies and a deeper understanding of the molecular and genetic bases of disease, the science of drug development has become even more complex.
- When the industry successfully develops a new product, the internally developed evidence is sometimes not as well accepted as evidence developed by other groups (e.g., academia and government).
- Although the need for additional sources of evidence and types of evidence is acknowledged, there is confusion and inconsistency regarding the standards and methodologies that should be used to obtain these data and evidence and the relative importance of these data in creating clinical guidance.
- The application of evidence in coverage decisions is inconsistent. Decisions should be based on all of the available evidence (albeit appropriately weighted), without arbitrary rules placed on the inclusion or exclusion of certain types of evidence.
- There is very little evidence on nonpharmaceutical interventions available, making the comparison of new products in this area with the available alternative interventions very difficult.

Evidence Available for Physician Point-of-Care Decision Making

The application of evidence in medical care is challenged in many ways. Physicians and other providers are overwhelmed with the vast amount of medical evidence constantly published and disseminated through publication in the medical literature. Additionally, clinical practice guidelines are often slow in adopting new evidence-based practices, and the dissemination of new guidelines and their recognition by healthcare providers are often delayed.

Without rapid access to new evidence at the point of care, physicians will continue to rely on the opinions of their colleagues and their own practice experience in patient care decision making. Unfortunately, current decision support methods focus on the enforcement of payment policies and the utilization of care rather than on support of the differential diagnosis and the treatment decisions that they make for their patients. Absent objective clinical evidence at the point of care, doctors may continue to overestimate the quality of care that they are providing. However, some evidence suggests that physicians are likely to change their clinical practices when they are provided with credible, actionable information about how the care that their patients receive compares with the recommended or best-practice care.

The move toward measuring medical outcomes, with healthcare providers receiving constant feedback on the quality of care that they provide (with incentives), will be key to improving the percentage of evidence-based care provided. Methods that provide up-to-date evidence through the use of decision support tools and methods that monitor patient outcomes in electronic medical records hold much promise for linking positive assessments to the rapid implementation of new clinical practice standards and the appropriate adoption of new technologies.

Information for Consumer Decisions

The large amount of patient-directed information in the marketplace can be confusing and misleading to many consumers unless it is actively filtered by well-trained healthcare professionals. Credible sources of consumer information need to be identified, and the information needs to be communicated in a form that allows patients to make educated decisions with their healthcare providers on the anticipated benefits and potential risks of a specific treatment.

Summary:
Healthcare Product Developers' Role in Evidence-Based Medicine

In summary, the healthcare product industry has a rich experience base and competency in the development and the dissemination of evidence about their products. However, the majority of evidence development in this sector is driven by the product learning curve and the regulatory requirements for approval. Evidence dissemination, a core capability for the sector, is limited to evidence consistent with the product label. Application of the evidence is essential for the safe and appropriate use of effective new interventions.

ACTIVITY CATEGORIES

The tasks of generating and helping to translate evidence into practice have long been core activities in pharmaceutical and medical device companies. However, the industry's approaches to these activities are evolving as it is asked to demonstrate the value of its products in a competitive, resource-constrained healthcare system. It is difficult to respond to this evolution, however, because there is little agreement about the right kinds of evidence and how the data should be generated. There are also barriers to the effective interpretation of the data and translation of the data into relevant, actionable, and patient-specific clinical information.

We believe that there is great value in evidence-based medical practice, but we are aware that developing and implementing systems that create and use such evidence is a very complicated process, and one that should be designed with careful thought and consideration. As key generators of evidence for the healthcare system, it is our view that we must consider all stakeholder perspectives in coming to consensus on what kinds of evidence are truly required for good decision making by regulators, payers, physicians, patients, and others. We also see a need for approaches to educating decision makers to help them understand and judge evidence in an objective manner and to place that information into the context of other medical procedures and tests. We advocate for decision support tools that will help with diagnosis, therapy selection, therapy adherence, and benefit design. This section will also include our assessment of some of the challenges associated with new standards for evidence, the barriers to overcoming them, and some suggested ways forward.

Opportunities in the Development of Evidence

To attain the vision of achieving a fully evidence-based healthcare system by 2020, the healthcare product sector can make significant contributions to a number of issues in the area of evidence development:

- *Explore standards for evidence development.* There is no consensus on the kinds of evidence that are best suited to guide various kinds of healthcare decisions. Although the randomized controlled trial has been considered a "gold standard" for health policy decision makers, other types of evidence may be more relevant for clinical decisions at the patient care level. Furthermore, there is little agreement about how outcomes metrics, comparators, and study designs should be standardized. This can reduce the reliability of the design and conduct of clinical studies and the application of their findings. Research must be prioritized to address questions judged to be the most valuable by all healthcare stakeholders.
- *Generate evidence that incorporates individual patient needs in the context of healthcare systems decision making.* To meet the needs of regulators, payers, healthcare professionals, and patients, a balance must be struck between generating broad-based evidence of safety

and efficacy in studies with a controlled population and generating evidence of high relevance to particular individuals and subgroups in the real-world setting. In addition, variations in clinical responses and patient preferences need to be acknowledged and considered.

• *Develop new methodologies and standards for application of the evidence.* Randomized controlled trials comparing one treatment modality with another are very costly and require significant investments by product developers, patients, and providers. Alternative methodologies and standards for their use, including large and robust observational studies that use validated sources, such as electronic health record systems, should be explored. These new approaches can also be used to evaluate other (nonpharmaceutical) products and services, such as medical and surgical procedures, behavioral interventions, and nutritional supplements. The establishment of standards for methodologies other than the randomized controlled trial, including systematic reviews, should also be explored. Such studies will need to address issues of potential confounding because of the selection of patients receiving particular therapies based on characteristics (sometimes unmeasured) that are related to outcomes. In the absence of high-quality comparative information, methods for capitalizing on other information, for example, genomics, need to be developed to facilitate a scientific process for identifying the most appropriate management for patients.

Standards of Evidence

The data required for regulatory review and approval by FDA are often not sufficient to meet all of the stated needs of insurers, patients, and other stakeholders; and those data rarely answer questions of effectiveness apart from efficacy. A clear and harmonized set of standards for evidence development that are consistently and appropriately applied will facilitate clear expectations for the quality of that evidence and broader agreement about the conclusions drawn from it. Despite the availability of guidelines from many different organizations (e.g., specialty and primary care professional organizations and federal agencies) and methods for the evaluation of utilization and outcome, no clear standards for guidelines on providing means for providers and consumers to understand the labyrinth of medical information and best recommendations for current care have been defined. These standards for evidence development should reflect input from a wide variety of stakeholders.

The healthcare product sector can provide insight into the evidence that is of greatest importance to patients, providers, and payers in making treatment choices and can apply its expertise with research design standards to these additional studies.

- The healthcare product sector's long experience with and considerable capacity for developing evidence for regulatory authorities has created a deep understanding of methods for the design and implementation of clinical trials and the strengths and weaknesses of such trials in meeting those evidentiary standards.
- The healthcare product sector also has experience in developing and implementing appropriate standards for the development of medical evidence and can define standards to support the development of evidence on the basis of other measures of product effectiveness with limited bias and error.
- Finally, the sector understands how patients and providers make decisions, including what kinds of information that they find important and how that information can be effectively communicated.

Individual Patient Needs in the Context of Healthcare System Decision Making

Even the highest-quality comparator trials often have rigid entry criteria and, consequently, have restricted and uniform patient populations that may limit the applicability of the findings of the trial to larger patient populations.

Depending on the available resources, the industry can contribute to the following:

- ensuring that the evidence is relevant to a broad range of patients and to specific populations,
- developing data with different patient populations who experience realistic follow-up consistent with that which today's healthcare system provides, and
- conducting longer-term evaluations of patients experiencing concomitant medical conditions and health interventions.

Although this is an important endeavor, there are trade-offs between developing evidence and supporting the healthcare product industry's continued ability to bring innovative products to market. This is particularly true given that the evidence required for product approval often differs from the evidence that payers, healthcare professionals, and other decision makers are now requesting. Indeed, the creation of customized clinical programs for each different type of healthcare organization, institution, or payer that answer questions relevant to every patient subpopulation is neither realistic nor affordable. There is likely to be a continued struggle to find the right balance, as will be discussed below in the "Challenges" section.

New Methodologies and Standards for Their Application

The goal to create the best evidence for product use will always demand high standards for the creation of unbiased evidence on the basis of rigorous scientific methods and quality. This goal will continue to be the standard for regulatory authorization throughout the world. The performance of randomized placebo-controlled trials that control for bias, confounding factors, and systematic error is the core requirement for the demonstration of safety and efficacy for regulatory approval.

Observational data evaluations are important additional tools that help provide an understanding of treatment practice and that support the benefits and safety of a product. The data sources underpinning these evaluations hold some promise; however, many observational studies (particularly those used primarily for administrative claims) have inherent limitations, including incomplete information about the total medical care experience (e.g., patient follow-up) and questionable accuracy, quality, and validity. The following are considerations in the use of observational data and other methodologies:

- The validity of data sources needs to be confirmed and reported to improve quality and accuracy. The healthcare product sector can contribute to the setting of standards for the quality of the data sources used for observational studies to ensure quality output. These standards can build on the work already completed by AHRQ on standards for registries and will need to be established in partnership with the other healthcare sectors.
- The use of observational data requires adjustment for confounding, missing data, and possible systematic bias. Techniques that allow such adjustments to be made exist, but they need to be applied in a rigorous fashion with transparency and with clarity about the assumptions that have been made to allow confirmation through scientific studies. The sector can contribute to the generation of standards for the conduct of observational studies along the lines of the good clinical practice level standards currently used for randomized controlled trials.
- The published literature describes a host of other methodologies. These include simple or practical clinical trials, real-world studies and the application of various technical procedures, such as predictive modeling and Bayesian analysis. The healthcare product sector

can contribute to the further development and eventual use of these evolving methodologies through the use of its already established infrastructure for clinical product development.

Little direct work has been done to understand the therapeutic responses of subsets of patients or to describe (and predict) individual variations in response to therapy. However, as scientific knowledge on the molecular nature of disease states has evolved, there has emerged a greater opportunity to define and study responses to therapy with narrower, more clearly defined patient populations. These approaches to development and commercialization, known as personalized medicine or stratified medicine, challenge the standards of traditional business economics but have the potential to make evidence-based medicine more patient-centric. Nevertheless, challenging statistical issues arise when subgroups of patients who are likely (or unlikely) to respond or have an adverse reaction to a particular therapy are identified.

The research community, healthcare systems, and patients have invested tremendous amounts of time and effort in the development of evidence. Moving toward the 2020 vision of having 90 percent of the health care provided be evidence based by 2020 will require unprecedented cooperation among the sectors if this process is to be efficient and still create meaningful evidence to guide patient-centric decision making.

Opportunities in the Interpretation of Evidence

The responsibility for ensuring integrity in healthcare decisions is broadly distributed in U.S. society. Without a shared understanding of how this evidence is being interpreted, the development of new evidence may result in little or no benefit to patient care. A dialogue is needed to establish principles governing how evidence is to be integrated into healthcare coverage decisions. This has immediate import when these coverage decisions include the denial of access to medicines to disenfranchised populations or the swift introduction of a new technology for which early evidence shows that it provides superior benefit. It is also important over the long term as the requirements of ongoing medical innovation are considered. This process, designed to balance societal and individual needs (which can potentially conflict), must be governed by transparency and full disclosure; in addition, it must be informed by the views of all the stakeholders. The following opportunities should be considered in the interpretation of evidence:

- Syntheses and interpretations of evidence should involve clinical and methodological experts, consider all potentially useful evidence, and use methods that are reproducible by others.

- The healthcare product industry can become more active in informing clinicians, payers, and patients about the proper interpretation and the limitations of various types of evidence. This would include educating the public, policy makers, and physicians about the uncertainties related to making decisions based on the statistical outcomes of studies with (potentially) nonrepresentative populations.
- The industry can assist with the development of best practice standards for evidence integration to address the complexity of clinical decisions and evaluating the trade-offs of different study designs.
- All stakeholders can participate in the initiation of a research agenda to conduct research on the interpretation and application of evidence in healthcare decisions and the actual practice of medicine.
- All stakeholders can also participate in an exploration of the importance of patient-consumer inclusion in the development, translation, and dissemination of evidence for healthcare decision making.

Opportunities for the Application of Evidence

The rate of translation of the available evidence into clinical practice is slow, and the translation of evidence is often challenged by gaps in the evidence. New evidence does not always translate into new behaviors among physicians and patients, in part because of the volume of new evidence, patient nonadherence, gaps in care, and a lack of decision support tools. The use of evidence in health policy decision making, coverage and reimbursement decisions, and patient care decisions requires different approaches to evaluating the evidence. All stakeholders must have a better understanding of the means of application of the evidence if they are to incorporate the evidence into their own decision-making processes. Finally, the practice of evidence-based medicine must allow the diffusion of innovation in medical practice.

There are important opportunities to improve the application of evidence in medical practice and decision making that focus on the creation of the specific evidence required for decision making, effective communication of the clinical action that is needed, and systems that make the information available and easy to implement at the point of care as well as for policy and population management. These opportunities include:

- Development and implementation of a research agenda to improve the creation and the translation of evidence-based guidelines into clinical practice. There is a need to identify the areas in which real-world evidence on the therapeutic use of medications needs to be generated to support the data needs of medical societies responsible for the creation of clinical practice guidelines. Again, this process should consider a wide variety of evidence, scientific reviews of the effectiveness of a product, consultations with many stakeholders, and the specific needs of the populations to be served (and should perhaps include benefits that are not included as part of most effectiveness evaluations, e.g., improved adherence or improved tolerability). These discussions will also need to address potential conflicts of interest. In addition, it is important that these guidelines be updated in a timely fashion so that clinical practice is not locked into being based on earlier standards, as the performance metrics may badly lag behind the state of the art.

- Development of general principles for applying evidence to foster predictable decisions, such as for coverage and reimbursement. The various healthcare system stakeholders should partner with payers to develop processes for setting coverage and payment policies that are seen to be open, transparent, and trustworthy in their consideration of a wide variety of evidence, including a scientific review of the effectiveness of a product, consultation with many stakeholders, and the specific needs of the populations served.

- Support for educational initiatives for physicians and other providers in applying evidence to patient care decisions, including consumer-based decision making. The funders of medical education should partner with continuing education providers to focus education on evidence-based care. Pharmaceutical industry promotions can focus on areas that support the recommendations of clinical practice guidelines and evidence-based care. Collaborations with healthcare systems, academia, and health information technology organizations will be required to accelerate the use of health information technology in health care and to bring evidence-based information to point-of-care decision making. Additionally, methods of communicating evidence to consumers must be explored to better assist consumers with their healthcare decision making.

- Promotion of a learning environment in healthcare practice. The various healthcare sectors can work collaboratively to promote a learning environment in healthcare practice in which healthcare practitioners apply the best available evidence, measure quality and outcomes, and recirculate the new evidence so generated to inform the practice of care. The healthcare manufacturing sector can support this learning environment by supporting quality improvement programs that measure medication use against defined quality indicators (that go beyond mere process) and informing healthcare plans and providers to ensure the appropriate use of medications and the quality of care provided by medications.

- Promotion of national quality improvement of medication use. A partnership with national quality improvement groups and quality improvement personnel in health plans can be created to obtain agreement on a strategy for measuring performance at the health plan, physician, and pharmacist levels; to collect and aggregate data in the least burdensome way; and to report meaningful information to consumers, physicians, and stakeholders to inform their choices and improve outcomes. This may include the development of performance measures for medication use, such as those endorsed by the National Quality Forum, and the design and approach to the measurement and reporting of results.

Challenges in Accelerating the Development, Interpretation, and Application of Evidence

The healthcare product industry can help advance the appropriate use of evidence; however, no one sector can move very far forward alone. With that in mind, some ongoing challenges remain as the various healthcare sectors try to align their efforts toward achievement of a common goal while focusing on areas in which the greatest gains in the quality of patient care and the efficiency of the healthcare system can be achieved.

Focus of Evidence-Based Medicine Activities on the Entire Spectrum of Health Care

The entire spectrum of healthcare delivery and overall treatment must be considered in order to achieve the greatest efficiency and impact. A narrow focus on any single portion of healthcare delivery, "because it's where the data is," will fail to produce the greatest savings or impact on quality of care and is likely to hamper innovation in that sector.

Rather than a narrow focus, there needs to be an explicit process to prioritize these expanding areas of research. The goal of the prioritization should be to identify the areas of greatest improvements in quality and impact on the total healthcare system and should ensure that the most valuable questions are being considered from the perspective of all healthcare stakeholders. The goals defined in Section 1013, Priority Topics for Research, of the Medicare Prescription Drug, Improvement, and Modernization Act of 2003 offer an opportunity but also highlight the ongoing uncertainty of how the gaps in research that can inform decision making and analysis can be identified and addressed. The current input process that allows stakeholders to question developments in the AHRQ Comparative Effectiveness Program provides a good starting point in this regard.

Standards for Evidence Development

If there is no standardization in research, in particular, guidelines for methodology selection and conduct of the chosen study, it will be impossible to prioritize resources and build a credible, widely trusted process for developing and appropriately using new forms of evidence.

Different stakeholders have a wide range of needs for various types of evidence as well as a similar range in how they interpret evidence. For example, it appears that payer organizations use the Academy of Managed Care Pharmacists standard dossiers of evidence in a variety of ways, with some requiring more and different kinds of evidence and others making little use of any evidence that a manufacturer provides. Given resource limitations, it will not be possible for the healthcare product sector to generate an evidence base that will meet a limitless range of needs. The harmonization of evidence standards will facilitate the understanding and use of data. Although a single set of standards will not likely be applied to every study and decision, appropriate and predictable variations in standards should be allowed for different purposes. Nevertheless, those standards should be consistent with one another and not require expensive, nonproductive parallel efforts, for example, one set of requirements for WellPoint, another for Aetna, and yet another for the Centers for Medicare and Medicaid Services. Decisions about how these issues should be addressed must reflect input from the full spectrum of stakeholders, each of which needs to consider the importance of the input from the other stakeholders.

Standards for Evidence Application

Once evidence is generated, a more comprehensive standard is needed to ensure that the evidence is appropriately applied. There is a lack of transparency in how interpreters of evidence (including physicians, payers, patients, and policy makers) use the evidence.

Transparency in this process is necessary to ensure that it is widely accepted and that the decisions are subject to quality checks through public scrutiny. In addition, the establishment of principles governing how evidence is integrated into coverage decisions will facilitate this process. The interpreters of the evidence also have various competencies and needs that they bring to understanding evidence, further complicating what evidence will bring to improving value. Finally, the development of appropriate methodologies for communicating comparative effectiveness research to other stakeholders in the healthcare system, especially patients, is a challenge (e.g., the current activities at AHRQ [Agency for Healthcare Research and Quality, 2007a] and Consumers Union Best Buy Drugs [Consumer Reports Health, 2007]) and represents an area in which the healthcare product sector can make a significant contribution.

Healthcare Information Technology

The use of health information technology has a great potential to make health care more transparent and evidence based and to provide clinicians with up-to-date decision-making support when treating their patients. In addition, the use of electronic data sources could accelerate the development of new evidence in real-world settings.

The establishment of a viable, interoperable health information technology infrastructure may, in fact, be a prerequisite for implementation of the learning healthcare system envisioned in the 2020 vision. There are enormous challenges to the implementation of a national health information technology architecture, and addressing those challenges is outside the scope of this chapter. Nonetheless, solutions to those challenges may be critical.

Personalized Health Care

The healthcare system of 2020 will encounter entirely new challenges as a result of the targeting of therapy for patients for whom a genuine benefit or the avoidance of harm can be achieved on the basis of molecular diagnostic testing.

Assessment of the clinical validity, reproducibility, and utility of molecular diagnostic tests, in conjunction with the demonstration of the effectiveness of an associated treatments, poses new challenges in the development of evidence but also holds great promise for making evidence-based medicine more patient-centric. By 2020 the healthcare system will likely be dealing with not only therapies for existing conditions but also preventive therapies and associated diagnostics to effectively avoid (or delay) the onset or escalation of disease. Standards of evidence for such preventive approaches have not yet been considered.

Health Care's Capacity for Sustainability in Evidence-Based Medicine

The nation's capacity for clinical research is currently inadequate to provide the information needed for regulatory approval and effectiveness research goals. Randomized controlled trials, on which the healthcare system currently depends, take too much time and are too expensive, and their findings are not always generalizable.

A key to advancing progress in meeting the near-term need for expanded requirements to generate evidence is the development of a sustainable evidence development and evidence application capacity for the private and public sectors involved in these efforts. The way forward will require collaboration among the various healthcare sectors to carefully consider research priorities and methods and the policies involved in decision making and the application of evidence to achieve sound medical care.

The economics of innovation in product development are such that the additional expense to the industry of producing evidence beyond that currently required by regulatory agencies is not sustainable from a financial perspective, especially if payers do not value the incremental benefits of new products. If the standards for evidence development are not realistic, the incentives provided to create genuine innovation could be substantially reduced, particularly for innovations for the treatment of uncommon conditions. This, in turn, could change the economics of innovation and affect the business models.

Strengthening the national capacity for additional effectiveness research will need to be addressed through the establishment of definitions for evidence development standards for different types of decisions. Ultimately, the process of generating and applying the best evidence will be the natural and seamless components of medical care itself.

Several concepts embedded in the healthcare product sector's recommendations for collaboration will contribute in the near term to efforts to create this capacity to generate and apply evidence:

- All stakeholders should be involved in establishing research priorities and setting standards for evidence development.
- Transparency and consistency (of standards) in processes, data requirements, methods of assessment and interpretation, and criteria for decision making are needed.
- Health policy decisions should be based on all of the available evidence (albeit, appropriately weighted), without arbitrary rules on the inclusion or exclusion of certain types of evidence. Several research designs should be explored to determine whether the findings of that research are adequate for healthcare decision making, including practical clinical trials, clinical registries, observational studies, and model development.
- A balance between population-based evidence and the evidence needs for an episode of care (i.e., the individual's interaction with his or her physician) is critical. Evaluations should consider the evidence on variations in individual responses to a treatment to ensure that an adequate variety of treatment choices are available to meet individual patient needs.

- Until (and if) consensus is reached on standards of evidence interpretation, the interpretation of evidence should be open to appeal through an independent, transparent, and facile process.
- The assessment of the safety and efficacy of a treatment should be separate from considerations of the clinical effectiveness of a treatment.
- The process of health technology assessment should be linked to implementation of the health technology in healthcare systems such that positive assessments then lead to the rapid implementation of decisions and the appropriate adoption of new technologies.

LEADERSHIP COMMITMENTS AND INITIATIVES

The healthcare product industry, as the supplier of healthcare products, can add far more value to healthcare delivery and the appropriate use of medications and devices than has yet been realized. The sector has demonstrated broad experience in the development of evidence on the safety and efficacy of medications and devices and has been involved in the promotion of the safe and effective use of therapeutics.

The tasks of developing and translating evidence into practice are the core capabilities of the industry. The scientists, clinicians, and technologists that the sector employs have broad experience and considerable knowledge in designing randomized controlled trials and are gaining experience in the conduct of practical clinical trials, observational studies, and registries. Additionally, many industry employees have expertise in statistical analysis, database aggregation and synthesis, and the communication of results to healthcare professionals and patients. It is important to recognize the dynamic nature of evidence development, beginning with the conduct of randomized controlled trials for regulatory purposes and continuing through the collection of data from real-world experiences in the postmarketing phase. Collaboration across this continuum will be a future requirement as the evidence base for the safe and effective use of a therapeutic product is established and monitored.

Unfortunately, a general misalignment of incentives in health care has promoted inefficiencies that have led to a lack of trust between the industry, the public, and the other healthcare sectors, including payers and providers. Although the industry is always concerned for patient health, competition within the industry has often relied not only on the productivity of its R&D pipelines but also on marketing. At the same time, the reputation of the industry has fallen on the basis of public concerns about the accuracy and the transparency of the evidence that the industry provides and the way in which companies employ evidence when they market their products to physicians and consumers.

The industry has made important strides in establishing healthcare compliance guidelines and a code of ethics in the promotion of products to physicians and consumers. Additionally, the transparency of clinical trials data has evolved with the implementation of the Clinical-Trials.Gov website and participation by the industry in communicating the results of clinical trials on the safety and efficacy of medications and devices.

In the past, healthcare sectors have missed opportunities to add value in healthcare delivery because of a lack of cooperation and partnering. In supporting the emerging evidence-based healthcare model, collaboration with the healthcare products industry, which is designed to improve overall patient value by using the right therapeutic products at the right time for the right patient, will be a big step forward to promoting evidence-based quality care.

Areas for Collaboration

Collaboration among Roundtable members will be critical in achieving the goal that, by the year 2020, 90 percent of clinical decisions will be supported by accurate, timely, and up-to-date clinical information, and will reflect the best available evidence.

The nature of the barriers and possible solutions and priorities for action will be addressed by open discussions that focus on key areas of collaboration and a program of activities to address them. The priority areas for collaboration are described in the next section.

NEXT STEPS

Evidence Development

- The development of standards of evidence for product approval, health policy decision making, and patient care decisions will allow consensus on the types of evidence that are best suited to inform various kinds of healthcare decisions. The role of healthcare product developers in achieving this goal will be to participate with other healthcare sectors, in particular, patients, healthcare delivery organizations, clinical research and evaluators, insurers, and regulators, in discussing the total cost of care and the overall value derived from greater research on evidence-based medicine. These discussions will result in a more prioritized approach to evidence-based research.
- To develop evidence that incorporates individual patient needs, a balance between generating broad-based evidence for safety and efficacy in a controlled population and generating evidence with a

high degree of relevance to particular individuals and subgroups in the real world is required. To help reach this goal, healthcare product developers and partners from healthcare delivery organizations, clinical researchers, and the insurer sector should engage in discussions on evidence requirements. These discussions should focus on the healthcare policy point of view and that of the consumer-patient.

Evidence Interpretation

- Collaborative dialogue is needed to establish principles governing how evidence is integrated into coverage decisions, especially when these decisions include the denial of access to medicines by disenfranchised populations or the swift introduction of a new technology with evidence of a superior benefit. Proposed sector partners include consumer-patient groups, healthcare delivery organizations, clinical investigators and evaluators, and insurers. From these discussions, healthcare product developers can become proactive, informing clinicians, payers, and patients about the proper interpretation and the limitations of the evidence generated.

- Education about the uncertainties of decision making by the use of evidence from studies conducted with nonrepresentative populations is another area for collaborative work. Healthcare product developers can educate the public, policy makers, and physicians about the residual uncertainties that any individual making decisions on the basis of statistical outcomes from studies conducted with potentially nonrepresentative populations may have. The partners needed in this effort include patients-consumers, healthcare delivery organizations, clinical investigators-evaluators, and insurers.

- The development of best practice standards for evidence interpretation is needed to inform practice, measure quality, and improve how evidence is integrated into coverage decisions. In partnership with consumers-patients, healthcare delivery organizations, clinical investigators-evaluators, and insurers, healthcare product developers can assist with the development of best practice standards for evidence integration by initiating a transparent research agenda on the basis of the interpretation and application of the evidence.

- Understanding the proper role of evidence in healthcare decision making at the patient care level versus the proper role of evidence at the health policy level requires collaborative work by product developers, consumers-patients, healthcare delivery organizations, clinical investigators, and insurers. The industry can contribute by engaging in a research agenda around policy-level decision-making and its impact on patient-level care.

Evidence Application

- The development of a process for setting coverage and payment policies that are open, transparent, and trustworthy as a result of the consideration of a wide range of relevant evidence can be achieved through industry collaboration with healthcare professionals, healthcare delivery organizations, and insurers. Work might include the development of appropriate policies, and product developers could provide relevant research, whenever applicable.

- The development and implementation of an agenda for research that provides real-world data about medications and the specific needs of populations that inform the creation of clinical practice guidelines could be performed in collaboration with healthcare professionals, researchers, healthcare delivery organizations, and insurers. The developers of healthcare products could gain a better understanding of the real-world data requirements of the developers of clinical practice guidelines.

- Refining methods of communicating evidence to consumers to assist them with their decision making is another opportunity for collaboration. Relevant partners would include healthcare professionals and consumers-patients. The industry can contribute knowledge about consumer behaviors relevant to medication use.

- The development and implementation of an agenda of research on the systems changes and behavioral approaches needed to improve the translation of evidence-based guidelines into clinical practice and factors influencing adherence to regimens is another important area for improving the application of evidence. To collaborative discussions and work involving healthcare professionals, healthcare delivery organizations, and insurers, healthcare product developers can contribute knowledge about the behaviors affecting adherence to guidelines and standards of medical practice.

- Healthcare product developers are also positioned to help support quality improvement programs that measure medication use against defined quality indicators and inform health plans and healthcare providers to ensure the appropriate use of medications and the quality of care provided by medications. Overall, this will require partnerships with national quality improvement groups and quality improvement personnel in health plans and healthcare systems to develop quality measures for medical practice that reinforce the appropriate use of evidence. The industry can engage with quality measure developers to focus on key medication use indicators of importance in guiding medication use. Additionally, measurement of medication use indicators in different types of studies can be addressed. Work might include collaboration with patients and consumer groups, healthcare delivery organizations, and insurers.

REFERENCES

Advanced Medical Technology Association. 2007. *Medical technology innovation process.* http://www.advamed.org/MemberPortal/About/NewsRoom/MediaKits/medical technologyinnovation.htm (accessed May 12, 2008).

Agency for Healthcare Research and Quality. 2007a. *Effective health care home.* http:// effectivehealthcare.ahrq.gov/ (accessed May 12, 2008).

———. 2007b. *Evidence-based practice program.* http://www.ahrq.gov/clinic/epcix.htm (accessed May 12, 2008).

BlueCross BlueShield Association. 2007. *Technology evaluation center.* http://www.bcbs. com/betterknowledge/tec/ (accessed May 12, 2008).

Cochrane Collaboration. 2007. *The Cochrane Collaboration.* http://www.cochrane.org/ (accessed May 12, 2008).

Consumer Reports Health. 2007. *Best buy drugs.* http://www.crbestbuydrugs.org/ (accessed May 12, 2008).

DiMasi, J. A., R. W. Hansen, and H. G. Grabowski. 2003. The price of innovation: New estimates of drug development costs. *Journal of Health Economics* 22:151-185.

ECRI Institute. 2007. *ECRI Institute website.* http://www.ecri.org/Pages/default.aspx (accessed May 12, 2008).

Kravitz, R. L., N. Duan, and J. Braslow. 2004. Evidence-based medicine, heterogeneity of treatment effects, and the trouble with averages. *Milbank Quarterly* 82(4):661-687.

Lomas, T., T. Culyer, and C. McCutcheon. 2005. *Final report: Conceptualizing and combining evidence for health system guidance.* Ottawa, Ontario, Canada: Canadian Health Services Research Foundation.

McGlynn, E., S. Asch, J. Adams, J. Keesey, J. Hicks, A. DeCristofaro, and E. Kerr. 2003. The quality of health care delivered to adults in the United States. *New England Journal of Medicine* 348(26):2635-2645.

National Institute for Health and Clinical Excellence. 2007. *National Institute for Health and Clinical Excellence, National Health Service of the United Kingdom website.* http://www. nice.org.uk/ (accessed May 12, 2008).

Oregon Health and Science University. 2007. *Drug effectiveness review project.* http://www. ohsu.edu/drugeffectiveness/ (accessed May 12, 2008).

Pharmaceutical Research and Manufacturers of America. 2005a. The cost of innovation. PhRMA member companies. In *Pharmaceutical industry profile 2007*, p. 5. http://www. phrma.org/files/Profile%202007.pdf (accessed May 12, 2008).

———. 2005b. R&D by function, PhRMA member companies, 2005. In *Pharmaceutical industry profile 2007*, Appendix, Table 5, p. 45. http://www.phrma.org/files/Profile%202007. pdf (accessed May 12, 2008).

———. 2005c. The R&D process: Long, complex and costly. PhRMA member companies, 2005. In *Pharmaceutical industry profile 2007*, p. 6. http://www.phrma.org/files/ Profile%202007.pdf (accessed May 12, 2008).

9

Clinical Investigators and Evaluators

Coordinator

Richard Platt, Harvard Medical School and Harvard Pilgrim Health Care

Other Contributors

*Carolyn Clancy, Agency for Healthcare Research and Quality;
Elizabeth DuPre, AEI-Brookings Joint Center for Regulatory Studies;
David Helms, Academy Health; Rae-Ellen Kavey, National Heart, Lung,
and Blood Institute; Cato Laurencin, University of Virginia;
Mark McClellan, Brookings Institution; Patricia Pittman,
AcademyHealth; Jean Slutsky, Agency for Healthcare Research and
Quality; Don Steinwachs, Johns Hopkins University*

SECTOR OVERVIEW

The discussion in this chapter reflects the perspectives of clinical investigators and evaluators in determining whether, how well, for whom, and at what cost prevention and treatment strategies work and on methods for ensuring their use. Its major focus is on evidence generation, which must occur in clinical and community settings rather than under tightly controlled experimental conditions. The authors of this chapter note that appropriately targeted clinical research has driven rapid changes in prevention and treatment practices; examples include the management of diabetes and the use of postmenopausal hormone replacement therapy. They also note that the topics addressed here form a continuum with population healthcare practices, especially primary prevention, that address many of the same clinical conditions. Many of the same considerations apply to those activities, and a complete plan to create a learning healthcare system should be developed in concert with the population healthcare stakeholders.

Evidence generation and evaluation in real-life situations span health services research and clinical research, including effectiveness, efficacy, and implementation research. The term "effectiveness research" refers to the examination of the benefit of an intervention when it is used under ordinary circumstances, including evaluations with broader patient populations and in broad healthcare delivery settings, and the term "comparative effectiveness research" refers to the evaluation of the relative risks and benefits of competing therapies (Learning What Works Best, 2007). Both of these terms are used in contrast to the terms "efficacy studies," which evaluate the impact of a therapy under the optimal conditions. The term "implementation research" refers to the assessment of methods used to promote the application of knowledge in routine practice and, hence, to improve the quality of care. It looks specifically at the determinants and outcomes of different processes and strategies by using theories and models derived from clinical research, program evaluation, and behavioral and organizational and management research. These types of inquiry span the domains of health services research and clinical research.

"Health services research" is often used as an umbrella term to refer to the multidisciplinary field that studies how social factors, financing systems, organizational structures and processes, healthcare technologies, and personal behaviors affect access to care, the cost and quality of health care, and ultimately, health and well-being. Its domains include individuals, families, organizations, institutions, communities, and populations (Lohr and Steinwachs, 2002). In 2007 an estimated 13,000 individuals were engaged in health services research; and these individuals were from many different disciplines, including epidemiology, biostatistics, physiology, decision theory, sociology, psychology, cognitive science, communications, and economics (Institute of Medicine, 1994; Moore and McGinnis, 2007). One current interdisciplinary focus is on bringing applied research closer to clinical practice, the so-called second translational block of bedside-to-practice research. Such research aims to improve the scientific basis for clinical practice as well as accelerate the identification and adoption of best practices and will be an increasingly important dimension of health services research design and analysis (Ricketts, 2007).

The term "clinical research" refers to the study of the safety and effectiveness of a particular intervention or set of interventions for patient outcomes. Just as the patient outcomes assessed may be broad, ranging from disease end points to levels of satisfaction, the interventions may also range from a diagnostic test or specific treatment to the organization of the interventions or prevention strategies. As a result, the clinical investigators (e.g., physicians, nurses, dentists, nurses, dentists, pharmacists) who make up a substantial proportion of health services researchers, may self-identify as clinical investigators rather than health services researchers.

The impact of clinical research depends on the effective dissemination and adoption of the findings of that research. Currently, dissemination often depends on publication in peer-reviewed journals and the incorporation of these published findings into clinical practice guidelines and other clinical decision-making aids. Many different organizations and disciplines publish and develop guidelines, and the approaches that the various guideline developers use vary considerably. Groups such as the Grading of Recommendations Assessment, Development and Evaluation Working Group and Appraisal of Guidelines Research and Evaluation have formed to develop standards for the syntheses of clinical evidence and the development of clinical practice guidelines (Learning What Works Best, 2007). Information about clinical practice guidelines can be found at the National Guideline Clearinghouse (http://www.guidelines.gov) and the Guidelines International Network (http://www.g-i-n.net).

Infrastructure and Support

Most researchers and research are funded on a project-by-project basis. Public-sector support comes largely from the U.S. Department of Health and Human Services, which includes the National Institutes of Health (NIH), the Agency for Healthcare Research and Quality (AHRQ), the Centers for Disease Control and Prevention (CDC), the Centers for Medicare and Medicaid Services (CMS), and the Food and Drug Administration (FDA), and from the Veterans Health Administration (VHA). AHRQ's Effective Health Care Program includes its Evidence-Based Practice Centers, which synthesize existing information; the DEcIDE (Developing Evidence to Inform Decisions on Effectiveness) centers, which conduct research to fill knowledge gaps; and the Eisenberg Center, which communicates findings. AHRQ also supports the Centers for Education and Research on Therapeutics. Additionally, AHRQ supports practice-based research networks to foster research that provides generalizable findings and the Accelerating Change and Transformation in Organizations and Networks. NIH's Clinical and Translational Science Awards (CTSA) Consortium includes as one of its goals the conduct of research in practice settings and the dissemination of research findings to clinical practice (Thornton and Brown, 2007), although the magnitude of its support for these CTSA activities has not yet been determined. NIH's Division for Application of Research Discovery and its Roadmap project include programs that develop translational and clinical research. Additionally, several individual NIH institutes support robust programs in health services research.

CDC's Division of Healthcare Quality Promotion leads a variety of research programs, including ones that target care in hospitals; its Immunization Safety Office is the home of the Vaccine Safety Datalink, which has developed novel methods for the routine use of the healthcare data that it collects to assess vaccine safety. CDC, which is the nation's principal health statistics agency, also maintains several national data resources, including vital statistics, data from health examinations, and data from health interview surveys.

Other public agencies also conduct health services research. CMS sponsors research and demonstration programs to align payment with quality. FDA supports postmarketing programs to assess the safety and, to a lesser extent, the benefits of therapeutic agents. VHA supports an array of clinical research and technology assessment programs, including its Quality Enhancement and Research Initiative, and it actively uses the information derived from its electronic medical records to inform both health policy and clinical practice.

In the private sector, academic organizations, healthcare product developers, insurers, healthcare delivery organizations, and professional societies also sponsor research. Several groups perform technology assessments; examples include BlueCross BlueShield Association's Technology Evaluation Center, the ECRI Institute, Hayes, Inc., the Institute for Clinical and Economic Review, and The Cochrane Collaboration. The HMO Research Network is a consortium of 15 health plan-based public-domain research groups that work cooperatively on effectiveness and other research (Learning What Works Best, 2007).

Funding Levels and Trends

It is difficult to ascertain the total national expenditure on clinical effectiveness research, but the total annual appropriations to the federal agencies noted above that are specifically identified for health services research total about $1.5 billion annually (Coalition for Health Services Research, 2006). Data are not currently available on the direct expenditures on clinical effectiveness research that private organizations make. In a review of health services research projects that began between 2000 and 2005, Thornton and Brown found that 34 percent were funded by foundations, 19 percent by AHRQ, and the remainder by NIH and other federal agencies (Thornton and Brown, 2007). Funding by foundations and NIH increased steadily over this period, with NIH becoming the lead federal funder, whereas the number of projects funded by AHRQ and other federal agencies decreased. These trends are independent of those for health services research that is identified as clinical research, data for which are not readily available.

Whatever the specific annual total, the national investment in clinical effectiveness research (health services research plus relevant clinical research) is less than half a percent of all healthcare expenditures (Kupersmith et al., 2005; Moses et al., 2005; Sung et al., 2003). The amount for comparative effectiveness research is even smaller.

ACTIVITY CATEGORIES

The work of clinical investigators and health services researchers may include evaluations of specific healthcare interventions, evaluations of interventions that improve individual and population health, cost-benefit analyses, decision analysis and modeling, and organizational studies conducted to reduce a healthcare organization's liability risk or to determine whether a healthcare organization meets accreditation standards. They may be quantitative or qualitative and include studies with a variety of experimental designs, surveys, focus groups, and record reviews. The principal activities of the clinical investigation and evaluation sector relevant to the development and application of evidence fall into these broad research and evaluation categories:

- clinical trial design, implementation, and coordination;
- registry design, management, and coordination;
- database development and use, including hypothesis testing and data mining;
- evidence synthesis;
- development of standards of evidence;
- development of methods to stimulate the adoption of evidence-based practice;
- evaluation of the application of evidence in clinical practice;
- methodology development; and
- modeling and simulation studies.

Current Methodological Approaches

Some of the methodological approaches are illustrated in Figure 9-1. Study designs are categorized as experimental or nonexperimental. Conventional controlled experiments, including randomized clinical trials, are generally considered to generate the most reliable results and may be particularly well suited to the evaluation of new approaches to treatment or prevention; but they are often costly and slow, and their findings lack generalizability to broad populations, subpopulations (including elderly individuals and children), and the practice environment. Practical clinical trials are controlled trials that are designed to reflect the real world rather than ideal practice, and cluster randomized trials—which randomize practice groups or other groups larger than individuals—are being explored as opportunities to improve both generalizability and efficiency. Studies with quasiexperimental designs (natural experiments) evaluate different levels of exposure to a treatment or prevention strategy, for instance, different levels of exposure resulting from differences in coverage or other factors thought

Basic Study Models

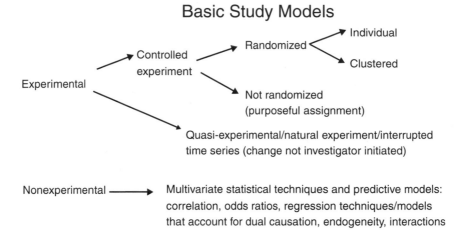

FIGURE 9-1 Basic study models.
SOURCE: Study Models in Health Services Research. Working document. Methods Council Meeting. AcademyHealth. June 8, 2008.

to be unrelated to a clinical outcome. Nonexperimental studies evaluate the routine delivery of care. These latter methods typically attempt to identify and compensate for confounding that occurs because variation in treatment choice is usually related to severity of illness or other factors that influence the outcome apart from the treatment.

The choice of research method depends on the specific issue or question under consideration, ethical concerns, resource availability, the acceptability of different forms of investigation for decision makers, and other factors. When a tightly controlled, randomized study is feasible, economical, and timely and can yield results that are generalizable to most of the population of interest, the consensus is that this approach is preferred (DeVoto and Kramer, 2006). However, many questions of central importance cannot be addressed in this manner. The inability of conventional randomized clinical trials to address many questions is due, in part, to the inherent limits of their external validity (e.g., related to factors such as restricted recruitment) as well as to the heterogeneity of treatment effects that results from different baseline risks or the heterogeneity in the response that individual patients exhibit (Kravitz et al., 2004). Often, randomized controlled trials fail to capture the longitudinal data that are important for obtaining an understanding of the true impacts of different interventions over time. The United States has devoted little funding or effort to the development or implementation of practical or clustered randomized trials; nor has the country yet assessed their potential to generate reliable, real-world evidence quickly and inexpensively.

Different study designs answer very different questions, and the broad range of questions requiring attention requires an array of study designs and methodologies. Because knowing that an intervention works under ideal circumstances (efficacy) is necessary but not sufficient for evaluating what is appropriate for patients in real-world practice settings, some contend that answers to these questions require an update of the traditional evidence hierarchy and its emphasis on the randomized trial (Atkins, 2007). A learning healthcare system will need both randomized controlled trials, especially pragmatic or practical trials that are broadly applicable, as well as other methods.

Challenges

Five major challenges confront the development of the knowledge needed to support a learning healthcare system. First, the limited support for research and development in this arena is an overriding constraint. Underinvestment is evidenced by the fact that the United States devotes less than one-tenth of a percent of its total healthcare expenditures to understanding how well health care works and how to improve it, an amount that is small compared with the amounts invested to understand other major segments of the economy. Underinvestment is also evidenced by the fact that more than 90 percent of the federal investment in healthcare-related research is applied to the development of new therapies rather than to understanding how well various strategies work in practice or how to ensure that the right preventive or therapeutic regimen is offered to the individuals who need it. We do not believe that too much is being invested in the development of new treatments and specifically do not suggest that resources be redirected from those used for the discovery of new therapies.

Second, it is difficult to use many of the existing data, even when they exist in electronic form, because of the fragmentation among organizations that control the data, variations in the ways in which different organizations interpret the Health Insurance Portability and Accountability Act (HIPAA), the various interpretations of regulations governing the use of these data for research by institutional review boards (IRBs), and the proprietary concerns of data holders.

Third, there are important limitations to the existing data. This is the case for both the data collected for administrative purposes and the clinical information in electronic medical records. Examples of these problems include misclassification of the data, which is sometimes inherent because of the different coding systems used and which is sometimes caused by errors and biases in the application of those systems, and missing data, which may include medical history data or which may result from the lack of collection or recording of information during routine medical care. Lack of generalizability of the populations served is another serious problem, particularly among those cared for by tertiary care facilities that tend to treat sicker, more complicated patients, with different intervention patterns.

Fourth, there are substantial barriers to determining what treatments and strategies do and do not work in many clinical settings. This is true both for randomized clinical trials and for other types of research. These barriers include a sense that research is a specialized activity that should involve a limited number of individuals in a few locations, restrictive policies, and logistical and financial obstacles.

Fifth, and finally, a full understanding of the strengths and weaknesses of the different research methods, ways in which to strengthen them, and the situations in which they are best applied is lacking. It is clear, however, that the findings of many randomized trials that are considered the "gold standard" lack generalizability because they are performed with highly nonrepresentative, referral-filtered populations.

LEADERSHIP COMMITMENTS AND INITIATIVES

The research and evaluation sector wishes to underscore the importance of establishing evidence generation, that is, learning what works and what does not work, as a normal part of health care. Such an emphasis is consistent with long-held medical values, as articulated, for example, in the Oath of Maimonides: "Grant me the strength, time, and opportunity always to correct what I have acquired, always to extend its domain; for knowledge is immense and the spirit of man can extend indefinitely to enrich itself daily with new requirements" (The Oath of Maimonides, 1793).

To accomplish this, the research and evaluation sector has identified advances that are needed and that are described in the following sections.

Invest in Applied Research and Development

Individuals and society will benefit from increased investments in applied research to develop new evidence about treatment effectiveness and to make better use of existing knowledge. Support should increasingly focus on linking researchers to decision makers and organizations (purchasers, payers, delivery systems, healthcare institutions, clinicians, patients, and the public) interested in participating in these activities. Examples of activities in need of increased support include assessments of primary prevention strategies and the comparative effectiveness of treatments in clinical use and the testing of ways to eliminate disparities in health care. The investment in research and development required is large in absolute terms but small in relation to total healthcare expenditures. An annual investment of 1 percent of medical spending (the equivalent of a few weeks of medical cost inflation) would yield an amount comparable to the current NIH budget for 1 year. The sector specifically recommends that this research and development investment be made in addition to current biomedical research spending. To advance this issue, a deliberative process should be undertaken to (1) develop a framework for allocating and using a sustained multi-billion-dollar public and private investment in healthcare research and development and (2) identify funding options.

The national investment should include specific provisions to redesign and expand the training of investigators in ways that reward the skills and creativity needed to implement the necessary research portfolio.

Reengineer Healthcare Delivery to Facilitate Structured Learning About Best Practices

Enhancing the efficiency and value of health care requires the ongoing development of comparative data on the benefits, risks, and costs of treatment alternatives. Much of the information required cannot be obtained from conventional randomized clinical trials. In some cases, this is because clinical trials require more time and resources than are available. More importantly, such trials do not address the effect of a treatment in typical populations under the conditions of its actual use. Conventional clinical trials also provide little information about the safety of new drugs, biologics, and devices. Specific methods for addressing these needs are discussed below.

Use the Information Collected During the Routine Delivery of Health Care to Assess Outcomes

The use of data for the systematic assessment of outcomes of care should be construed as routine. The goals for the use of these data would be to (1) inform better decision making about the effectiveness of the prevention strategies and treatments currently in use, (2) understand how different strategies and treatments work in diverse populations, and (3) make efficient use of resources. This use of existing data should be contrasted with the conventional notion of "research" that is both extraordinary and which poses risk beyond that entailed by regular care. It will be important to improve the ability to use different kinds of healthcare data, including claims data, data from electronic medical records, data from registries, vital statistics data, and self-reported information. For many purposes, it will be necessary to use information about very large populations. It will therefore be essential to develop governance and oversight procedures that encourage the holders of confidential and proprietary data to allow their use for approved purposes. Accomplishing this will require the participation of a broad array of stakeholders.

Consideration should also be given to whether it is necessary to use the same rules and oversight mechanisms for these secondary uses of data that are applied for the protection of human subjects of conventional experimental research. Because research and development shares many characteristics with healthcare operations, consideration should be given to whether the rules governing the use of data for operations can apply in some circumstances.

The value of the systematic assessment of outcomes might be linked more directly to the growing public interest in the disclosure of healthcare costs and outcomes. To the extent that public reporting becomes more established, it will be worthwhile to ensure that the methods of assessing the outcomes and adjusting for case mix are sufficiently scientifically valid to allow understanding of comparative effectiveness.

Specific actions that will facilitate the broader use of healthcare data concern the interpretation of HIPAA regulations, the ways in which IRBs oversee observational research, the priorities of purchasers, and the roles that payers play. Suggestions include the following:

Expand the range of HIPAA-compliant assessments of outcomes   Determine whether HIPAA allows the use of medical care information to characterize treatments and outcomes. Specifically, can assessments of benefits, risks, and costs be defined to be healthcare operations within the context of HIPAA? This interpretation of HIPAA could be particularly suited to assessments that can be performed within covered entities for local use and reported in summary fashion for pooled analysis. An important first step will be to clarify the ways in which outcomes assessments can be performed so that they are in compliance with HIPAA regulations.

Facilitate approval of research restricted to review of medical records   Studies of benefit and risk typically require fully representative participation that is impossible when individual informed consent is required. There is a need for the better standardization of practices between IRBs and for the review process to have improved efficiency when multiple IRBs have oversight. Improving efficiency will require preservation of the understanding of the local context and the protection of special populations, particularly disadvantaged and vulnerable individuals. Clarification of the understanding of the Common Rule provision for the waiver of informed consent for record review studies is needed. Although the Common Rule allows waivers of consent in this situation, they are not uniformly granted, and many holders of clinical information unilaterally require individual authorization for the release of information, even when both the controlling IRB and the HIPAA privacy board waive the consent requirement. Additional steps needed include (1) standardization of IRB applications and reporting forms to expedite submissions to multiple IRBs; (2) the creation of regional or national IRB consortia to streamline inter-IRB communication and the coordination of the review of proposals presented to multiple IRBs; and (3) the development of national standards for training for IRB staff and reviewers, in the interest of creating a more uniform interpretation of standards.

Authorize public and private payers to create evidence about benefits and risks Establishing assessment of the benefits and risks of specific preventive and therapeutic regimens and strategies as a normal activity of the healthcare delivery system will blur the distinction between practice, quality improvement, and research. It will require greater interactions among regulators, payers, providers, and investigators. It may also require revision of the regulations and contract provisions that govern CMS and private payers. Some payers, including CMS, are constrained in their ability to make an assessment of benefits and risks a condition of payment. CMS's recent efforts to link coverage to evidence development, participation in clinical trials, or inclusion in a registry have been a step in the right direction but are too limited for many needs. Additionally, many private payers are limited by contracts with their purchasers in the ways in which they can guide care. For private payers (e.g., health plans), discussions among purchasers, payers, and regulators are needed to increase the ability to learn about the comparative benefits, safety, and costs of regimens. Both public and private payers and funders of research need to engage policy makers at the national and local levels on the importance of creating a regulatory and financing environment that supports robust research on comparative effectiveness and the benefits and harms of different healthcare interventions. This engagement must occur in a manner that is transparent and deliberative, and the reasoning behind decisions should be apparent. It should include a broad range of stakeholders, specifically including patients and the general public.

Consider advance coverage approaches In some situations, it may be worthwhile to provide advance coverage for new therapies for a subset of individuals as a temporary measure to inform decisions about whether the therapy should be adopted as a standard covered item. Advance coverage means that a purchaser or, possibly, a payer pays for a new therapy or prevention strategy for some individuals before it covers the same therapy for the population as a whole. In every case, this selective coverage would be limited to therapies that are approved by FDA. Because coverage is extended to a limited number of individuals and only the purchaser or payer is allowed to decide whether the treatment should be covered, this practice does not deprive individuals of treatments to which their insurance coverage entitles them. The period of coverage for only some individuals would typically be limited to the minimum period needed to acquire the needed information, after which it would be available to all individuals or would not be covered. Advance coverage could be used in two ways: (1) for participants in conventional clinical trials for the assessment of efficacy (CMS has used this approach in some situations as part of its Coverage with Evidence Development Policy [Tunis and Pearson, 2006]) and (2) for groups (for example, practices, health plans, or geographic areas) to assess the population-level effectiveness of a new therapy or prevention strategy.

Advance coverage for selected groups will allow direct assessment of the population-level effectiveness of a new therapy or prevention strategy, because it would be possible to compare outcomes among the people who were eligible for the new treatment with those among comparable people who were not eligible. This kind of information is rarely available now and will be extremely valuable in providing an understanding of the overall benefit and cost of a new therapy. Nevertheless, the use of accelerated coverage for some members of society will require the development of a consensus that this is fair and ethical.

To explore the stakeholder perspectives, a broadly representative stakeholder group should explore whether and under what circumstances it will be useful and acceptable to use advance accelerated coverage for the purpose of understanding the benefits and risks of therapies and thus informing decisions about whether to make the therapy available for the entire covered population. The Center for Medical Technology Policy[1] is one organization that convenes multistakeholder groups to develop and implement advance coverage as one of several strategies for evidence generation.

Advance coverage is an especially attractive method for evaluating disease prevention and health promotion activities, activities that often benefit by active collaborations among the healthcare delivery system, purchasers, payers, community organizations, and public health agencies. For example, there would be value in evaluating the effectiveness of the widespread use of an arthritis self-management program that has been shown to decrease pain and the need for physician visits (Theis et al., 2007).

Expand the Use of Both Conventional and Pragmatic Randomized Clinical Trials Comparing Approved Treatments

A principal use of both conventional and pragmatic randomized clinical studies will be to evaluate approved therapies for which information is needed about both efficacy and effectiveness compared to other modalities

---

[1]See http://www.cmtpnet.org.

for similar indications. Such studies can also be used to evaluate therapies for which information about the efficacy and effectiveness of a therapy in special populations, such as children, elderly individuals, and members of specific ethnic groups, is needed. For example, note the success of pediatric oncology in making participation in clinical trials normal behavior for clinicians and patients, and contrast that behavior with the lack of a similar practice of clinical inquiry among other medical specialties.

A goal, then, is to make randomized clinical trials commonplace and to transform both patients' and providers' views about the desirability of participating in them. Ideally, both patients and providers would inquire about the availability of clinical trials before initiating treatment. To obtain clinically useful results, the inclusion criteria should be broad and the trial should replicate the conditions of the actual use of the treatment to the greatest extent possible. In addition, data collection requirements should be minimized. These are attributes of practical or pragmatic trials (Tunis et al., 2003). Considerable work will be necessary to refine these methods.

These changes will require a strong partnership with clinical care sites that commit to institutional participation in applied clinical research as their standard operating procedure. Academic medical centers can be major venues for research addressing inpatient care, and large ambulatory-care practices will be the logical sites for research addressing outpatient care. This institutional participation need not occur throughout an institution; for instance, selected intensive care units (ICUs) or surgical subspecialty sites within a hospital might choose to participate in multicenter research collaborations that routinely test agreed-upon interventions. Some of these interventions will be large simple clinical trials that randomize individual patients. Other trials might be evaluations of unit- or practice-level changes in practice. An example of the latter might be an ICU's participation in a randomized study of different unit-wide protocols for ventilator care. In this example, the entire unit would adopt a specific protocol as its standard operating practice for the duration of the study. Such protocols would, of course, need to meet all applicable IRB requirements for cluster-randomized studies.

The likelihood of success will be enhanced by the broader adoption of protocols that minimize data collection requirements. However, no matter how simple the protocols are, it will be necessary to provide a new infrastructure to support organizations' participation in these new research collaboratives. Most importantly, success will require a change in the culture and the expectations of clinical care delivery so that at least some communities of providers and healthcare institutions and their patients expect to participate in ongoing systematic evaluations of commonly used clinical practices and therapies.

To accelerate this transition, clinicians, healthcare delivery sites, and clinical investigators must work together to design a more robust clinical trials program that takes advantage of the existing clinical care infrastructure. This work can build on but does not need to be limited to the work of the Practice-Based Research Networks, the various related AHRQ initiatives, the U.S. Department of Veterans Affairs' Cooperative Studies Program, the NIH Roadmap project and CTSA Consortium, and other research networks.

Improve Data Sources, Access, and Utility

It will be important to address the nonrepresentativeness of the populations for whom data from clinical studies are available. Nonrepresentativeness is sometimes immediately evident, for instance, a lack of children and adolescents in institutions that care only for adults. Other times it is not so clear, for instance, with regard to representation by individuals who are part of minority, vulnerable, and disadvantaged populations. Examples of opportunities to progress in this area include the development of (1) improved methods for understanding which populations are represented in the healthcare datasets used for research; (2) an improved ability to collect and link different kinds of healthcare data, including claims data, pharmacy dispensing information, electronic medical records, laboratory test results, vital statistics registries, cancer registries, and self-reported information, including data in personally controlled health records; (3) an improved capability for collecting patient-reported outcomes of treatments, perhaps by taking advantage of the anticipated diffusion of personal medical records and methods developed in the NIH-funded Patient-Reported Outcomes Measurement Information System (PROMIS) initiative (NIH PROMIS Initiative, 2007); (4) an improved ability to collect and link nonmedical data, such as census data, motor vehicle department data, and consumer information; and (5) an improved capacity for biobanking (the collection and storage of tissue samples and genetic data). Both tissue and genetic data will be important, but genetic information is essential to taking full advantage of the potential for fully personalized medicine.

Addressing the infrastructure, governance, and policy issues at play will be critical. Priority issues include (1) the need to support the development of database architectures and governance procedures that address these data needs (both architecture and governance procedures will need to respect the privacy needs and the proprietary interests of the data holders) and (2) the need to develop regulations that balance privacy and proprietary concerns without restricting the generation of essential knowledge.

Invest in Improving Research Methods

Innovation is needed to improve the quality of research and accelerate the translation of knowledge into practice. New methods as well as interdisciplinary agreements in areas of dispute around existing methods are needed. Specific needs include better methods of prioritizing and assessing gaps in the evidence; determination of the best uses of observational data and randomized trials that are both simpler and yield more generalizable results; and methods for the translation of research into practice.

Use the Full Range of Methodologies and Research Tools

The use of methods and tools other than conventional randomized clinical trials should be expanded to develop evidence (AHRQ, 2007; Institute of Medicine, 2007). The proceedings of an AHRQ workshop, Comparative Effectiveness and Safety: Emerging Methods, provides an overview of some of the opportunities (AHRQ, 2007). It should also be acknowledged that the current evidence hierarchy is inadequate to address certain essential healthcare questions. Areas of particular importance that cannot be addressed by randomized controlled trials of individuals include the assessment of safety in the postmarketing environment and the population-level effects of coverage decisions. Therefore, the level of evidence needs to be matched to the situation. This may require the development or refinement of a taxonomy that classifies evidence for its utility for supporting both clinical and health policy decision making (Teutsch et al., 2005). Clinicians, healthcare delivery sites, and clinical investigators must be engaged in the development of improved methods for observational research.

Specific research methods other than conventional randomized trials include

- *Pure observational studies that use data obtained during the routine delivery of care.* Analytical methods for these studies include time series analysis, logistic regression analysis, propensity score analysis, analysis with marginal structural models, doubly robust estimator analysis, and instrumental variable analysis. Research will be needed to assess the powers of these and other methods to identify and reduce bias and confounding.
- *Quasi-experimental designs (natural experiments).* These use similar data as above, but exploiting differences in utilization between segments of the population, for instance because of differences in coverage, abrupt secular changes in practice, or other factors unrelated to outcome.
- *Registries.* These can contribute essential information that is not collected during routine care. These will be most useful when they are combined with data obtained during the routine delivery of care.
- *Practical or pragmatic simple trials.* To the greatest extent possible these should occur under conditions of representative clinical

practice and should minimize cost; such trials require broad inclusion criteria, minimal exclusion criteria, and a minimal number of outcomes assessments.

- *Cluster randomization.* This includes selective advance access (with coverage) to new therapies for segments of a population or the selective delayed imposition of new coverage policies and the provision of encouragement or incentives to some segments of the community to alter their therapeutic decisions.
- *Mathematical modeling.*

Improve Methods to Prioritize Research on Gaps in Evidence for All Segments of the Population

In addition to understanding the situations in which evidence is most needed, better methods are needed to understand the benefits and risks of a therapy among individuals who are not typically included in research studies, including individuals who are members of vulnerable populations and groups with complex clinical and social needs. It is not necessary to fill all research gaps for knowledgeable decision making. Setting realistic and rational priorities to conduct research in areas with knowledge gaps is essential for the equitable use of research investments.

Research on Methods for Translation of Research into Practice

Many dissemination strategies result in little or no change in physician behavior or health outcomes. Studies of more complex and more costly interventions like audit and feedback, message prompts, and educational outreach visits suggest potential changes in physician behavior and health outcomes; but interpretation of the results is often complicated by a high risk of bias, before-and-after assessments of outcome measures, a lack of head-to-head assessments of different methods, small sample sizes, unadjusted variations in the intensity of the intervention, and an absence of process evaluations. Potential areas for research include

- the development and evaluation of innovative approaches to changing physician behavior on the basis of adult learning principles, including consideration of financial benefit for compliance;
- the design of rigorous trials to evaluate changes in professional practice;
- the development and evaluation of innovative approaches to changing consumer-patient behavior on the basis of adult learning principles, including the use of evidence, decision support, and adherence enhancing tools; and

- coordination of the release of major new guidelines with the simultaneous initiation of research to evaluate predefined practice outcomes; for this, consider the use of methods for the collection, evaluation, and use of data that are not published through the peer-review process as part of the evidence base.

Specific follow-up activities that might catalyze the needed action include (1) convening of a broad-based task force composed of multiple stakeholders, including patients plus experts in evidence-based medicine and behavior change, to design research initiatives to increase the rate of adoption of recommended practices, possibly including differential reimbursement for compliance with guidelines, and (2) convening of a conference of guideline developers to develop recommendations for clinical trials to assess the implementation of guidelines combined with the release of guidelines, similar to the Guidelines International Network annual research meeting, which was held in Toronto, Ontario, Canada, in 2007 and in which guideline implementation was the overarching theme.

As recommendations, policies, and procedures are developed to broaden the participation of many stakeholders in developing evidence and evaluating practice, it will be important to minimize the administrative burdens of these activities on the participating organizations and individuals.

NEXT STEPS

The clinical investigators and evaluators sector puts most emphasis on the need to establish assessments of the benefits and risks of specific preventive and therapeutic regimens and strategies as a normal part of health care.

To accomplish this, cross-sector collaboration should focus on the priority action items identified below.

Invest in Applied Research and Development

The following actions are needed for investment in applied research and development:

- Establish a process to (1) develop a framework for using a sustained multi-billion-dollar public and private investment in health-care research and development and (2) identify funding options.
- Ensure the development of programs of investigator training that foster the levels, skills, and creativity needed to implement the necessary research portfolio.

- Introduce into all healthcare professional educational curriculums training in the philosophy and skills necessary to imbue the ethic that each caregiver is part of the evidence development process.

Make Better Use of Information Developed During the Routine Delivery of Health Care to Assess Outcomes

The following actions are needed to make better use of the information during the routine delivery of health care to assess outcomes:

- Support the development of database architectures and governance procedures that address these data needs. Both architecture and governance procedures will need to respect privacy needs and the proprietary interests of the data holders.
- Develop regulations to protect privacy and proprietary concerns.
- Clarify ways in which outcomes assessment can be performed efficiently but still adhere to HIPAA regulations.
- Clarify the understanding of the Common Rule provision for the waiver of informed consent for record review studies. Standardize IRB applications and reporting forms to expedite submissions to multiple IRBs.
- Create regional or national IRB consortia to streamline inter-IRB communication and coordination of the review of proposals presented to multiple IRBs.
- Develop national standards for accessible training for IRB staff and reviewers, in the interest of creating more uniform interpretation of standards.

Authorize Public and Private Payers to Create Evidence About Benefits and Risks

The following actions are needed to authorize public and private payers to create evidence about benefits and risks:

- Both public and private payers and funders of research need to engage policy makers at the national and local levels about the importance of creating a regulatory and financing environment that supports robust research on comparative effectiveness and the benefits and the harms of different healthcare interventions.
- Stakeholders should explore the appropriate circumstances for the use of accelerated coverage.

Expand the Use of Different Types of Clinical Trial Randomization Comparing Approved Treatments

The following actions are needed to expand the use of different types of clinical trial randomization comparing approved treatments, including practical and pragmatic, cluster randomized trials, and the use of other novel approaches to affecting statistical randomization in large databases:

- Engage clinicians, healthcare delivery sites, and clinical investigators so that they may articulate the needs for a more robust clinical trials program that takes advantage of the existing clinical care infrastructure.
- Engage all stakeholders so that they may address the appropriateness of the more widespread use of such trials and the situations in which they can be integrated into both prevention and treatment.

Invest in Improving Research Methods

The following actions are needed for greater investments in improving research methods:

- Engage clinicians, healthcare delivery sites, and clinical investigators in the development of improved methods for observational research.
- Convene a broad-based task force composed of multiple stakeholders, including patients, the public at large, and experts in evidence-based medicine and behavior change, to design research initiatives to increase the rate of adoption of evidence-based medicine, possibly including differential reimbursement for compliance with guidelines.
- Convene a conference of guideline developers to develop recommendations for trials to assess guideline implementation combined with the release of guidelines.

REFERENCES

AHRQ (Agency for Healthcare Research and Quality). 2007. Comparative effectiveness and safety: Emerging methods. Special Issue dedicated to Harry Guess. *Medical Care* 45(10 Suppl 2):S1-S172.

Atkins, D. 2007. Creating and synthesizing evidence with decision makers in mind: Integrating evidence from clinical trials and other study designs. *Medical Care* 45(10 Suppl 2): S16-S22.

Coalition for Health Services Research. 2007. *Federal funding for health services research.* http://www.chsr.org/AHfundingreport1206.pdf (accessed May 12, 2008).

DeVoto, E., and B. Kramer. 2006. An evidence based approach to oncology. In *Oncology: An evidence-based approach*, edited by A. E. Chang, D. F. Hayes, H. I. Pass, R. M. Stone, P. A. Ganz, T. J. Kinsella, J. H. Schiller, and V. J. Strecher. New York: Springer. Pp. 3-13.

Institute of Medicine. 1994. *Health services research: Opportunities for an expanding field of inquiry—an interim statement*, edited by S. Thaul, K. N. Lhor, and R. E. Tranquada. Washington, DC: National Academy Press.

———. 2007. *The learning healthcare system*. Washington, DC: The National Academies Press.

Kravitz, R. L., N. Duan, and J. Braslow. 2004. Evidence-based medicine, heterogeneity of treatment effects, and the trouble with averages. *Milbank Quarterly* 82(4):661-687.

Kupersmith, J., N. Sung, M. Genel, H. Slavkin, R. Califf, R. Bonow, L. Sherwood, N. Reame, V. Catanese, C. Baase, J. Feussner, A. Dobs, H. Tilson, and E. A. Reece. 2005. Creating a new structure for research on health care effectiveness. *Journal of Investigative Medicine* 53(2):67-72.

Learning What Works Best. 2007. *The nation's need for evidence on comparative effectiveness in health care*. http://www.iom.edu/Object.File/Master/43/390/Comparative%20Effectiveness%20White%20Paper%20(F).pdf (accessed May 12, 2008).

Lohr, K. N., and D. M. Steinwachs. 2002. Health services research: An evolving definition of the field. *Health Services Research* 37(1):7-9.

Moore, J., and S. McGinnis. 2007. The health services researcher workforce current stock. Paper presented at AcademyHealth's Health Services Researcher of 2020 Summit, Washington, DC.

Moses, H., III, E. R. Dorsey, D. H. Matheson, and S. O. Thier. 2005. Financial anatomy of biomedical research. *JAMA* 294(11):1333-1342.

NIH PROMIS Initiative. 2007. *Functional components: Network structure*. http://www.nihpromis.org/Web%20Pages/Network%20Structure.aspx (accessed May 12, 2008).

The Oath of Maimonides. 1793. http://www.library.dal.ca/kellogg/Bioethics/codes/maimonides.htm (accessed May 12, 2008).

Ricketts, T. 2007. Developing the health services research workforce. Paper presented at AcademyHealth's Health Services Researcher of 2020 Summit, Washington, DC.

Sung, N. S., W. F. Crowley, Jr., M. Genel, P. Salber, L. Sandy, L. M. Sherwood, S. B. Johnson, V. Catanese, H. Tilson, K. Getz, E. L. Larson, D. Scheinberg, E. A. Reece, H. Slavkin, A. Dobs, J. Grebb, R. A. Martinez, A. Korn, and D. Rimoin. 2003. Central challenges facing the national clinical research enterprise. *JAMA* 289(10):1278-1287.

Teutsch, S. M., M. L. Berger, and M. C. Weinstein. 2005. Comparative effectiveness: Asking the right questions, choosing the right method. *Health Affairs* 24(1):128-132.

Theis, K. A., C. G. Helmick, and J. M. Hootman. 2007. Arthritis burden and impact are greater among U.S. women than men: Intervention opportunities. *Journal of Women's Health (Larchmt)* 16(4):441-453.

Thornton, C., and J. D. Brown. 2007. The demand for health services researchers in 2020. Paper presented at AcademyHealth's Health Services Researcher of 2020 Summit, Washington, DC.

Tunis, S. R., and S. D. Pearson. 2006. Coverage options for promising technologies: Medicare's "coverage with evidence development." *Health Affairs* 25(5):1218-1230.

Tunis, S. R., D. B. Stryer, and C. M. Clancy. 2003. Practical clinical trials: Increasing the value of clinical research for decision making in clinical and health policy. *JAMA* 290:1624-1632.

10

Regulators

Coordinator

Janet Woodcock, Food and Drug Administration

Other Contributors

Mark Benton, State of North Carolina Department of Health and Human Services; Nancy Derr, Food and Drug Administration; Mark Gibson, Oregon Health and Science University; Karen Milgate, Centers for Medicare and Medicaid Services; Jane Thorpe, Centers for Medicare and Medicaid Services

SECTOR OVERVIEW

This chapter presents perspectives on two ways that the regulators sector—in particular, state and federal healthcare regulators, the Food and Drug Administration (FDA) and the Centers for Medicaid and Medicare Services (CMS)—can contribute to accelerating progress in the delivery of health care that is evidence driven. Although FDA and CMS regulate different aspects of health care—FDA regulates the marketing and use of medical products, whereas CMS regulates reimbursement for healthcare products and services for two of the largest healthcare programs in the country (Medicare and Medicaid)—both agencies share a critical interest in the safety and effectiveness of pharmaceuticals, medical devices, and healthcare services.

The Institute of Medicine (IOM) Roundtable on Evidence-Based Medicine is focused on furthering the use of the best available evidence in clinical decision making, that is, evidence that will help provide an understanding of which diagnostic or treatment intervention, among an array of possible options, is best for a given patient. For medical products, this can happen only if the system for identifying, quantifying, and qualifying the evidence that is gathered on the product throughout its life cycle is formalized. As the nation moves toward the personalization of treatment, it is critical that ways to improve the evidence base be found. Making use of existing and emerging information management technologies (i.e., standards and information management systems) will be critical to efforts to formalize an evidence-based system of healthcare practice. Key to this effort, however, is combining the strengths and resources of the many stakeholders involved.

As this chapter explains, FDA's contribution to this effort will primarily be in its ability to improve the quality and the type of evidence generated during the early phases of a medical product's life cycle, as well as to improve the development, communication, and use of risk and efficacy information throughout the product's life cycle. CMS's key contribution, which will occur at both the federal and state levels, lies in its ability to leverage the broad healthcare system through initiatives and incentives that advance evidence-based medicine.

Overview of Regulator Roles

The following paragraphs describe the roles of FDA and CMS in evidence-based medicine. Although these two agencies are very different types of regulators, they share a keen interest in both the safety and the effectiveness of medical products and services and in informing and minimizing the risks associated with the diagnostic and therapeutic choices made in the delivery of health care. Medical product use can be seen as a continuum that begins with the discovery of a candidate product; moves through product development, testing in clinical studies with humans, and FDA marketing approval for specific indications; and proceeds to postmarketing use for the approved indications, including possible subsequent approval for other indications. Throughout this life cycle, substantial data are collected and analyzed to evaluate whether a product is safe and effective for its indicated use. In the premarketing phase, statutes and regulations require that a product's safety and efficacy profile be carefully monitored and that the data be carefully quantified and qualified. Once a product goes on the market, however, the generation of further evidence about a product's safety and effectiveness is not structured. To achieve the IOM Roundtable's goal of achieving medical care that is more solidly based on the evidence, the careful quantification and qualification of evidence related to medical products needs to be extended throughout the life cycles of products.

Food and Drug Administration

The FDA has regulatory responsibility for drug and biological products and medical devices, beginning in the premarketing phase and lasting for the duration of a product's life cycle. Before a product is marketed, FDA oversees and advises the sponsor on the development of the data submitted in the marketing application to demonstrate the safety and efficacy of regulated products. FDA reviews the collected data submitted in marketing applications and makes approval decisions on the basis of safety and efficacy data. After a product is marketed, FDA is responsible for monitoring both the safety and the effective use of the product. In fulfilling its regulatory responsibilities, FDA carefully assesses the data that inform the use of regulated products and that can have a significant influence on the design of studies intended to delineate the attributes of a regulated product. In this role, FDA is also active in facilitating the implementation of advances in the biomedical, product development, and regulatory sciences. As discussed later in this chapter, it is in the latter role that FDA has the best opportunity to contribute to improving the evidence on which clinical decision making is based, but its work to improve monitoring of a product's use is also key.

Recognizing the pipeline problem—that is, the slowdown during the past decade in the development of new and novel medical products—FDA launched (FDA, 2007a) its Critical Path Initiative (CPI) in 2004. This initiative is a long-term effort to modernize the ways in which regulated products are developed, evaluated, manufactured, and used. As part of this initiative, FDA has launched, often in partnership with others, a series of projects[1] to modernize the scientific tools (e.g., in vitro tests, assays, computer models, qualified biomarkers, and innovative study designs) and harness the potential of bioinformatics to improve the ways in which it evaluates regulated products and to help better predict the safety, effectiveness, manufacturability, and use of those products throughout their life cycles. Many of these efforts will result in the improvement of the quantity, quality, and utility of primary clinical effectiveness data as well as facilitate the analysis of secondary clinical effectiveness data.

The white paper developed as background for Roundtable deliberations, Learning What Works Best: The Nation's Need for Evidence on Comparative Effectiveness in Health Care, describes two broad categories of clinical effectiveness research. The first category, primary clinical effectiveness research, which comprises direct comparisons between interventions or between an intervention and no therapy, includes a range of randomized clinical trial designs as well as observational and cohort studies. Primary clinical effectiveness research delivers the principal data that product developers rely on to demonstrate the safety and effectiveness of an intervention. The second category, secondary clinical effectiveness research (or evidence synthesis), is defined as the structured assessment of evidence from multiple primary sources

---

[1]See, for example, the list of more than 40 Critical Path Initiative activities initiated in 2006. More are in planning, and this list was to have been updated at the end of 2007 (http://www. fda.gov/oc/initiatives/criticalpath/).

mostly for the purpose of reaching conclusions about an intervention(s) that cannot be deduced from the individual studies alone (e.g., meta-analyses). FDA more typically uses data from secondary clinical effectiveness research to understand safety issues related to a regulated product.

As explained in more detail below, FDA's statutory authority may not always permit the agency to require significant primary clinical effectiveness research that both is comparative and provides a sound basis for understanding how a new intervention is best used among the existing treatment options. Typically, the primary focus of the major efficacy studies intended to support the approval of new products is the development of data that establish that an intervention has a beneficial clinical effect (i.e., that it is effective and safe for a given use in a defined population). The findings obtained from types of study designs that are the most effective and efficient at establishing that an intervention has a clinical benefit—prospective, randomized comparisons of the new intervention and a control intervention— are often not broadly generalizable to populations beyond the populations enrolled in the study (e.g., the findings might not apply to younger or older patients or to patients with different stages of a disease). In addition, the efficacy findings might not contribute much to the understanding of how the intervention differs from among an array of options. FDA can, however, implement or facilitate a range of activities that can improve the quantity, quality, and utility of primary clinical effectiveness data generated for regulatory purposes. FDA is doing that under the CPI.

Centers for Medicare and Medicaid Services

With expenditures of approximately $650 billion in 2006 and with more than 90 million beneficiaries, CMS plays a key role in the overall direction of the healthcare system. It is CMS's mission to ensure effective, up-to-date healthcare coverage and to promote quality care for its beneficiaries. CMS's mission is to achieve a transformed and modernized healthcare system in which patients and doctors together can make informed decisions about the most effective medical care, based on timely access to the latest evidence, in a way that delivers the highest-value care. This will help to ensure the right care for the right patient at the right time.

CMS is undertaking a number of efforts that support the IOM Roundtable goal. Among those that are particularly relevant to evidence-based medicine are the implementation of SMART health care (science-driven opportunity for management of personal health through affordable, reliable, and targeted care), encouragement of the use of secure electronic health records and personal health records, advancements in the use of electronic prescribing, and the creation of new disease management programs. CMS is also emphasizing prevention, implementing pay-for-performance systems to promote better-quality and more efficient care, establishing an integrated data repository, and modernizing health information capabilities. Finally, CMS is encouraging health plan and drug plan sponsors to improve the coordination of care and to develop innovative approaches to improving the quality of care for its beneficiaries. These activities directly or indirectly support the development, collection, quantification, and qualification of evidence and encourage the application of evidence to guide the delivery of care.

Evidence is therefore an anchor in CMS operations. CMS uses evidence when making national coverage determinations, when determining whether CMS paid correctly for an item or service, and when determining whether an item or service was provided or performed in a quality manner. CMS is keenly interested in encouraging the development of better evidence and in ensuring that evidence-based medicine is used through a variety of regulatory and other incentives. In addition to the efforts noted above, CMS's Coverage with Evidence Development protocol, the clinical trials policy, and the use of registries support this work.

CMS recognizes that collaborative partnerships with a variety of organizations, individuals, and institutions are necessary to support quality measurement efforts. For example, CMS works closely with the Agency for Healthcare Research and Quality (AHRQ) as well as the National Committee for Quality Assurance and other public–private quality alliances, such as the AQA alliance (formerly known as the Ambulatory Quality Care alliance), the Hospital Quality Alliance, and the National Quality Forum to develop, adopt, and implement quality measures. Through such collaborations, CMS is working to help create and sustain a better environment for the provision of high-quality, personalized care to every person every time.

State Medicaid Programs

Within broad national guidelines set by federal statutes, the states have flexibility in determining the final form of the program in their own jurisdictions. This flexibility includes determining what eligibility criteria are used to control access to coverage under the Medicaid program and to determine which services will be provided for those who are covered. Although there are certain federally mandated benefits (established by CMS), such benefits can be waived for demonstration and research purposes. For example, under such waivers, Utah has developed an approach that emphasizes preventive and primary care and has a very limited hospital benefit. Oregon has developed a priority list, which is linked to its budget that determines which services that it covers. In the formation of each of these programs, the states used clinical evidence and outcomes-based research to inform the decisions that shaped the policies.

Similar to the federal government's role in Medicare, the state's role in Medicaid is that of a large purchaser. In fact, Medicaid programs sometimes cover more lives than any other single insurer in a given state. Because of limits in the Medicare program, many low-income adults over age 65 years are often covered by both Medicare and Medicaid. Until the passage of Medicare Part D (the prescription drug benefit under Medicare), these "dual eligibles" depended on Medicaid to help them purchase prescription drugs, and because Medicare has a limited long-term care benefit, many adults over age 65 years depend on Medicaid to provide community and institutionally based long-term care. Across this spectrum of healthcare services, the states are moving steadily toward the greater use of clinical evidence to guide their policies.

A primary difference between Medicare and Medicaid has to do with their funding sources. Medicare is funded solely by the federal government. Medicaid is funded jointly by the federal government and states through a system that uses matching funds. States establish overall spending levels and then state treasuries are required to fund a predetermined share of the cost on the basis of the state's economic well-being. The federal government then covers its share of the costs incurred. Because states determine the spending level, cost is an important consideration for policy makers in the state system than in the federal system. A delicate balance must be struck between the needs of residents who cannot afford to finance their own care, the demands of healthcare institutions and providers, and the need for policy makers to be good stewards of public resources in light of the limited amount of taxation that the public will bear. Once again, the use of research evidence is helpful in making certain that maximum value is obtained for the limited resources available.

State Regulation of Medical Practice

The states directly regulate the practice of medicine and the healthcare workforce. This regulatory authority has its foundation in the 10th Amendment to the U.S. Constitution. Because these duties are not assigned to the federal government by the Constitution, this amendment provides the states the right to enact laws and regulations to protect the health and general welfare of their residents. Because the inappropriate practice of medicine could result in significant harm to the public, each of the 50 states, the District of Columbia, and each of the U.S. territories have enacted medical practices acts that define the practice of medicine and delegates the authority to enforce the act to a board composed mainly but not entirely of physicians. Although the structures of the state regulatory frameworks vary, the common elements that state policies oversee are the initial and ongoing licensing of physicians, including education requirements; examinations; continuing education; and physician conduct, including the appropriate treatment of patients and the regulation of physician conduct.

As the gatekeepers to all that the healthcare system has to offer, physicians play the pivotal role in whether or not the public will receive the benefit of the knowledge generated through initiatives that increase the amount of good-quality evidence. If physicians are unable to access the information or do not choose to incorporate existing knowledge into their practices, the enhanced knowledge will not translate into better health outcomes for patients. In a perfect world, the rapid adoption and use of the best available clinical evidence would be the community norm; however, there is reasonable evidence that this does not always happen. State regulators are increasingly turning their attention to ways in which they can help physicians keep up with the changes that are sweeping through their profession.

State Insurance Regulation

The states are the primary regulators of health insurance in the United States, just as they are the primary regulators of the practice of medicine. However, states regulate only commercial (including nonprofit) health insurance that is purchased from health insurance companies or commercial managed care health plans. This distinction is important, because the Employee Retirement Income Security Act (ERISA) preempts state regulation of employee benefit plans that self-insure, which includes approximately 60 percent of employment-based health insurance coverage.

In addition to ERISA, the federal government has passed several other pieces of legislation that affect narrow but important elements of health insurance for both commercial offerings and self-insured employers. These include the Consolidated Omnibus Budget Reconciliation Act (1986), which requires that certain individuals who have lost their employment-based insurance coverage be given the opportunity to purchase a continuation of that coverage for a limited time; the Health Insurance Portability and Accountability Act, which limits how long insurers can exclude coverage of preexisting conditions for new enrollees; and two other laws that require coverage for minimum hospital stays for newborn children and their mothers and reconstructive breast surgery for women who have had breast cancer. These laws are enforced by the U.S. Department of Labor. The states govern virtually all other features of health insurance. This authority encompasses everything from requirements relating to financial solvency to access to health insurance coverage policies and the oversight of certain clinical issues. Because healthcare organizations and providers depend on insurers for much of their revenue, the regulatory actions of the states play a major role in not only how medical services are financed for millions of Americans but also how health care is delivered in any given location.

Health insurance companies doing business in a given location must meet state requirements. The most fundamental requirement is financial solvency. Regulations require companies to have sufficient fiscal resources and reserves to fund care for conditions found while they are covering a given patient. In addition, state regulations may control everything from what questions can be asked of a person applying for coverage to which services must be included in a policy and which are optional and to whether or not the premiums charged are reasonable. Clinical evidence influences a subset of these activities, primarily the definition of mandatory services for inclusion in policies and the determination of when covered services must be provided.

ACTIVITY CATEGORIES

Premarketing Review of Drug and Device Products

Large quantities of primary clinical data are generated pursuant to FDA requirements to demonstrate the effectiveness and safety of drug and biological products and medical devices before marketing. Typically, multiple clinical studies of various sizes, designs, and purposes support a marketing application. These may include, for example,

- studies intended to determine the pharmacokinetic properties of a drug (absorption, metabolism, and excretion);
- studies intended to determine the pharmacological effects of a drug (its mechanism of action, structure-activity relationships, drug interactions);
- studies intended to determine or optimize dosing;
- small randomized trials to obtain preliminary evidence of safety and effectiveness in individuals with the disease of interest; and
- large randomized trials comparing the new intervention with a control(s) intervention; these are intended to establish that the drug meets the statutory standards for safety and effectiveness necessary to obtain marketing approval.

Clearly, FDA and its regulations affect the quality, quantity, and utility of primary clinical effectiveness data generated for regulatory purposes. However, as the authors of the IOM's white paper *Learning What Works Best: The Nation's Need for Evidence on Comparative Effectiveness in Health Care*, point out, there is often somewhat of a disconnect between the evidence that will most efficiently demonstrate the safety and effectiveness for the purpose of obtaining marketing approval and the evidence that would be best suited to clinical decision making about how to make the best use of a new intervention in clinical practice, that is, understanding which intervention among an array of options is best for a given patient. The primary use for many of the data generated to support a marketing application is to elucidate the various product-specific characteristics of the intervention that must be known before its marketing, and those data have somewhat limited utility for determining how the intervention fits into the medical armamentarium.

Various organizations have suggested that studies conducted to better understand the optimal use of multiple related interventions might best be coordinated by an independent entity capable of identifying evidentiary needs, prioritizing those needs, and funding research to address the priorities on behalf of a broad coalition of affected parties.

Postmarketing Monitoring of Drug and Medical Device Products

During the postmarketing phase of a product's life cycle, FDA oversees a mostly passive safety surveillance system—that is, it largely depends on spontaneous voluntary reports from healthcare professionals and patients of suspected adverse events noted during standard patient care—but it may also require the development of additional clinical data after a drug is marketed (so-called Phase IV studies). Manufacturers are required to report to FDA adverse events reports it receives.

Postmarketing Surveillance

FDA's postmarketing drug safety surveillance program receives more than 400,000 adverse event reports per year. FDA's initiative to increase the submission of these reports electronically is progressing successfully. Currently, FDA receives approximately 54 percent of total adverse event reports from drug manufacturers electronically; 79 percent of manufacturer reports concerning events with a serious outcome not included among the possible adverse events listed on the product label are reported electronically. The internationally standardized electronic format has resulted in the timely electronic receipt of safety information, enhancing FDA's ability to make informed decisions more quickly. Furthermore, agency costs have substantially decreased with the electronic receipt of reports.

To enhance the ability to better capture safety signals within the Adverse Event Reporting System (AERS), FDA uses data-mining techniques in its review of AERS data. Data mining is a tool that helps detect safety signals that might otherwise not be recognized or identified in a more timely fashion than by the review of spontaneous case reports. Data mining identifies adverse events in the AERS database occurring with the use of a particular drug more frequently than would be expected. Such signals can then be pursued with more intensive case evaluation. It is important to realize that data mining looks at associations in the database between drugs and adverse events. It makes no inference regarding a causal role for the drug in the development of the adverse event.

Phase IV Commitments

FDA often requests, as a condition for approval, that additional studies (called Phase IV studies) be conducted after approval for the purposes of

- comparing two drugs (e.g., comparison of the new drug with a standard therapy);
- comparing a new drug plus standard therapy with standard therapy alone;
- evaluating long-term efficacy (e.g., when premarketing studies evaluated only short-term efficacy);
- evaluating drug use or dosing in pediatric populations;
- evaluating the use of a drug in geriatric populations;
- evaluating the use of a drug in patients with renal or hepatic failure;
- optimizing dosing regimens;
- evaluating the interactions of a drug with drugs that are likely to be administered concomitantly; and
- evaluating a specific safety concern that arose during drug development.

Data from Phase IV studies make an important contribution to the knowledge base about a drug and often contribute to understanding how a drug is being used. However, their utility is still somewhat limited, in that they ordinarily do not provide the kind of comprehensive evidence that would facilitate optimal therapeutic decision making in situations with many therapeutic options. Discussed here are activities that will enhance FDA's evidence base for clinical decision making.

FDA Communication Activities

FDA oversees both the generation of evidence about the uses of medical products and the communication of that information to healthcare professionals and, to some extent, patients. Prescription drug labeling or prescribing information is the primary information tool for communicating drug information to healthcare professionals. Prescribing information focuses on a drug's indications (or uses), dosing, and safety concerns. It also describes the data that were the primary basis for FDA approval of the drug. In September 2005, FDA implemented a final rule that completely revised the content and format of the prescribing information for prescription drugs and biologics and was the most complete change that had been made in more than 50 years. The changes to the prescribing information, including a highlights or summary section, a table of contents, numbering of sections and subsections, and reordering of the content on the basis of the frequency with which healthcare practitioners refer to the different types of information in labeling, are intended to make the information therein more accessible, clinically informative, and easy to use. In addition, the new label format provides clinicians with a list of sections that have been modified or updated in the previous 12 months.

FDA also uses a variety of communication mechanisms to disseminate new information about medical products, in particular, emerging safety issues. In recent years, FDA has made efforts to disseminate emerging information about safety concerns before a complete regulatory review and action has been taken. On September 22, 2006, the IOM released a report entitled *The Future of Drug Safety—Promoting and Protecting the Health of the Public* (Institute of Medicine, 2006). The IOM report made a series of recommendations, including recommendations about how FDA could improve its drug safety program. In March 2007, FDA issued a response (FDA, 2007b) to that report, in which FDA outlined in detail what efforts were already under way and what efforts were planned to make FDA's drug safety and risk communications program more robust. Although these efforts are too extensive to be discussed here in detail, a few key life cycle efforts are briefly described.

Issues Related to the Medical Product Life Cycle

During the past decade, FDA has invested in a number of areas that are improving its ability to systematically monitor the use of a product over its entire life cycle. The safety of the medical products that FDA regulates has always been a key focus of FDA's commitment to its mission to protect and promote the public health, and monitoring of safety postmarketing is an important piece of any effort to strengthen the evidence base. A number of efforts are under way at FDA that, once they are implemented, will strengthen the nation's ability to identify the risks related to medical products and to collect, quantify, and qualify the risk information to help inform the growing evidence base. These efforts are being enhanced through the increasing use of emerging information technologies.

Safety and Effectiveness Information

Extensive information on the safety and effectiveness of medical products is available from many different sources, including medical product developers, healthcare practitioners, and healthcare payers, not to mention from FDA, CMS, the Veterans Health Administration (VHA), and others. The information is useful, however, only if it gets to those who need it when they need it. FDA is exploring ways to take advantage of the large amount of data that are available on product risk and effectiveness to enable the sharing of important safety and effectiveness data. To build a solid evidence base for medical products, FDA needs to develop not only a way to collect, quantify, and qualify relevant information but also a way to communicate key findings to point of care in the clinic. FDA is working to modernize the processes by which it collects, analyzes, and communicates to the public important risk information, including the creation of user-friendly information sheets for healthcare professionals on emerging safety issues and a periodic, World Wide Web–based newsletter for healthcare professionals on important drug safety information. FDA's MedWatch website and listserv disseminate critical health-related information on all FDA-regulated medical products and encourage participants to report possible adverse events to the agency through the website.

Harnessing Electronic Information Management Technologies

Electronic prescribing, electronic health records, and electronic adverse event reporting are all important areas whose development and use FDA is encouraging to improve evidence-based practice. At FDA, bioinformatics involves the design, development, and use of modern computer systems to efficiently and effectively manage the regulatory product information that FDA receives and communicates. FDA relies on the management of this information to assess a medical product's safety and effectiveness throughout its life cycle. The current bioinformatics infrastructure that supports the exchange of information about products is undergoing modernization.

Other FDA initiatives to move the agency into an electronic environment include standardizing the electronic submission of premarketing data, updating and improving the ability to receive and disseminate adverse event reports, and enabling manufacturers to update the registration and listing of their facilities and products electronically using the Internet. In 2007, FDA began requiring that labeling information be submitted to FDA electronically by use of an approved standard, Structured Product Labeling, which is making it possible to efficiently develop and maintain a large database of labeling information on prescription drug products on the Internet. Healthcare professionals and the public are now able to access the most current prescribing information, the professional label, cost free on the Internet at a National Library of Medicine-sponsored website called DailyMed (http://dailymed.nlm.nih.gov/dailymed/about.cfm).

Bioinformatics modernization requires improvements in three important information management domains: access, standards, and interface. Better access to information, more standardized information, and better interfaces to information (i.e., better tools to convert information into knowledge) are needed. As these improvements are made to the system, FDA is consulting extensively in the United States and internationally[2] with the regulated industry, relevant healthcare-related organizations, and the public to ensure that the vast information at its disposal can be shared across systems in a secure fashion when it is needed. FDA is also working closely with many other federal agencies, (e.g., CMS, VHA, and the National Institutes of Health [NIH], among others) individually and through the office of the National Coordinator for Health Information Technology to standardize and harmonize standards and systems. The potential advantages of this long-term effort to fulfilling the reality of a national electronic health environment are huge, with the potential for research being equally as large. For example, once product information is standardized and can be exchanged across systems, the search and analysis of datasets to try to learn something about a disease's pathogenesis or differential response because of, for example, genetic variation will become a routine undertaking. Modernizing the nation's bioinformatics infrastructure is costly, complex, and time-consuming. Nonetheless, it is a necessary step to creating a modern, efficient American health information system.

Standards Development

A necessary key component to modernizing the information management framework (and formalizing the creation of a national evidence base) is to develop, agree to, and implement nationwide shared standards. For example, today, medical product safety information is largely nonstandardized, making even the most basic analyses and data-mining efforts difficult and time-consuming. The lack of data standards also impedes the development of newer analytic tools. For example, although the definitions in the MedDRA (Medical Dictionary for Regulatory Activities) have emerged as

---

[2]FDA has been working closely with its international partners to harmonize processes and procedures. For example, the FDA meets regularly with the international community as part of the International Conference on Harmonization of Technical Requirements for Registration of Pharmaceuticals for Human Use and the International Cooperation on Harmonization of Technical Requirements for Registration of Veterinary Medicinal Products.

the worldwide regulatory terminology for the reporting of adverse events in the postmarketing setting, other important data elements in a typical safety report (e.g., the medication, ingredient, or device name) are not associated with standard terms or codes that can facilitate data mining and analysis. Furthermore, the lack of a standard format for the exchange of safety information means that information exchange among key stakeholders is often slow, cumbersome, and manually labor-intensive. These areas are the focus of continuing work.

Medical Care Coverage, Coding, and Payment

Several elements of CMS policy are key for activities related to the evidence base for medical care. At the most basic level, Medicare's payment systems affect the development and use of evidence for decisions relating to coverage, coding, and payment. For every new item or service, CMS must decide what it can and should pay for, how payment should be made through coding and coverage decisions, and how much it should pay. CMS also plays a role in encouraging the development of better evidence and in ensuring that evidence-based medicine is used through a variety of regulatory and other incentives.

Coverage

CMS relies heavily on clinical evidence in its coverage determination process. In determining whether to cover an item or service, CMS must make a determination of whether that item or service is reasonable and necessary for the treatment of Medicare beneficiaries. CMS may make coverage decisions in several ways. The first mechanism is the National Coverage Decision (NCD) process. Through the NCD process, CMS may grant, limit, or exclude Medicare coverage for an item or service. When an application for an NCD is approved, experts review the available scientific and clinical evidence to determine the effectiveness of the item or service in question. A judgment about the adequacy of the evidence for making coverage decisions depends on the methodological quality of the available research and the magnitude of the effect of an item or service on specific clinical outcomes. By using the principles of evidence-based medicine, the aggregate evidence is used to draw conclusions about whether the item or service under review is "reasonable and necessary for the diagnosis or treatment of illness or injury or to improve the functioning of a malformed body member." Pursuant to the Medicare Prescription Drug Modernization and Improvement Act of 2003 (MMA), CMS has also expedited its process for the consideration of new or expanded coverage.

NCDs actually account for a small portion of coverage decisions. Many coverage decisions are made by local contractors and are referred to as Local Coverage Decisions (LCDs). These decisions are processed faster and are less formal than the NCDs. Because of differences in the practice of medicine in different regions, communities, and institutions, it is often preferable not to have a single decision that uniformly applies to all providers. This may be due to insufficient information for determination of whether coverage should be provided on a national basis or to legitimate regional differences in the delivery of health care. LCDs often provide guidance to providers, suppliers, and beneficiaries in the absence of an NCD as well.

As authorized by the MMA, CMS has also developed the Coverage with Evidence Development (CED) protocol, which is intended to enable Medicare to provide payment for items and services under conditions that help ensure significant net benefits of the treatment for beneficiaries and that give rise to additional information. This evidence also assists doctors and patients in better understanding the risks, benefits, and costs of alternative diagnostic and treatment options. Consequently, the linkage of coverage to data collection will also help to ensure that individual patients are receiving care that is reasonable and necessary given their specific clinical situation.

CMS believes that systematic, protocol-driven data collection has the potential to increase the likelihood of improved health outcomes. The care provided under these protocols generally involves greater attention to appropriate patient evaluation and selection, as well as the appropriate application of the technology. These additional data may alter the course of patient treatment on the basis of the best available evidence and may lead a physician to reconsider the use of the item or service or otherwise alter a patient's management plan, potentially improving health outcomes. Two current applications of the CMS CED protocol include the implantable cardioveter defibrillator and positron emission tomography registries, which collect information about patients receiving these treatments.

On the basis of the recommendations from the Medicare Evidence Development and Coverage Advisory Committee, in July 2007, the clinical trial policy was expanded to include paying for the investigational clinical service if covered by Medicare outside a trial or required through an NCD (i.e., CED).

This change exemplifies the agency's commitment to providing access to services for beneficiaries by encouraging the conduct of research studies that add to the knowledge base about the efficient, appropriate, and effective use of products and technologies in the Medicare population, thus improving the quality of care that Medicare beneficiaries receive.

Coding

Coding of medical items and services is crucial to the functioning of the healthcare system. Medicare alone processes about 1 billion claims for items and services each year. On each claim, codes indicate what items or services were provided and why. The code sets most commonly used and recognized by the secretary of U.S. Department of Health and Human Services (HHS) as standards pursuant to the Health Insurance Portability and Accountability Act are the *International Classification of Diseases*, 9th edition (ICD-9), and the Healthcare Common Procedure Coding System (HCPCS). ICD-9 is used for diagnoses in all settings and for procedures in the inpatient setting. HCPCS is used for services and items in ambulatory-care settings.

Many areas of the ICD-9 code set are full, making it difficult to add new codes. CMS is considering whether to move to its successor, ICD-10. HCPCS consists of two subsystems: Level I and Level II. Level I is the Current Procedural Terminology (CPT) system and is maintained and updated by the American Medical Association. CPT codes identify the medical services that physicians and other healthcare professionals perform. CMS maintains and updates Level II codes and identifies products, services, durable medical equipment, prosthetics, orthotics, and supplies (DMEPOS). CMS is in the process of phasing in updates to the coding cycle and improving the process for the development of new codes.

Payment

Ultimately, CMS is responsible for reimbursing providers and suppliers for covered items and services under the Medicare program. In general, Medicare pays on the basis of fixed payment rates that are revised periodically (annually for most systems). However, as the cost of medical care continues to escalate, CMS is developing incentive programs that can be built into the payment system to encourage the delivery of high-quality, efficient care. Measuring and incentivizing high-quality care requires sound evidence to support those decisions. CMS is working with stakeholders to develop measures that can be used to measure quality and modify current payment systems to enable the use of the results of these measures to affect payment rates.

State Programs

Local Medicaid Coverage Decisions

Just as CMS must determine whether a service or device is reasonable and necessary for the treatment of Medicare beneficiaries, so must the states make those determinations for Medicaid patients. Although the NCDs and LCDs that CMS makes for the Medicare program can influence whether or not a service will be funded by Medicaid, the states are not required per se to duplicate the coverage. Typically, the NCDs have a greater impact because of the more inclusive and thorough process that accompanies the making of such a decision. However, these federal decisions cover only a fraction of the items that states must review and rule on, and often, the time frame over which the states must make these decisions is shorter than that at the federal level.

Because most Medicaid beneficiaries do not have significant disposable income, Medicaid programs are using evidence to determine which optional benefits will be included in the benefit design. Although it seems illogical, prescription drugs are still an optional benefit under Medicaid. Regardless, all Medicaid programs currently provide prescription drug coverage, but questions of which drugs should be covered and what purchasing strategies are the most appropriate for the needs of patients must still be answered. Although a small minority of states still uses coverage policies that limit the number of brand-name prescriptions or the overall number of prescriptions available to Medicaid patients, more than 40 states use some form of evidence-informed preferred drug list to make these choices. Similarly, decisions to cover certain preventive and restorative dental services are often made on the basis of research that demonstrates the cost-effectiveness of these interventions, especially for children and adolescents. Medicaid programs also annually determine which of the new HCPCS Level II codes for DMEPOS will be covered by the program.

Once the benefit design is complete, Medicaid program medical directors and other clinical staff use a wide variety of sources to obtain clinical evidence to inform their decisions on when it is appropriate to pay for a given intervention. Sources include secondary research (including literature reviews and policy analyses) conducted by state staff, consultant organizations, federal agencies, and international organizations such as the Cochrane Collaboration. States do not generally perform primary research through their Medicaid programs, although other public institutions such as medical schools and universities may. A number of states are involved in pay-for-performance and disease management initiatives, both of which draw on clinical research and system reorganization to improve the quality of care and, it is hoped, health outcomes.

State Insurance Regulation

Determining which services must be included in insurance coverage can be a controversial and highly political process in which clinical evidence plays an important but not conclusive role. Traditionally, a policy covers broad categories of services, such as physician services, laboratory and imaging services, and hospitalization. However, within these broad categories of coverage, many questions regarding the appropriateness of specific elements of care remain. These questions are usually resolved by attempting to determine whether or not the element of care is medically necessary. Such a determination includes a consideration of the effectiveness of an intervention in treating a given condition, a comparison of an intervention with other interventions that might be available, and the overall condition of the patient in question. The levels of evidence required to demonstrate medical necessity vary from state to state.

At the highest level, legislative action mandates what must be included in the insurance policies sold within a state. Screening mammograms, organ transplants, hospice care, and even access to off-label uses of medications for cancer patients are examples of services that state regulations often require. Occasionally, mandates such as those requiring access to autologous bone marrow transplants for patients with advanced breast cancer are enacted in the absence of good supporting evidence and are later repealed as better evidence becomes available. Mandates can also require insurers to provide access to certain practitioners. Examples of such mandates include chiropractors, physical therapists, and midwives. Evidence is often helpful in determining the questions of the scope of practice and competency that inevitably arise in these decisions. The rationale for insisting on good evidence of effectiveness before enactment of a mandate continues to grow because mandates almost always increase the cost of premiums, and cost is the primary reason that millions of Americans are unable to obtain health insurance coverage.

Once a service is included in health insurance coverage, regardless of whether its inclusion is due to mandates, market, or other considerations, there are still questions of when it is appropriate to use that service. In this case, states generally require a process for patients to appeal any denial of care based on appropriateness. A qualified third party with no direct interest in the outcome of the decision often conducts these processes. In these cases, statutes or regulations often call for using the best available evidence and include a ranking of evidence based on the commonly used hierarchy, starting with randomized controlled trials as the most desirable and moving to case series and expert opinion as the least helpful. In addition, there is a growing appreciation of the value of systematic reviews of the existing evidence on a given procedure. Treatment guidelines produced by medical specialty organizations connected to treatment for a given condition are also commonly invoked as evidence that can guide whether a given service should be provided to a given individual. It is also recognized that all guidelines are not created equal, and there is movement toward giving evidence-based guidelines primacy over guidelines based on primarily on consensus. NIH, AHRQ, the National Academy of Sciences, CMS, and

FDA are also frequently cited as trusted sources of evidence that can be used to guide decisions.

State Regulation of Medical Practice

Initial medical licensure   All states set out minimum requirements for the postgraduate training required before an individual is qualified to take one of the nationally recognized licensing examinations. Typically, 1 or 2 years is required for graduates of a medical school in the United States, and international medical graduates are required to obtain 1 to 2 years of additional training before qualifying for the examination. Those seeking licensure as an osteopathic physician are required to pass the Comprehensive Osteopathic Medical Licensing Examination, and those seeking the license of an allopathic physician are required to pass the United States Medical Licensing Examination. State policy determines the number of attempts allowed to pass these examinations. The states do not write these examinations per se but, nonetheless, deem the standards that they set as sufficient for bestowing a medical license. To the extent that these examinations require would-be physicians to understand how to assess and appropriately apply clinical evidence, they are a critical instrument for helping ensure that the many efforts to improve and produce clinical evidence actually succeed in affecting medical practice.

Continuing medical education   Most states require physicians to complete a minimum amount of continuing education to maintain an active medical license. Requirements run from 20 to 50 hours per year, and the types of activities qualifying as continuing medical education are set out by state policy. Often, the activities are required to meet criteria established by the American Osteopathic Association or the American Medical Association. In addition, certain subject matter has been specified by a number of states, including HIV/AIDS, pain management (a particularly thorny issue, given the issues surrounding opioid medications), and end-of-life palliative care. Less often, medical errors and risk management are specific subjects that must be covered. Clearly, these requirements provide a fertile ground for improving practicing physicians' knowledge of emerging evidence and encouraging them to improve their practice by applying the evidence appropriately.

Consumer information   Among the states, 47 have established policies that provide the public with easily accessible profiles of the doctors in the states. In some cases, this activity has been mandated by legislation, and in others, the regulating agency has established it on its own motion. Even those states that do not provide profiles make disciplinary actions taken by the state accessible to the public. Among the states that provide profiles, some include only educational qualifications and license status, whereas others provide a lengthy additional list of items from specialty qualifications to malpractice records, disciplinary proceedings, hospital privileges, and criminal convictions.

LEADERSHIP COMMITMENTS AND INITIATIVES

Several regulator sector initiatives, some of which are agency specific and some of which are collaborative, may have direct implications for enhancing the evidence that is used to support clinical decision making.

Food and Drug Administration

Many of the efforts described here have been launched under FDA's CPI. They are dependent on the availability of sufficient resources.

Reengineering and Streamlining the Clinical Trials Processes

FDA is engaged in or is planning a number of initiatives listed together under the headings of reengineering and streamlining the clinical trials process. Collectively, these initiatives are intended to facilitate adoption of new development and regulatory approaches to facilitate a better understanding of product performance (leading to better patient outcomes), hasten the implementation of personalized medicine, increase the quality and quantity of information that can be derived from clinical trials and other data analyses, and ease administrative and other burdens associated with the conduct of complex, multisite studies. For example, FDA and the Duke University Medical Center have launched a collaboration aimed at modernizing the way in which clinical trials are conducted. The collaborative will include broad representation from government, industry, patient advocacy groups, professional societies, and academia. The goal is to work together to develop new standards and identify new methods and technologies that will improve safety, boost the quality of information derived from clinical trials, and make the research process more efficient.[3]

Facilitating Development of More Personalized Interventions

Personalized medical interventions present significant challenges to a regulatory process that has historically been geared to evaluating interventions with fairly general populations. Increasingly, selecting the correct

---

[3]For more detail, see http://www.fda.gov/oc/initiatives/criticalpath/partnership.html.

intervention for a given patient will require use of a diagnostic to determine whether the patient is likely to respond to a therapy. FDA is very committed to providing guidance for scientists and the regulated industry to facilitate the development of drug and biological products that target specific subsets of a general disease and the concurrent development of a diagnostic needed to identify the subset to be treated. FDA is developing specific recommendations and plans to issue draft recommendations in 2008. Other initiatives discussed below are also relevant to the advancement of more personalized medical interventions. For example, the HHS Secretary's Personalized Health Care Initiative, in which FDA and CMS are participants, is designed to improve the safety, quality, and effectiveness of health care for every patient in the United States. By using genomics, the identification of genes and how they relate to drug treatment, personalized health care will facilitate the tailoring of medical care to a person's individual needs. Successfully speeding up insights on individual variation will require the ability to use networked health data, in effect, creating a network of networks to aggregate anonymous healthcare data to help researchers establish patterns and identify genetic definitions of existing diseases.

Developing New Biomarkers and Disease Models

Biomarkers are measurable characteristics that reflect physiological, pharmacological, or disease processes. Because changes in established biomarkers after a treatment may reflect a clinical response to a product, facilitating the development and qualification of the next generation of biomarkers is crucial to the successful implementation of more personalized medical care. For more personalized interventions, the selection of the patient population to be treated or the dose to be administered may rely on a diagnostic test for a biomarker that predicts whether a patient has responded or the rate of drug metabolism. New biomarkers are also needed to allow the earlier detection of potential toxicity in treated patients. Genomics, proteonomics, and metabolomics hold great promise as source of biomarkers; and FDA is committed to facilitating the application of these sciences to drug development. Several agencies, including FDA and CMS, are involved in the Biomarker Consortium, a broad-based group of interested parties devoted to identifying and qualifying the next generation of biomarkers.

Advancing Innovative Clinical Trial Designs

FDA is committed to the implementation of innovative trial designs. The current paradigm—an empirical clinical trial intended to assess patient improvement, lack of improvement, and the incidence of adverse reactions—often contributes little to understanding of the disease process and the drug's mechanism of action against that process. Innovative designs, in conjunction with new and better biomarkers, are needed to obtain more and better information. Innovative enrichment designs and adaptive designs, for example, will likely be needed to demonstrate the safety and effectiveness of a targeted drug therapy and the diagnostic that identifies the target population and to establish the clinical utility of the biomarker that the diagnostic tests for. Trials that define and measure variations in individual responses and that seek a correlation with biomarker status are necessary first steps toward providing the evidence base needed for personalized medicine. As new and innovative trial designs are implemented, it will also be important to develop standardized clinical trial designs and outcomes measures tailored to specific diseases or indications. Standardized designs will, among other things, help reduce variation and error and facilitate more informative cross-study analyses, which is important for evidence-based medicine. They will also improve the efficiencies of clinical trials and product development efforts for subsequent products.

Safety

Rapid advances in science and technology have increased the complexity of medical products, resulting in increased attention to safety-related issues by the broad healthcare community. In 2004 and 2005, FDA and HHS announced a series of steps intended to address drug safety issues. FDA created its Drug Safety Oversight Board (FDA, 2005) to, among other things, monitor emerging safety information. FDA also asked the IOM to convene a committee to assess the U.S. drug safety system and to make recommendations to improve risk assessment, surveillance, and the safe use of drugs. On September 22, 2006, after extensive interviews with FDA staff and public outreach, the IOM released a report entitled *The Future of Drug Safety: Promoting and Protecting the Health of the Public* (Institute of Medicine, 2006). The IOM report made substantive recommendations about how FDA could improve its drug safety program and about what actions other parts of government should take to create a more robust and comprehensive system for better ensuring the safe use of medical products. FDA responded to the report, expressing substantial agreement with most of the IOM recommendations and full commitment to strengthening its drug safety program just as rapidly and efficiently as the available resources allow. The response describes a series of initiatives that are among the highest priorities of the FDA commissioner (FDA, 2007b). One FDA goal that is particularly pertinent to the IOM Roundtable on Evidence-Based Medicine is harnessing the power of bioinformatics and other information management technologies to enable the sharing, tracking, and analysis of safety and effectiveness information in a secure fashion across systems.

Sentinel System Initiative

As the U.S. healthcare system moves into the twenty-first century, it is critical to modernize the way that the nation manages medical product safety information. Many activities are already under way to create a rational and systematic nationwide approach to managing the risks of medical product use. It is very important that FDA work with the healthcare community's public and private sectors—payers, healthcare practitioners, provider organizations, medical product manufacturers, academia, patients, the states, and other agencies in the federal government—to identify potentially serious problems resulting from the use of medical products (e.g., adverse reactions and effects, product use errors, and product quality problems) and get that information to the public as quickly as possible. With that goal in mind, FDA has begun exploring the possibility of working with the broad healthcare community to enhance the ability to identify problems with medical products and provide information to the healthcare community as quickly as possible. In collaboration with other agencies within HHS, the U.S. Department of Defense, and Veterans Affairs, FDA has begun to explore the feasibility of creating a distributed, electronic, national medical product safety system. Such a system ultimately could foster the seamless, timely electronic flow of medical product safety information from electronic databases and surveillance reporting systems through risk identification and analysis processes to healthcare practitioners and patients at the point of care while protecting patient privacy. It would help make information about the safe and effective use of medical products accessible to patients and healthcare professionals in a timely and efficient fashion. Such a system could be assembled through public–private collaborations and consist of existing systems, rather than creating new systems.

Uniform Terminology and Electronic Data Standards

FDA, NIH, and the Centers for Disease Control and Preventions (CDC) have been working with stakeholders through Health Level 7 on a national electronic standard for a medical product adverse event report, called the individual case safety report (ICSR).[4] ICSR will facilitate the timeliness and reduce the cost of reporting, aggregating, and analyzing possible medical product-related adverse events. An ongoing effort within Health Level 7

---

[4]In January 2007, Health Level 7 approved the ICSR standard as a draft standard for trial use.

will harmonize ICSR with other adverse event reporting formats, including the adverse event domain of the Clinical Data Interchange Standards Consortium[5] standard for adverse event data collected during clinical trials. The development and use of a harmonized adverse event reporting standard across the entire life cycle of a medical product can enhance the ability to integrate all adverse event information collected pre- and postmarketing and can facilitate the development of integrated adverse event repositories, such as the Janus data warehouse currently being developed jointly by FDA and the National Cancer Institute. This should enhance the analytic ability to detect and interpret medical product-related adverse events, regardless of their source. Similar efforts should be pursued in other bioinformation settings.

Centers for Medicare and Medicaid Services

CMS is seeking a balance in resources in which all participants in the healthcare system can continually learn about the available technologies so that the decisions that are most likely to improve health outcomes can be made. Currently, efforts to develop evidence are focused on getting access to the market. Once access is obtained, far less attention is devoted to ensuring that the evidence used to garner access is verified in clinical practice. When data are collected under pressure to gain rapid access to the market, rarely do those studies include long-term safety and effectiveness head-to-head comparators of a population similar to that of Medicare beneficiaries.

Life Cycle Evidence Development

One concept being considered to address this issue is life cycle evidence development (LED). The LED process represents a substantial culture change by way of continuous data acquisition, evaluation, and response to findings. As it is currently envisioned, the concept involves eight domains: identification of healthcare need, proof of concept, safety (both short and long term), effectiveness, comparative effectiveness, quality/appropriateness, and efficacy. The information needed for each domain will vary depending on the current state of information about the technology. At the moment, Medicare's involvement is primarily limited to effectiveness/comparative effectiveness and quality/appropriateness through Medicare's CED process and making claims data available to researchers. However, realizing

---

[5]The Clinical Data Interchange Standards Consortium is an open, multidisciplinary, nonprofit organization that has established worldwide industry standards to support the electronic acquisition, exchange, submission, and archiving of clinical trial data and metadata for medical and biopharmaceutical product development (http://www.cdisc.org).

the goal of LED involves the gathering of data on an ongoing basis by all providers and purchasers. Currently, data are gathered in disparate mechanisms. Sources include healthcare claims, information submitted by clinical trial investigators, manufacturers, professional societies, hospitals, physicians, federal agencies, technology assessments, registries, and other monitored data systems. This data gathering needs to be better coordinated so that current knowledge is available in a standard and open manner. In particular, for LED to succeed, hospitals and other providers of information need systems to coordinate the multiple entries of the same data into various internal databases, clinical trial databases, and other registries. The technology needed to develop common platforms is available, but the lack of national standards for data definitions and for defining the national architecture for such a system are barriers to creating such a platform. In determining effectiveness on a continuing basis, the healthcare system as a whole must determine what questions to ask and answer; agree on consistent definitions, data elements, and collection methods; and develop consistent statistical constructs that are applied across all reporting.

Chronic Condition Data Warehouse

The CMS Chronic Condition Data Warehouse (CCW) is a step forward in the coordination of data collection efforts and analysis across settings. CCW provides researchers with Medicare beneficiary claims and assessment data linked by beneficiary across the continuum of care. In the past, researchers analyzing Medicare data files were required to perform extensive analysis related to beneficiary matching, deduplication, and merging of the files in preparation for their study analysis. With the CCW data, this preliminary linkage work is already accomplished and is delivered as part of the data files sent to researchers.

Evidence-Oriented Payment Incentives

As noted above, CMS is also working to modify its payment systems to encourage the delivery of high-quality, efficient health care. Specifically, CMS is building incentives into its payment systems. These pay-for-performance programs include the Physician Quality Reporting initiative and the Hospital Value-Based Purchasing Plan. As set out in the Tax Relief and Health Care Act of 2006, CMS's Physician Quality Reporting initiative will award a 1.5 percent bonus (subject to a cap) to physicians who voluntarily report applicable consensus-based quality measures. In addition, since 2004, hospitals that voluntarily report specified quality measures are entitled to receive the full payment update. This information is also made available for beneficiaries on the CMS website. If the U.S. Congress passes legislation authorizing CMS to do so, CMS will also implement a hospital pay-for-performance program. Through this program, CMS will seek to align payment policy with the delivery of high-quality, efficient care. One of the core tenets of the program will be an ongoing process for developing, selecting, and modifying measures of quality and efficiency. An equally important element of this program will be continued public reporting of this quality information to beneficiaries.

State-Level Initiatives

Medicaid Local Coverage Decisions

States are working with each other, not-for-profit organizations, federal partners, and others to expand the use and availability of evidence in clinical and administrative decision making. Many states are in the process of designing and purchasing new Medicaid information systems. This presents an opportunity to enhance the ability of the states to capture data that can be helpful in informing policies and providing providers and patients alike with important clinical and policy information. This effort is a collaboration between states and their federal partners because the federal treasury pays for 90 percent of the cost of the information system. Similarly, CMS has recently awarded Medicaid transformation grants to a number of states. These grants are primarily focused on improving information systems to support clinical care.

Notable initiatives that combine the efforts of states and nonprofit organizations to improve the use of research evidence in policy making include the Milbank Memorial Fund's program that annually provides travel and tuition for policy makers to attend the Rocky Mountain Workshop on Evidence-Based Medicine and the Center for Health Care Improvement's initiative that seeks to improve the care of Medicaid patients with multiple comorbidities.

Elsewhere, states have joined together to produce evidence heretofore unavailable. A collaboration of 13 states and the Canadian Agency for Drugs and Other Technologies in Health are producing systematic reviews comparing the efficacy/effectiveness, safety, and effects of classes of drugs on subpopulations. This collaboration has recently expanded its work to include other questions that are important to administering preferred drug lists with the highest clinical integrity. The collaboration, dubbed the Drug Effectiveness Review Project, has completed systematic reviews of 28 classes of drugs as well as numerous updates to the reports on the basis of need dictated by new research. These reports are placed in the public domain.

Eleven other states have also joined together to create a similar collaboration to obtain high-quality evidence to inform other coverage decisions made by Medicaid programs. The subjects reviewed by the Medicaid Evidence-Based Decisions project run a continuum from the appropriate use of various medical procedures, such as bariatric and spinal surgery, to the establishment of which elements of disease management programs are most effective in improving care and saving money and comparison of strategies for obtaining the most value for the money spent in DMEPOS. Similarly, AHRQ has established a learning network for state Medicaid medical directors that allows them to share their evidence, experiences, and policies with each other and to nominate subjects for reviews performed through the Effective Health Care program at AHRQ.

Insurance Regulation

State insurance policy makers in both the legislative and executive branches continue to grapple with the challenges associated with determining which services are appropriate for inclusion in insurance coverage and under what conditions it is appropriate to pay for a covered service. Increasingly, their deliberations are shaped by the inclusion of research evidence. A growing understanding of the nature of good-quality clinical evidence and its strengths and limitations seems to be evident. Some states are even considering the implementation of policies that require vendors to demonstrate through the provision of scientific evidence that new interventions provide improved health outcomes compared with the outcomes obtained with existing treatments. This change could result in a considerable increase in the standards required for payment because many vendors can now provide only the findings of placebo-controlled studies as a basis for a treatment, and such studies often focus only on intermediate outcomes, such as changes in laboratory test results rather than true health outcomes.

Regulating Medical Practice

State regulators are playing a catalytic role in moving toward the use of a more consistent, relevant, and accessible approach to measuring and communicating information about a physician's competence throughout his or her career. Conceptualized as the National Alliance for Physician Competence, this approach seeks to integrate more fully the continuum of physician education, training, licensing, and certification. Its purpose is to assist physicians in achieving and maintaining the highest possible level of competence to improve the health and safety of patients and to demonstrate to the public that the medical profession has created processes that ensure that physicians are of high quality and are competent to render the care that they seek. The alliance's initial work will focus on identifying the appropriate metrics for measuring physician competence and conceptualizing a data management structure that supports the life-long learning of physicians, the need for physicians to fulfill continuing competence requirements, and the need for the public and other elements of the healthcare system to have ready access to information that demonstrates the competence of a physician. Research evidence will play a crucial role in providing an understanding of what makes a doctor a good doctor, how to measure competence, and how best to create the ability within the medical community to use the findings from clinical research to improve care.

Standards

A key element of regulating medical practice is creating a concise statement of what constitutes good medical practice that is meaningful to physicians and that resonates with the public. Toward this end, state medical regulators have joined together with colleagues and associates across the medical community to articulate such a standard. Now being circulated for public comment, the document *Good Medical Practice—USA* sets out six domains of skills, knowledge, and behaviors that define the elements that make up the appropriate and responsible practice of medicine. The domains include medical knowledge, patient care, professionalism, communication, system-based practice, and practice-based learning. The document calls for physicians to have the ability to critically appraise research and to appropriately incorporate research findings into self-assessment and practice improvement in each of these domains. This clear articulation of the objective of medical education and training will help prepare physicians to sort through and use the vast amounts of clinical evidence that will emerge from the efforts of other healthcare institutions.

In addition, a group of leading medical regulators from Canada and the United States are drafting a report on a survey of state and provincial licensing agencies about their current and desired activities for improving the quality of physicians' practice. The report will include an analysis of feasible new policies that will make the regulatory bodies more effective in improving quality and the cost of implementing such policies. The members of the group, convened by the Milbank Memorial Fund, were chosen by the federation of regulatory bodies in each country.

NEXT STEPS

Any meaningful effort to advance the application of evidenced-based medicine through the development of data that provide better information about therapeutic options and the implementation of those findings in clinical practice requires a coordinated national effort by the range of interested players. These players include governments and other third-party payers; the medical community at large and the various professional organizations that provide clinical practice guidance; NIH; CDC; VA; FDA; CMS; and the pharmaceutical, biopharmaceutical, and medical device industries. The regulator sector also recognizes that the resources that will be available to be devoted to evidence-based medicine initiatives are likely to be limited and, therefore, need to be used in the most cost-effective way to achieve the stated objectives. A carefully coordinated effort by all players is the only path forward.

Finally, the types of urgent public health questions requiring answers and the types of studies needed to provide those kinds of evidence-based answers (e.g., head-to-head comparisons of a particular form of therapy) are often not clearly within the mandate or financial interest of any one player acting independently. There needs to be, in addition to existing structures like the VA or cancer cooperative groups, additional consortia of investigators who conduct clinical trials who can rapidly be signed up, identify local site managers, and initiate studies. Models for this also exist (e.g., the International Studies of Infarct Survival in Europe and perhaps the Department of Clinical Research Informatics and the Thrombolysis in Myocardial Ischemia study in the United States). It seems at least possible that some health maintenance organizations with record systems that could greatly simplify patient selection and follow-up could become enthusiastic about answering the kinds of questions that might be posed.

The regulator sector believes that there are two initial areas in which immediate collaboration in the regulator sector could be transformative.

Create a National Think Tank and a National Problem List

The attempt to identify the areas with the greatest need for evidence should be termed the "national problem list." An entity, for example, a national think tank with broad representation from the healthcare community (including FDA, CMS, VHA, healthcare providers, industry, and others, perhaps under the sponsorship of the IOM) should be created and tasked with coordinating the development, prioritization, and management of the national problem list. This effort can succeed only if it reflects the views of the full range of people with healthcare interests:

- the medical community;
- professional organizations that prepare clinical practice guidelines;
- third-party payers, both private and governmental (CMS);
- government health organizations (CDC, NIH, FDA, VHA, Department of Commerce, AHRQ);

- the pharmaceutical, biopharmaceutical, and medical device industries; and
- patient groups.

Once it has identified the critical evidence needs, this organization would then be responsible for identifying and brokering the conduct of studies or other activities by parties with the capacity to support such studies or activities. In all likelihood, this would require the establishment of a consortium of entities with the ability to conduct the necessary research. For example, these could include entities with particular clinical expertise (e.g., in cardiovascular medicine, oncology, and diabetes treatment), expertise in clinical pharmacology (biomarkers), or technical expertise (e.g., information technology, data mining, and bioinformatics), in addition to the ability to conduct large-scale clinical trials.

The issue of financial support is complex. As acknowledged above, it is unlikely that any private entity will find it in its financial interest to support a particular study (in contrast to the effort as a whole, the success of which is in everyone's financial interest); and the resources of public entities such as the NIH, VA, and CMS are limited. Thus, there would undoubtedly have to be some financial entity that could collect and distribute funds (e.g., a foundation, consortium, or public–private partnership). The information that could be gleaned from these studies on effectiveness (or the lack thereof) and the best choices in health care could result in significant savings. Savings aside, the gains in the health of the public that could result from the findings of such studies could also be immense.

There are several proposals, in the U.S. Congress and elsewhere, to establish such an entity. An initial first step might be the creation of a coordinating entity to help identify priorities and design strategies for the establishment of an infrastructure to better support controlled studies and gather data on an ongoing basis.

Support the Sentinel Safety System Initiative

Cooperative work between FDA and the healthcare community— payers, healthcare practitioners, provider organizations, medical product manufacturers, academia, patients, the states, and the federal government— is important to enhance the ability to identify problems with medical products and provide information to the healthcare community as quickly as possible. Agencies within HHS, the U.S. Department of Defense, and VA have just begun to explore the feasibility of creating a distributed, electronic, national medical product safety network. Such a *sentinel system* would help make information about the safe and effective use of medical products accessible to patients and healthcare professionals in a timely and efficient fashion. The system could be assembled through public–private collaborations and connect to existing systems. Although this project is in an exploratory phase, it is consistent with Section 905 of the recently enacted Food and Drug Administration Amendments Act, which provides for such a network to enable postmarketing surveillance.

REFERENCES

FDA (Food and Drug Administration). 2005. *Drug safety oversight board meetings public summaries*. http://www.fda.gov/cder/drug/DrugSafety/DSOBmeetings/default.htm (accessed May 12, 2008).

———. 2007a. *FDA's critical path initiative*. http://www.fda.gov/oc/initiatives/criticalpath/ (accessed May 12, 2008).

———. 2007b. *The future of drug safety—promoting and protecting the health of the public: FDA's response to the Institute of Medicine's 2006 report*. Washington, DC.

Institute of Medicine. 2006. *The future of drug safety: Promoting and protecting the health of the public*. Washington, DC: The National Academies Press.

11

Insurers

Coordinator

John W. Rowe, Columbia University
(former Chief Executive Officer, Aetna)

Other Contributors

Carmella Bocchino, America's Health Insurance Plans;
George Halvorson, Kaiser Permanente; Carmen Hooker Odom,
State of North Carolina Department of Health and Human Services;
Mark McClellan, AEI-Brookings; Leslie Norwalk, Centers for Medicare
and Medicaid Services; Steve Udvarhelyi, Independence Blue Cross

SECTOR OVERVIEW

The Institute of Medicine's (IOM's) Roundtable on Evidence-Based Medicine seeks to transform the way in which medical evidence is generated and used to improve health care. This is a goal strongly supported by the insurer sector, as evidenced by this sector's continual evolution of tools and techniques designed to encourage excellence in medical practice and improve the value of the health care provided. This chapter describes the strategies already under way within the insurer sector (i.e., health insurance plans and public payers) and also sets out the insurer sector's sugggestions for furthering this necessary transformation through a shared and collaborative effort.

Insurer Sector Profile

The United States spends nearly 16 percent of its gross domestic product—or $2 trillion—on health care, more than any other developed nation. In 2005, private health insurance plans were the largest payers for health-care services, with payments from health insurance plans and other private spending, including consumers' out-of-pocket costs, accounting for almost

269

55 percent of total healthcare expenditures (approximately $1.09 trillion of the $2 trillion) (CMS, 2005). Employment-based coverage continues to be the primary vehicle for private coverage, with 155 million nonelderly workers receiving such coverage in 2005 (Claxton et al., 2006). The different health insurance plan types are all represented within employment-based coverage, with 60 percent of workers covered by preferred provider organization (PPO) networks, 20 percent by health maintenance organizations (HMOs), 13 percent by point of service (POS) plans, 4 percent by high-deductible health insurance plans with a savings option, and 3 percent by conventional plans (Claxton et al., 2006). The top 10 providers of private health insurance in the United States cover approximately 115 million lives enrolled in the health plans' fully and self-insured managed care products, including HMOs, PPOs, POS plans, Medicaid and the State Children's Health Insurance Program (SCHIP), Medicare, fee-for-service managed medical plans, and consumer-directed health plans. The enrollments in the different health plans include 27 million for WellPoint, Inc., 22 million for UnitedHealth Group, Inc., 14 million for Aetna, Inc., 12 million for the Health Care Service Corporation, 9 million for CIGNA Health Care, 9 million for Kaiser Permanente, 8 million for Humana, Inc., 5 million for Blue Cross Blue Shield of Michigan, 5 million for Highmark, Inc., and 4 million for the Health Insurance Plan of New York. Of these health plans, Kaiser Foundation Health Plan, Inc. and Blue Cross of California lead in HMO enrollment, at 5.6 million and 1.5 million enrollees, respectively (AIS Health, 2007).

Public spending—including that by the Medicare, Medicaid, SCHIP, U.S. Department of Defense, and U.S. Department of Veterans Affairs (VA) health benefits programs—accounted for the remaining 45 percent of total healthcare expenditures (CMS, 2005). In 2007, there were 43.5 million people enrolled in either Medicare Part A or Part B, or both, which included 8 million enrollees participating in a Medicare Advantage plan (CMS, 2007a). Approximately 7.9 million veterans received benefits through VA (2006); and another 9.2 million active-duty personal, retirees, and dependents received care under TRICARE (2005) (U.S. Department of Veteran's Affairs Office of Public Affairs Media Relations, 2007; U.S. Government Accountability Office, 2007). During 2006, almost 7 million children were enrolled in SCHIP at any one time, and in 2005, 58 million people received at least one health benefit through Medicaid (Congressional Budget Office, 2007; Kaiser Family Foundation, 2007).

The private health insurance plan sector is represented by America's Health Insurance Plans (AHIP), a trade association that represents the full spectrum of health insurance plans, and the Blue Cross and Blue Shield Association (BCBSA), a licensing entity that represents those health insurance plans that are licensed to use Blue Cross and Blue Shield service marks in exclusive service areas.

America's Health Insurance Plans

AHIP is the national association that represents nearly 1,300 companies providing health insurance coverage to more than 200 million Americans within the group and individual health insurance markets as well as government programs. Their members offer medical expense insurance, long-term care insurance, disability income insurance, dental insurance, supplemental insurance, stop-loss insurance, and reinsurance to consumers, employers, and public purchasers. AHIP represents 90 percent of all the accident and health insurance business in the United States; and AHIP members include commercial insurance companies, most Blue Cross Blue Shield plans, managed care organizations, self-funded plans, PPO networks, third-party administrators, disease management organizations, and reinsurers.

AHIP's goal is "to provide a unified voice for the health insurance industry, to expand access to high quality, affordable health care for all Americans, and to ensure Americans' financial security through robust insurance markets, product flexibility and innovation, and an abundance of consumer choice." The organization represents member interests on legislative and regulatory issues at the federal and state levels and with the media, consumers, healthcare professionals, and employers (America's Health Insurance Plans, 2004).

Blue Cross and Blue Shield Association

BCBSA is the national federation of the 39 independent and locally operated Blue Cross and Blue Shield companies, which collectively provide healthcare coverage for more than 98 million Americans. BCBSA is a leading supplier of business strategy, technical support, healthcare services, and consulting expertise for its member companies. BCBSA and the Blue Cross and Blue Shield companies work to strengthen the movement to greater transparency in health care by providing increased detail about healthcare trends, quality, cost, and best practices (BlueCross and Blue Shield Corporation, 2007).

Today's Environment and Challenges for Change

For much of the 1990s, healthcare costs rose at a slower rate than they had during the previous decade. After a period of relatively low cost growth in the mid-1990s, costs began to rise again, resulting in a health insurance premium growth that peaked at 13.9 percent in 2003 (Claxton et al., 2007). Not surprisingly, the number of uninsured Americans grew during this same time period, rising from 14 percent in 2000 to 15.3 percent in 2005. Although the growth in premiums has slowed over the last three consecutive years (2003 to 2006), healthcare costs continue to outpace inflation and place significant pressure on the cost of insurance coverage, as evidenced by the approximately 46 million Americans who remain uninsured.

Although a wide range of drivers of rising costs have been suggested, there are several that are generally agreed to be key contributors. These generally agreed-upon drivers include new treatments and higher-priced technologies; the increased bargaining power of providers; increased consumer demand; an aging population; and chronic conditions associated with obesity, smoking, and substance abuse.

Accompanying these rising healthcare costs and, many would argue, contributing to these costs is the fact that medical care has become notorious for wide regional variations in treatment, the significant underuse and misuse of recommended best practices, and an undue reliance on treatments of little or no value. Research has consistently shown that Americans receive healthcare services in accordance with the latest scientific evidence only about half of the time. A 2003 RAND study reported that, on average, Americans receive the recommended medical care less than 55 percent of the time, with little difference shown when the care provided is divided into preventive care (54.9 percent), acute care (53.5 percent), and care for chronic conditions (56.1 percent). Research by John Wennberg and others has concluded that evidence-based medicine plays virtually no role in governing the frequency of use of supply-sensitive services and that most of the care provided is driven by other factors, such as the numbers of physicians and hospital beds in a given market, and the widely held assumption that more medical care means better care (Wennberg, 2007).

Additional research conducted over the last two decades by Wennberg's group has effectively demonstrated the wide variation in care received by patients across the country. For example, one study demonstrated that care was consistent with evidence-based guidelines less than 20 percent of the time in 10 of the 306 hospital referral regions in the United States and in only 8 regions was care consistent with medical evidence more than 80 percent of the time (Wennberg and Cooper, 2007). Despite such research, there continue to be examples of treatments widely adopted and used outside the boundaries of supporting evidence that are later found to offer no advantages to existing treatments (e.g., the use of drug-eluting stents for the treatment of coronary artery disease) and, in some cases, to even be harmful (e.g., rofecoxib [Vioxx]).

Legislative and regulatory processes have also contributed to some of the problems of overuse, underuse, and regional variation. The provision of high-dose chemotherapy following an autologous bone marrow transplant (HDC/ABMT) is a prime example of the influence that legislative and regulatory processes can have. In the 1990s, physicians began performing HDC/ABMT for women with late-stage breast cancer, often forgoing standard chemotherapy treatment. Given that there was virtually no good evidence supporting the safety and effectiveness of HDC/ABMT, many health insurance plans denied coverage for the procedure. In response, physicians, patients, and policy makers successfully lobbied state legislatures to pass legislation mandating that health insurance plans provide coverage for this treatment. It was not until 1999 that the preliminary results of five clinical trials for HDC/ABMT showed that the treatment was no better in extending survival than standard treatment and, in fact, posed higher risks of toxic side effects. In addition, because this treatment had become so widely used before its effectiveness had been assessed, many women declined to enroll in clinical trials for HDC/ABMT for fear of being assigned to the standard treatment control group. It took years longer than it might have to gather the evidence showing that HDC/ABMT is an ineffective, risky, and expensive procedure.

The current trends in both cost and quality, coupled with the influence and expectations of legislators, regulators, consumers, and purchasers, have resulted in an environment fraught with significant challenges to the promotion of evidence-based decision making. Yet those same challenges represent the very reasons why such a transformation is necessary. A healthcare system that relies on evidence-based decision making will (1) improve the quality of healthcare delivery; (2) maximize the value and effectiveness of the nation's investment in health care; and (3) help guide providers, consumers, health insurance plans, and purchasers in making decisions pertaining to treatment and benefit design.

ACTIVITY CATEGORIES

Private Sector

From individual health insurance plan efforts to health insurance plan consortium activities, such as those of the HMO Research Network,[1] to industry-wide initiatives led by AHIP and BCBSA, the private health insurance plan sector has led the way in adopting strategies to improve the value of health care by using medical evidence to enhance both quality and affordability. The widespread adoption of these strategies also helps stimulate the interest in and development of further evidence.

---

[1]The HMO Research Network is a consortium of 15 HMO organizations that have formal, recognized research capabilities with a mission to use its collective scientific capabilities to integrate research and practice for the improvement of health and health care among diverse populations. Its database includes information on more than 12 million covered lives. More information can be found at http://www.hmoresearchnetwork.org/.

Below are selected examples of how medical evidence is used in developing medical policy, benefit design, network design, and provider reimbursement arrangements.

Pharmacy Management

Health insurance plans use pharmacy and therapeutics (P&T) committees—which comprise physicians, pharmacists, and other healthcare professionals—to research the scientific evidence on what works and review the available cost and comparative effectiveness data to determine which drugs should be placed on formularies.

Utilization Management

Early in their evolution, health insurance plans relied on utilization management programs as a tool to promote evidence-based care and the cost-effective use of healthcare resources. These programs screened recommended care against evidence-based guidelines to reduce unnecessary variations in practice and to identify care that was inappropriate or unsupported by the medical evidence. However, pressure from consumers, providers, and legislators forced health insurance plans to significantly curtail their utilization management programs, which has led to continuing issues with healthcare quality and which has prompted health insurance plans to seek alternative ways to promote quality and cost-effective care.

Coverage of New Technologies and Services

Drawing on the latest scientific findings on effectiveness and value, health insurance plans use internal staff and processes to guide the creation of medical policy, including decisions about coverage. Many health insurance plans conduct their own assessments of new technologies and services or commission external technology assessments by academic or private groups to help inform their internal deliberations. All health insurance plans base their medical policies on evidence, with each creating its own method for gathering evidence and weighing it in relation to the values of various stakeholders to seek high-quality and efficient care. Recognizing that there is inadequate evidence to determine the appropriate role for experimental or investigational interventions, health insurance plans have promoted the more rapid development of new evidence by covering routine care costs for patients enrolled in clinical trials that are appropriately designed to study experimental and investigational interventions and not covering the costs when patients are not enrolled in such trials.

Disease Management and Wellness

Health insurance plans have developed a new generation of tools to ensure that the coordination of care and that the delivery of evidence-based medicine are complementary, particularly for individuals with multiple chronic or complex conditions, because these individuals are often treated by multiple healthcare professionals. Through their use of health risk assessments, health insurance plans can offer patients and providers customized tools that they can use to modify behavior, encourage the use of preventive care, monitor potential medication interactions, and improve health. As part of this approach, many health insurance plans have reduced or eliminated altogether the cost sharing for maintenance drugs or preventive services that reduce the likelihood of hospitalization, such as asthma controller medications. Additionally, many health insurance plans have incorporated fitness benefits more widely into their benefit designs. By profiling the actual care received and comparing it with evidence-based recommendations, identifying gaps, and working to close those gaps, health insurance plan disease management and wellness programs maximize an opportunity to advance nationally recommended preventive services, among other types of recommended care.

One of the most successful models of disease management and wellness programs relies on health coaching to promote behavior changes. Under this model, patients who have been identified as being at risk for a disease or complications from a chronic disease are offered the opportunity to work with a healthcare professional trained as a health coach. The health coach helps the patient make life style changes that improve his or her health, increase compliance with physician treatment plans, and address unmet health and social service needs.

Despite the conclusion from a recent Congressional Budget Office analysis that it is too early to estimate the impact that disease management programs are having on overall healthcare spending, the market response to disease management suggests that health insurance plans and employers are finding that disease management provides good value. A national study that used data from a large health insurance plan in 10 urban areas found that overall costs were significantly lower for full-year program participants with diabetes than for nonparticipants with diabetes, and the purchasers of the disease management program saved more than was spent. The most important source of savings was a 22 to 30 percent reduction in hospitalization, which was beneficial for both patients and providers (Villagra and Ahmed, 2004). A study that evaluated the impact of a heart disease management program on hospital service utilization, as well as the potential costs savings over and above the cost of delivering the program, found that participants experienced 46 percent fewer inpatient days and 49 percent lower inpatient costs than the control group, but no significant differences in the rates of emergency department utilization were reported between the two groups (Wheeler et al., 2003).

Pay for Performance

Both public and private health insurers have begun to offer financial and other incentives to providers for delivering higher-quality care. Performance is measured by the use of selected evidence-based standards and performance measures as a method to potentially reverse the perverse incentives of current payment models that lack any recognition of quality performance. By aligning incentives to encourage improvements in patient care, some health insurance plans have already begun to see rising rates of preventive care and improvements in key indicators of patient health. Some studies of pay-for-performance programs have shown an increase in the quality of care received. In one study, the most significant improvements in quality were seen among physician groups with the lowest baseline performance (Rosenthal et al., 2005). Some private insurers are targeting incentives to reward physician groups not only for high absolute performance but also for relative improvements (Rosenthal et al., 2006).

Work with provider professional societies and certification boards in the design and implementation of pay-for-performance programs has resulted in added success and support of these programs. In fact, a 2004 poll of physicians found that 71 percent of physicians supported payments based on the quality of care (Rowe, 2006). Additional support from purchasers, such as the Leapfrog Group, which represents large employers and public purchasers who work to engage consumers and clinicians in improving healthcare quality, led the Medicare Payment Advisory Commission to recommend that Medicare adopt performance-based payment (Galvin et al., 2005).

In a 2007 comparison of the results of the Centers for Medicare and Medicaid Services' Premier Hospital Quality Incentive Demonstration (HQID) and the Hospital Quality Alliance's (HQA's) public reporting initiative, researchers found that hospitals whose public reporting was tied to financial incentives had greater improvements in the quality of care than hospitals that only publicly reported quality data. Although both groups of hospitals showed improvements in each of the individual and compound performance measures, the pay-for-performance hospitals (HQID) that were offered a 1 to 2 percent bonus for achieving high levels of performance compared with the performance of their peers showed a 2.6 to 4.1 percent improvement in quality over a 2-year period (Lindenauer et al., 2007).

Value-Based Purchasing and Benefit Design

Value-based purchasing and benefit design is a strategy that both purchasers and health insurance plans use to base decisions regarding coverage and payment policies on the value of the treatments or the services provided compared with the underlying costs of those treatments (Clancy, 2006). Under value-based purchasing strategies, value is judged on the basis of a comparison with the best existing alternative and not on the basis of a comparison with a placebo or no treatment. Additionally, value is judged only when marginal benefits can be viewed in the context of marginal additional costs. This analysis of benefits and costs occurs not only at the individual patient level but also because it involves issues of implementation, staffing, and quality assurance within systems of care.

Although the detractors of value-based purchasing and benefit design argue that decisions regarding healthcare coverage should not include costs, others point to the escalation of healthcare spending as an outcome of not considering cost in relation to the amount of additional benefits that new technologies and treatments can provide. Value-based purchasing and benefit design can help break the pattern of wasteful spending and increase the quality of the care provided by basing decisions on both clinical and cost-effectiveness, without leading to all-or-nothing coverage decisions.

Both public and private insurers are already using methods, such as tiered drug formularies and premium networks, that allow consumers to make personal healthcare choices according to what benefits they desire and what risks and costs they are willing to incur. Patients who see physicians outside of the premium network or who take medications in a higher formulary tier may have to pay more in terms of deductibles and or copayments, but the value-based judgment is theirs to make. CMS has already implemented multiple value-based purchasing initiatives (e.g., programs, demonstration projects, pilot programs, and voluntary reporting efforts) in hospitals, physician offices, nursing homes, home health services, and dialysis facilities. Currently under development and scheduled to be launched in 2009 is a value-based purchasing program for Medicare hospital services that will measure and reward performance for the care provided in hospital outpatient settings (CMS Hospital Pay-for-Performance Workgroup et al., 2007).

A recent example of a private insurer working with purchasers and providers to implement value-based purchasing occurred at the Virginia Mason Medical Center in Washington. The insurer completed an analysis of high-quality providers in Seattle and found that the costs in several of Virginia Mason's subspecialty departments far exceeded the cost benchmarks for the region. To remain the insurer's high performance network, Virginia Mason worked with the insurer and four of its largest employer clients to implement a cost-reduction strategy. The strategy focused on a set number of conditions and services. The initial results showed a reduction in costs for purchasers and patients, with no adverse impact on patient outcomes (Pham et al., 2007).

Continued progress in the area of value-based purchasing should include the development of a common understanding of the noncost components of value, such as patient preferences and personal values.

State Medicaid Programs

Rising costs have also led state Medicaid programs to place a greater emphasis on value. For example, rising drug costs and decreasing amounts of state funding for Medicaid programs have led states to look for methods by which they may control pharmacy costs, in particular. The Drug Effectiveness Research Project (DERP) is a collaboration of public and private organizations, including 15 state Medicaid programs, that have joined together to share the cost of conducting systematic evidence-based reviews of the comparative effectiveness and safety of pharmaceuticals in many widely used drug classes. The collaboration can then use the results of these systematic reviews to develop public policies or preferred drug lists.

DERP reports contain no cost data and do not recommend specific purchasing policies, which allow partners to use global information to make local decisions on what would be best for the beneficiaries within their states. DERP is a self-governing project, with member organizations voting to set priorities, determining which drug classes will be reviewed, and developing key questions and inclusion criteria for each drug class review. In some states, DERP reports are the sole source of evidence for the support of drug coverage decisions, whereas other states use multiple sources. Some states use DERP reports to validate their own evidence-based clinical reviews or those that contractors develop for them (Hoadley et al., 2007).

Like most large-scale programs, DERP is not without controversy. Some have maintained that DERP reviews tend to include only randomized controlled trials (RCTs), to the exclusion of observational studies (Neumann, 2006). Proponents of DERP counter that DERP reviews do favor RCTs as the "gold standard" of clinical studies, but observational studies are also used to assess the safety of medications. Supporters also consider DERP one of the more transparent research projects ongoing, citing the fact that DERP publishes draft key questions and draft reviews for public comment before finalization (Gibson and Santa, 2006).

The success of DERP led to the formation of a similarly structured project, the Medicaid Evidence-Based Decision Project, which is also a collaboration of state Medicaid programs whose purpose is to better inform clinical coverage issues and benefit design beyond pharmaceutical use. Initiated in June 2006, state collaborators receive access to systematic reviews of the existing evidence on treatments and procedures, assessments of current and new healthcare technologies, support in designing evaluations of products when there are evidence gaps, and access to an information clearinghouse (Oregon Health and Science University, 2007). Medicaid programs have used the work of relevant government agencies, such as the Agency for Healthcare Research and Quality (AHRQ) through its Evidence-Based Practice Centers and DEcIDE (Developing Evidence to Inform Decisions about Effectiveness) projects.

Furthermore, some state Medicaid agencies have established independent advisory entities that provide access to the latest evidence for policy decisions. Several state Medicaid programs have also undertaken innovative pilot efforts to improve the quality of care based on principles that originated in the private sector. A number of states have implemented pay-for-performance strategies, such as physician profiling incentive programs in Maine and provider profiling incentive programs in Massachusetts (Llanos et al., 2007). Other states have implemented disease management initiatives through homegrown efforts or commercial vendors. One such demonstration program, Community Care of North Carolina, has had significant success in asthma and diabetes programs, which have been demonstrated to be cost-effective and to have increased the quality of care that they provide according to set performance measures. Savings have been estimated to be $3.5 million for asthma care and $2.1 million for diabetes care (Community Care of North Carolina, 2003; Ricketts et al., 2007).

Medicare Program

Medicare's Quality Improvement Organization (QIO) program, created in 1982, was developed with the purpose of improving the quality and efficiency of services delivered to Medicare beneficiaries. The QIO program consists of 41 organizations that hold 53 contracts with CMS to provide services in each state, territory, and the District of Columbia. The QIOs work with stakeholders, including consumers and physicians, hospitals, and other caregivers, to improve care delivery systems to ensure that patients get the right care at the right time, with particular attention paid to patients from underserved populations. In addition, QIOs work with physicians and other stakeholder organizations to measure and report on performance and to help with the adoption of healthcare information technology (CMS, 2007d). Announced in 2005 for a 3-year period, the 8th Statement of Work for QIOs focuses on reporting, improving, and rewarding quality within four care settings: nursing homes, home health agencies, hospitals, and physician offices (CMS, 2007c).

Medicare also continues to focus more attention on the use of evidence in coverage, reimbursement, and compensation policies. In 1999 Medicare published a notice in the *Federal Register* describing for the first time the steps that it follows in the coverage process. The agency also established an independent committee of experts and stakeholders, the Medicare Coverage Advisory Committee, which meets in public to consider complex and controversial coverage-related topics. The progress of all national coverage decisions can be tracked on the CMS website, which also contains detailed documents that summarize all scientific evidence, expert input, and other information that was considered during the policy-making process. CMS's Coverage and Analysis Group performs rigorous evidence-based reviews of new medical technologies and services to support national coverage decisions. As part of its decision-making process, CMS may also request formal technology assessments from AHRQ.

The Medicare program has also been an innovator in exploring new ways to generate evidence to support its coverage and reimbursement policies. On July 12, 2006, CMS released a guidance document that describes new policies involving national coverage decisions (NCDs) that require the collection of additional patient data as a condition for reimbursement, known as Coverage with Evidence Development (CED). There are two subtypes of CEDs: Coverage with Appropriateness Determination (CAD) and Coverage with Study Participation (CSP).

Under the first subtype, CAD, providers are required to submit additional patient data to databases or registries specifically designed to include data for that treatment at the time that they submit their standard claims data. This supplemental patient data are needed to show that the treatment is being administered appropriately to the correct population noted in the NCD. Under CSP, coverage is linked to participation in clinical studies that produce evidence to guide appropriate care in the future.

The new CED policy requires the development and capture of additional patient data beyond standard claims data as a condition for payment. By doing so, the policy will make available additional clinical information, which will contribute to the medical evidence about a particular healthcare item or service. Private health insurance plans may become more engaged with CED-type initiatives in the future to support this approach to evidence generation (Atkinson, 2007). One such example is the use of a CED approach by a health plan for computed tomographic coronary angiography. By using a collaborative model, the plan is partnering with qualified providers who will contribute data to a registry. Practice patterns will then be analyzed and used to support providers' efforts to develop, apply, assess, and improve standards for the judicious use of this technology.

Additionally, in December 2006, President George W. Bush signed the Tax Relief and Health Care Act of 2006 (TRHCA). Section 101 under Title I of TRHCA authorized CMS to establish a physician quality reporting system, a voluntary pay-for-reporting program for physicians who treat

Medicare beneficiaries known as the Physician Quality Reporting Initiative (PQRI). PQRI enables eligible physicians to receive a financial incentive, totaling 1.5 percent of allowed charges for covered Medicare physician fee schedule services, if they report patient data on 3 of a set of 74 quality measures (CMS, 2007b). Medicare has also developed similar pay-for-reporting programs for hospitals and home health agencies.

LEADERSHIP COMMITMENTS AND INITIATIVES

Strategies for Setting a Higher Bar: Improving Quality Through Better Generation, Dissemination, and Implementation of Medical Evidence

Although the insurer sector has played a leadership role in the ongoing evolution toward a more value-based healthcare system, the quality, cost, and access problems that continue to plague the healthcare system clearly indicate that more can—and must—be done. Several innovative strategies merit expansion and adoption within the private and public sectors to further this evolution.

Set a Course to Support Innovation Essential to the Advancement of Health Care

Systemwide changes are necessary to create the foundation of medical evidence on which a full continuum of quality improvement efforts can be supported. The first crucial step in creating a foundation of medical evidence is to improve the process by which evidence is generated. There currently exists a significant lack of reliable information about what works best—a gap that helps to raise healthcare costs while potentially lowering the quality of health care. Compounding this problem is the fact that a consistent method for evaluating evidence does not currently exist. Despite the clear need to address these issues, the United States is virtually alone among developed nations in not having an entity dedicated to comparing the effectiveness and value of new drugs, devices, and medical procedures with those currently being used.

One model, which is under consideration by the insurance sector, leading economists, and policy makers, is the creation of a new entity, a Comparative Effectiveness Board (CEB), to provide Americans with a trusted source from which they can get up-to-date, objective, and credible information on which healthcare services are the most effective and provide the best value. The CEB would be responsible for (1) comparing the clinical and cost-effectiveness of new and existing drugs, devices, procedures, therapies, and other healthcare services; (2) assessing alternative uses of treatments currently in practice; and (3) distributing this information in a useful format so that patients, clinicians, and payers can make more informed choices among healthcare options. By establishing a sustainable capacity to generate and provide information on the comparative effectiveness of healthcare services and technologies, work can then be done to strengthen the use of this information in everyday medical practice, that is, what works, what works best, and what yields the best value for patients.

It is important to point out that the results of the CEB's evaluations not only will identify those interventions that offer very little marginal benefit at high cost but also will identify those interventions that are cost-effective but currently being underused or whose true value to the healthcare system may not yet be widely recognized. For example, there is currently little evidence to help differentiate the mortality benefit of different treatments for early prostate cancer. Some newer forms of radiation therapy for prostate cancer cost four to five times as much as other forms of treatment. At the same time, statins are considered to be highly effective and cost-effective at reducing cholesterol levels, yet they continue to be underused. Disease management represents another area in which the CEB's evaluations could help promote the use of a technique that improves health outcomes while reducing overall healthcare costs.

The next steps in this new course of action will involve integrating the information that the CEB generates into benefit designs, medical policies, and provider and patient decision-making tools. Health insurance plans have already adopted a range of strategies designed to promote evidence-based benefit design. The development and dissemination of CEB evaluations will provide a reliable resource while allowing health insurance plans the autonomy they need to make coverage decisions and benefit designs on the basis of what best suits their members. One prominent example of the use of evidence-based recommendations is health insurance plans' approach to the coverage of preventive services supported by authoritative review of medical evidence by AHRQ's U.S. Preventive Services Task Force. As mentioned earlier, health insurance plans' use of P&T committees to evaluate and review pharmaceutical cost-effectiveness data for formulary development has become standard practice as well.

Increased research on comparative effectiveness will also enable the greater use of innovative strategies to link cost sharing to value (Braithwaite and Rosen, 2007). Comparative effectiveness research will promote efficiency by identifying treatments and procedures that provide the most benefits for the cost incurred. The results of this type of research can then be used to tie different levels of cost sharing to value. For example, by establishing different levels of cost sharing for different prescription drugs on the basis of their safety, efficacy and value, health insurance plans' use of tiered formularies has been successful in stemming the rise in spending on prescription drugs. Increased data on comparative effectiveness for other services and technologies will enable an expansion of the tiering techniques beyond prescription drugs with the promise of further cost savings and value-based decision making. Tiered cost sharing also has the potential to allow consumers to make individual healthcare choices on the basis of what works best for them, as opposed to the current style of payer-based coverage systems that tend to be binary: either 1 for "it works" or 0 for "it does not work" (Denny et al., 2007; Health Industry Forum, 2007).

Some have called for the expansion of existing federal agencies, such as AHRQ or the National Institutes of Health, to assume responsibility for such functions; however, the task at hand is so critical to improving the U.S. healthcare system that others, including many in the insurer sector, believe that a new entity should be charged with this responsibility. Such an entity should be a public–private partnership and should be funded through public sources and supplemented by support from private sources through mechanisms that will provide stability and independence from political pressures. Whereas the CEB will not be a federal agency, it must use the expertise and skills of the existing federal agencies to establish methodological standards for comparative research, conduct the necessary research, and help disseminate the results.

As an interim and, in fact, complementary step, the capture of additional patient data in the course of clinical care for assessment of the appropriateness, utilization, and impact of particular healthcare services for which evidence may be lacking is another worthwhile strategy. Participants within the healthcare system must work together to identify and evaluate other data sources that could be used in the development of evidence. There currently exists an unrealized potential to use nontraditional data sources in the development of evidence. Collaborations among stakeholder groups should consider the appropriateness of data in registries, claims data, and population-based measures for use in the generation of additional evidence. For provider decision making to benefit from the development and capture of additional patient data, barriers to appropriate data sharing within the healthcare system must be minimized. Privacy and security standards must be implemented in a way that recognizes the benefits of data sharing in assessing the appropriateness of particular treatments for specific patients.

Invest in the Workforce Needed to Conduct Comparative Effectiveness Research

Plans for a CEB designed as a public–private partnership—and with it a significant increase in comparative effectiveness research—depend on adequate investment in the training of researchers so that they have the skills to perform this kind of work. The skills needed include those necessary to support the two main types of comparative effectiveness research:

systematic review of clinical and cost-effectiveness and the design, conduct, and analysis of pragmatic clinical trials.

- *Systematic review of clinical and cost-effectiveness.* The performance of systematic reviews, decision modeling, and cost-effectiveness analyses by researchers will be needed to augment the production of important comparative effectiveness reports. Specifically, researchers with skills in clinical epidemiology, decision analysis, meta-analytic statistics, and health economics will be required. Currently, few postgraduate training centers provide top-level training in these domains within collaborative or multi-disciplinary training programs. In particular, training in clinical epidemiology, often offered to physicians in postgraduate research training programs, rarely includes or is linked to programs of training in health economics and decision analysis. Funding to support the establishment and greater integration of these training programs is needed.
- *Design, conduct, and analysis of pragmatic clinical trials.* Greater investment is needed to help train clinical researchers to understand and adopt the findings of pragmatic or practical clinical trials. Study design along traditional lines is often taught to clinical researchers, but greater cross-fertilization from healthcare services research and from disciplines that employ quasiexperimental and qualitative research designs is needed because comparative effectiveness trials often cannot be randomized controlled trials because of practical and ethical constraints.

Reinforce FDA's Capacity to Assess the Long-Term Safety and Effectiveness of New Drugs

As the principal federal agency with jurisdiction for the approval of new drugs, devices, and biologics, FDA has a significant role to play in assessing safety and effectiveness. Approaches for improving FDA's review of new drugs were recently recommended by the IOM Committee on the Assessment of the U.S. Drug Safety System in its September 2006 report *The Future of Drug Safety: Action Steps for Congress* (Institute of Medicine, 2006). Below are several suggestions that are consistent with many of the IOM's recommendations and also some new ideas for reforming FDA to meet twenty-first century demands.

The law governing the approval of new drugs (Prescription Drug User Fee Act) places a priority on increasing the speed of the drug approval process. Yet data on long-term drug safety are typically lacking (Wood, 2006). To better balance the need to get new drugs to market quickly with the need for information on long-term drug safety, congressional action specific to postmarketing safety goals is needed. For example, to further achieve the balance between speedy approvals and postmarketing safety, a portion of the funds collected from drug user fees should be dedicated to safety and effectiveness evaluations once a new drug has been approved for use.

Additionally, FDA's enforcement abilities should be expanded to better enable the agency to require drug manufacturers to make labeling revisions and to perform additional clinical trials to ensure postmarketing safety. Health insurance plans and employers can play an important role in integrating the results of these postmarketing studies by regularly updating their formularies and reimbursement policies to integrate the new data that may emerge as a result of those studies.

As part of the reauthorization of the Federal Food, Drug, and Cosmetic Act, key congressional members have introduced the Food and Drug Administration Revitalization Act and the Safer Drug Assessment Technology Advancement Act to improve the underlying science of drug safety decision making and to strengthen FDA's ability to inform patients and providers about drug safety and effectiveness.

Strengthen FDA's Review of Certain Devices and Capacity to Track Device Safety

The less-stringent 510(k) approval process of FDA for certain new devices requires manufacturers to show only that a new device is similar to an existing, approved device and does not raise any new concerns about safety or effectiveness. Narrowing the range of medical devices that can be deemed similar and allowing only devices that have truly insignificant changes to previously approved devices to use the 510(k) process will help reduce some of the unanticipated failures or complications seen with these devices. All other devices should be evaluated through the same rigorous process used for the approval of new drugs.

FDA has not had the ability to track failed or unsafe devices once they are in the marketplace. This was evident during the recent recall of failed implantable cardiac defibrillators, when an alert notifying physicians that certain implantable cardiac defibrillators were found to fail to trigger when they were needed by patients was released. To address this void, a unique device identification system that would mark each device with its own unique identifier should be implemented. Such a system would greatly improve FDA's ability to track the safety and performance of medical devices and would make tracking far easier for devices that have been recalled.

Focus and Coordinate Research Efforts to Address Identified Gaps in Evidence and Factors That Drive Physician Decision Making

Given that gaps in evidence can lead to variations in medical practice and put patients at risk, identifying key areas that need further research will serve to address this known evidence gap and aid clinicians in their decision making. No one entity is currently accountable for the development of a long-term strategy that can be used to address this deficiency. Because the U.S. Department of Health and Human Services (HHS) is the fiscal manager of federal dollars for research, HHS's fiscal responsibility should be coupled with the task of developing a strategy to prioritize the research agenda needed to address known gaps in evidence and safety. In this new role, HHS, in collaboration with the CEB recommended above, can help ensure that research is conducted in areas that currently lack sufficient research findings yet have the potential to significantly improve patient outcomes. One important benefit of this enhanced emphasis on the evidence gap will be to draw attention to the fact that a significant portion of modern medicine is not supported by medical evidence and that more work needs to be done to align current medical practices with medical evidence.

In addition to identifying and promoting research in these priority areas, HHS's role should include enhanced communication with the public about those studies under way to address these priority areas. Such public information and education will advise both consumers and providers of the lack of reliable evidence on these conditions or treatment protocols and provide them with the ability to track this information throughout the study period. Similar to the information that the National Cancer Institute releases on its website highlighting the current cancer clinical trials that are under way and providing information on patient eligibility, trial protocols, and the current status of the trial, HHS could, for example, coordinate the release of public information on any postmarketing approval studies—studies conducted after FDA approval of drugs, devices, and biologics—currently under way, the goals for such studies, and their expected completion dates.

Better Dissemination of Actionable Information at the Point of Care and Transparency of Performance and Information Used to Make Decisions

In the majority of U.S. economic markets, entities compete on the basis of price and quality and consumers make their decisions on the basis of reliable, accurate information. For a variety of reasons, this has never been the case in the healthcare market. Instead, many consumers, having little other information to go on, tend to equate higher costs with higher quality—although this is often not the case. In recognition of this problem, the IOM in its 2001 report *Crossing the Quality Chasm* stressed that transparency should be a key element of any strategy to improve clinical quality and achieve better value in the healthcare system (Institute of Medicine, 2001). A healthcare marketplace that empowers consumers to make informed choices on the basis of both cost and quality will result in a healthcare system that offers improved value to consumers and encourages innovation and continued evolution.

The private sector has led the way in developing a uniform approach to the disclosure of relevant, useful, understandable, and actionable information to facilitate consumer decision making. The key stakeholders among the different disciplines, including health insurance plans, physicians, hospitals, consumers, and employers, have convened broad-based, national alliances (AQA Alliance and HQA) to determine a more effective strategy for measuring, reporting, and improving physician and hospital performance. The leadership of AQA and HQA has recently formed a new national entity, the Quality Alliance Steering Committee (QASC), whose purpose is to better coordinate the promotion of quality measurement, transparency, and improvement in care across all care settings. CMS has been an active member of both alliances and is working to use the recommendations from AQA and HQA and the measures endorsed by the National Quality Forum as part of the PQRI, the hospital public reporting project (Hospital Compare), and hospital demonstration projects on value-based purchasing. The private sector has also begun building the capacity to analyze certain agreed-upon episodes of care (e.g., pregnancy), in addition to specific services (e.g., labor and delivery), to allow consumers to make more comprehensive and informed assessments of the health care that they receive.

In an effort to eliminate duplicative efforts to measure and report on performance, AQA has launched a pilot project at six sites across the country that would combine public- and private-sector data to measure and report on physician-level practice. These sites, which will eventually include an aggregation of data from commercial sources and the Medicare program, are now called "value exchanges." In an effort to encourage the development and growth of public–private collaborations under this project, HHS has established two levels of recognition for participants in these initiatives. Partnerships in the early stages of development are designated "community leaders," and more advanced collaborations are designated as "value exchanges" and will be invited to participate in a nationwide learning network, sponsored by AHRQ, that will provide access to expert faculty, lessons about successful quality improvement, and reporting to consumers.

This comprehensive approach being undertaken to promote better assessments of performance will make it far easier to identify opportunities for quality improvement, result in valid and consistent measures of quality and efficiency that can be used to improve care throughout the healthcare system, and provide important information to patients in making health-care decisions. Only by improving performance assessment and making the results of those assessments available to consumers in both the private and public sectors can systemwide improvement be achieved.

Another important research need that deserves specific attention relates to the accurate display of cost information for consumers. More focus has been placed on asking consumers to make informed healthcare choices, either in choosing an efficient provider or in comparing their treatment options; the medical community has little understanding of how best to share information on cost by either specific procedure or episode of care. This is especially difficult in an industry in which the consumer has been isolated from the true costs of health care. With the rise in popularity of consumer-directed health plans and the desire of the consumer to receive the highest-quality health care for the lowest price, the importance of this type of research should not be discounted (Buntin et al., 2006).

Achieve Data Consistency to Allow Easy Sharing of Information Among Various Stakeholders

In addition to emphasizing the need for information to aid consumers with making decisions about their health care, the IOM's 2001 report *Crossing the Quality Chasm* also identified the need for better information to aid physicians, hospitals, and other healthcare professionals with the identification of gaps in quality and to assist them in comparing their performance with that of similar practicing providers. The lack of consistency in the available information makes comparisons of providers and health care difficult while the public is becoming increasingly aware of gaps in care and safety for themselves and their family members (American Health Information Community, 2007). Many different private- and public-sector groups have attempted to step up to the challenge by designing models for assessing performance and aggregating and reporting data. Although some progress has been made, the proliferation of multiple, uncoordinated, and sometimes conflicting initiatives has had significant unintended consequences for different stakeholders. Duplicative efforts unnecessarily burden physicians, other clinicians, and health insurance plans with different data requests, shifting the focus away from quality and efficiency improvement. When divergent information is collected and publicly reported, it creates confusion among consumers, detracts from efforts by employers to design programs that meet the needs of their employees, and diverts limited resources and focus away from achieving systematic improvements in health.

Through AHIP, the health insurance plan sector is working to implement a national strategy to aggregate data from multiple health insurance plans and other sources to produce and report on an increasingly sophisticated set of quality and cost measures throughout the country. This national strategy will build on the foundation provided by existing quality measurement efforts, such as the AQA alliance and HQA efforts mentioned above, as well as the efforts of individual health insurance plans. The data aggregation method may also be applied to address other issues related to monitoring and improving medical practice, such as tracking drug utilization and safety and developing better evidence on medical treatments.

Promote Optimal Care by Emphasizing Evidence-Based Coverage and Reimbursement Strategies

As mentioned above, health insurance plans have adopted a range of strategies designed to encourage evidence-based decision making. In addition to creating medical policies that reflect scientific findings on effectiveness and value, health insurance plans routinely provide information to patients encouraging them to receive preventive benefits supported by medical evidence. Health insurance plans have also capitalized on their ability to advance nationally recognized preventive services through their disease management and wellness programs. Additionally, health insurance plans provide feedback to individual practitioners about their performance and alerts about potential drug interactions. They also offer incentives to practitioners to practice medicine in a manner that is consistent with the medical evidence and that yields high-quality health care. The use of such pay-for-performance strategies represents a mechanism that aligns incentives in a way that encourages ongoing improvement in the quality of care that is provided and should continue to be pursued.

Although the reimbursement practices of public programs preclude a direct corollary with those of private programs from being made, coverage and reimbursement policies in public programs offer immediate opportunities for policy reform. For example, because of its tremendous influence on the adoption of healthcare technologies and treatments, the U.S. Congress should give CMS the explicit authority to use the available data on comparative effectiveness and cost-effectiveness in determining its coverage policies. Similarly, empowering CMS to set reimbursement rates for new technologies more in alignment with the added (or marginal) value of a new technology over established alternatives will help constrain unsustainable trends in increased cost and improve overall quality. Parallel efforts by other federal agencies that have a role in establishing coverage policy, such as VA and the Office of Personnel Management, as well as by state agencies responsible for administering state Medicaid programs, should also be considered.

In addition to modernization of state Medicaid coverage and reimbursement policies, state enactment of coverage mandates must be addressed. A number of states have enacted laws requiring the systematic review of benefit mandates and the extent to which such mandates are consistent with the medical evidence. By nature, a mandate is static and unable to reflect changes in the practice of medicine that may make the mandate obsolete or even harmful to patients. Yet mandates do exist and may persist in the future. The continued establishment and use of independent state advisory bodies, such as external review organizations and state cost-containment boards, to evaluate the consistency of state mandates with the latest medical evidence are essential and will provide valuable information to policy makers, clinicians, and consumers.

Invest in Infrastructure Development, Deployment, and Use

The transparent collection, analysis, and dissemination of information on the latest medical evidence, performance, and comparative effectiveness at the point of care will require further investment in several key areas of the healthcare infrastructure. First, significant investment will be needed to build the early systems that can aggregate administrative data and electronic health record information in a reliable fashion. Second, for this information to reach clinicians and patients, new research and investment in methods of information synthesis and dissemination will be needed. An important impetus to restructuring the U.S. healthcare system is the presence of the American Health Information Community (U.S. Department of Health and Human Services, 2007); the work of QASC, HQA, and the AQA Alliance in seeking to reach common standards for data stewardship and aggregation; and the work of multiple vendors, clinicians, and other stakeholders.

Additional resources must also be directed toward efforts to translate the results of clinical research into best practices. Providers will need to look for ways to redesign their business practices so that they allow the easy adoption of new evidence. An interoperable healthcare system will ensure that appropriate, reliable information is available to guide medical decisions at the time and place of care, help reduce preventable medical errors, improve quality, and advance the delivery of evidence-based medical care. In doing so, it will create a more effective marketplace, create greater competition, reduce overall healthcare costs, and create a value-based healthcare system.

NEXT STEPS

Opportunities for Collaboration

The insurer sector is well positioned to play an integral role in a national effort to improve the generation, dissemination, and implementation of medical evidence. The current state of the quality and the affordability of health care in the United States demand nothing less than a concerted and collaborative commitment to improving the value of health care.

All of the progress that has been made to date has been achieved through partnerships and collaborations across the healthcare system. The AQA Alliance and HQA initiative to determine a more effective strategy for measuring, reporting, and improving physician and hospital performance is an excellent example of the type of broad-based coalition necessary to drive change and improvement.

Just as AHIP and BCBSA represent the health insurance plan sector, different groups also represent providers, consumers, employers, and other stakeholders. Countless organizations representing different stakeholders have been involved in collaborative and cooperative efforts with the health insurance plan sector on a variety of healthcare issues.

Collaboration among providers, insurance plans, consumers, purchasers, and manufacturers must increase to take advantage of these opportunities. Several specific areas in which continued progress would greatly benefit from enhanced collaboration between health insurance plans and other stakeholders are as follows:

- Efforts to develop benefit language compatible with medical evidence-based innovative benefit designs (e.g., tiered benefits for procedures, devices, and diagnostics and incentives for consumers to take up therapies supported by evidence) will require collaborations among health insurance plans, purchasers, and state regulators.
- The creation and the design of the proposed CEB will require collaboration among all stakeholders in the healthcare system to help identify for evaluation priority areas that will have the greatest potential to improve the quality of health care.
- Public awareness and education efforts to communicate the underlying goal of evidence-based medicine and comparative effectiveness as being one of care improvement and not access reduction will require collaboration among health insurance plans, consumer groups, purchasers, manufacturers, and providers.
- The continued evolution of performance-based payment models that recognize and reward hospitals, physicians, and other clinicians for adopting evidence that results in improved outcomes and appropriate resource use will benefit from collaboration among health insurance plans, purchasers, providers, and consumers.
- Efforts to develop a more transparent and consistent approach to judging evidence in the context of medical policy decision making will require the broad-based involvement of health insurance

plans, manufacturers, experts in evidence-based medicine, patients, employers, and government. The development of a consensus around what constitutes "value," focusing particularly on the non-cost components of value, will require collaboration among these stakeholders.

- The development of a new format for technology appraisals that allows the integration of ratings of clinical and cost-effectiveness that can support value-based insurance benefits and guide decision making by patients and clinicians toward higher value could benefit from collaboration among health insurance plans and other stakeholders and the Institute for Clinical and Economic Review.
- The exploration of further application of CED initiatives in circumstances in which further evidence generation is needed to assess important remaining questions about the safety and comparative effectiveness of new technologies could be achieved through collaboration among CMS, health insurance plans, and other private-sector entities, such as the Center for Medical Technology Policy.
- The current paradigm for building evidence and value may have limited application in the future as personalized medicine becomes more in demand. Evidence on demographics, genomics, patient preferences, and other factors will need to be considered. This will require collaboration among providers, payers, and manufacturers to make sure that the necessary information on treatment options is available to allow improved quality at both the individual and the aggregate levels.
- Reform of the medical liability system, so that the resolution of disputes is based on scientific evidence, will require the collaboration of groups representing virtually all of the healthcare system's stakeholders.

The heightened level of attention being paid to issues of healthcare cost, quality, and access signifies an opportunity for stakeholders within the healthcare system to come together and develop the necessary road map for the transformation to a more evidence-based system. The IOM Roundtable has provided a much needed forum for the discussion and development of this road map, and the insurer sector looks forward to continued active participation in this overall effort to drive progress.

REFERENCES

AIS Health. 2007. *AIS directory of health plans*. http://www.aishealth.com/Products/dhp.html (accessed December 9, 2007).

American Health Information Community. 2007. *Quality workgroup. Quality workgroup full vision summary. January 31, 2007.* http://www.hhs.gov/healthit/ahic/materials/qual_vision_summary.pdf (accessed March 15, 2007).

America's Health Insurance Plans. 2004. *America's Health Insurance Plans website.* http://www.ahip.org (accessed May 12, 2008).

Atkinson, W. 2007. The impact of CED on private payers. *Biotechnology Healthcare* 24:24-30.

BlueCross and BlueShield Corporation. 2007. *BlueCross and BlueShield Corporation website.* http://www.bcbs.com (accessed May 12, 2008).

Braithwaite, R. S., and A. B. Rosen. 2007. Linking cost sharing to value: An unrivaled yet unrealized public health opportunity. *Annals of Internal Medicine* 146(8):602-605.

Buntin, M. B., C. Damberg, A. Haviland, K. Kapur, N. Lurie, R. McDevitt, and M. S. Marquis. 2006. Consumer-directed health care: Early evidence about effects on cost and quality. *Health Affairs* 25(6):w516-w530.

Clancy, C. M. 2006. *Arming health care consumers: Testimony before the Joint Economic Committee, May 10, 2006.* Washington, DC.

Claxton, G., I. Gil, B. Finder, B. DiJulio, S. Hawkins, J. Pickreign, H. Whitmore, and J. Gabel. 2006. *The Kaiser Family Foundation health research and educational trust (HRET) employer health benefits: 2006 annual survey.* http://www.kff.org/insurance/7527/upload/7527.pdf (accessed June 1, 2007).

Claxton, G., J. Gabel, B. DiJulio, J. Pickreign, H. Whitmore, B. Finder, P. Jacobs, and S. Hawkins. 2007. Health benefits in 2007: Premium increases fall to an eight-year low, while offer rates and enrollment remain stable. *Health Affairs* 26(5):1407-1416.

CMS (Centers for Medicare and Medicaid Services). 2005. *2005 CMS national health expenditures data; web tables.* Baltimore, MD. http://www.cms.hhs.gov/NationalHealthExpendData/downloads/tables.pdf (accessed May 21, 2007).

———. 2007a. *CMS Management Information Integrated Repository (MIIR).* Baltimore, MD.

———. 2007b. *Physician quality reporting initiative: Overview.* Baltimore, MD. http://www.cms.hhs.gov/pqri/01_overview.asp (accessed May 28, 2007).

———. 2007c. *Quality improvement organizations: 8th round statement of work contract.* Baltimore, MD. http://www.cms.hhs.gov/QualityImprovementOrgs/downloads/8thSOW.pdf (accessed June 27, 2007).

———. 2007d. *Quality improvement organizations: Overview.* Baltimore, MD. http://www.cms.hhs.gov/QualityImprovementOrgs/ (accessed May 15, 2007).

CMS Hospital Pay-for-Performance Workgroup, RAND Corporation, Brandeis University, Booz Allen Hamilton, and Boston University. 2007. *U.S. Department of Health and Human Services Medicare hospital value-based purchasing plan: Development issues paper.* Washington, DC.

Community Care of North Carolina. 2003. *Progress report: Asthma initiative.* http://www.communitycarenc.com/PDFDocs/AsthmaProgressReport.pdf (accessed May 15, 2007).

Congressional Budget Office. 2007. *The state's children health insurance program.* Washington, DC. http://www.cbo.gov/ftpdoc.cfm?index=8092&type=1 (accessed May 30, 2007).

Denny, C. C., E. J. Emanuel, and S. D. Pearson. 2007. Why well-insured patients should demand value-based insurance benefits. *JAMA* 297(22):2515-2518.

Galvin, R. S., S. Delbanco, A. Milstein, and G. Belden. 2005. Has the Leapfrog Group had an impact on the health care market? *Health Affairs* 24(1):228-233.

Gibson, M., and J. Santa. 2006. The drug effectiveness review project: An important step forward. *Health Affairs* 25(4):W272-W275.

Health Industry Forum. 2007. *Comparative effectiveness forum: Executive summary.* Waltham, MA: Brandeis University-Heller School for Social Policy and Management.

Hoadley, J., J. Crowley, D. Bergman, and N. Kaye. 2007. *Understanding key features of the Drug Effectiveness Review Project (DERP) and lessons for state policy makers.* Washington, DC: National Academy of State Health Policy.

Institute of Medicine. 2001. *Crossing the quality chasm: A new health system for the 21st century.* Washington, DC: National Academy Press.

———. 2006. *The future of drug safety: Action steps for congress.* Washington, DC: The National Academies Press.

Kaiser Family Foundation. 2007. *Medicaid enrollment in 50 states: A June 2005 data update.* Washington, DC. http://www.kff.org/medicaid/upload/7606.pdf (accessed May 21, 2007).

Lindenauer, P. K., D. Remus, S. Roman, M. B. Rothberg, E. M. Benjamin, A. Ma, and D. W. Bratzler. 2007. Public reporting and pay for performance in hospital quality improvement. *New England Journal of Medicine* 356(5):486-496.

Llanos, K., J. Rothstein, M. Dyer, and M. Bailit. 2007. *Physician pay-for-performance in Medicaid: A guide for states.* Hamilton, NJ: Center for Health Care Strategies. http://www.chcs.org/publications3960/publications_show.htm?doc_id=471272 (accessed May 21, 2007).

Neumann, P. J. 2006. Emerging lessons from the drug effectiveness review project. *Health Affairs* 25(4):W262-W271.

Oregon Health and Science University. 2007. *Medicaid evidence-based decisions project (MED).* Portland, OR. http://www.ohsu.edu/ohsuedu/academic/som/phpm/med/index.cfm (accessed May 12, 2008).

Pham, H. H., P. B. Ginsburg, K. McKenzie, and A. Milstein. 2007. Redesigning care delivery in response to a high-performance network: The Virginia Mason Medical Center. *Health Affairs* 26(4):w532-w544.

Ricketts, T., S. Greene, P. Silberman, H. Howard, and S. Poley. 2007. *Evaluation of Community Care of North Carolina asthma and diabetes management initiatives: January 2000-December 2002.* Chapel Hill, NC: The Cecil G. Sheps Center for Health Services Research, University of North Carolina at Chapel Hill.

Rosenthal, M. B., R. G. Frank, Z. Li, and A. M. Epstein. 2005. Early experience with pay-for-performance: From concept to practice. *JAMA* 294(14):1788-1793.

Rosenthal, M. B., B. E. Landon, S. L. Normand, R. G. Frank, and A. M. Epstein. 2006. Pay for performance in commercial HMOs. *New England Journal of Medicine* 355(18):1895-1902.

Rowe, J. W. 2006. Pay-for-performance and accountability: Related themes in improving health care. *Annals of Internal Medicine* 145(9):695-699.

U.S. Department of Health and Human Services. 2007. *The American Health Information Community.* Washington, DC. http://www.hhs.gov/healthit/community/background/ (accessed May 14, 2007).

U.S. Department of Veteran's Affairs Office of Public Affairs Media Relations. 2007. *Facts about the Department of Veterans Affairs.* Washington, DC. http://www1.va.gov/OPA/fact/docs/vafacts.pdf (accessed May 21, 2007).

U.S. Government Accountability Office. 2007. *Military health care: TRICARE cost-sharing proposals would help offset increasing health care spending, but projected savings are likely overestimated.* Report to Congressional Committees. Washington, DC.

Villagra, V. G., and T. Ahmed. 2004. Effectiveness of a disease management program for patients with diabetes. *Health Affairs* 23(4):255-266.

Wennberg, J. 2007. *The care of patients with severe chronic illness: A report on the Medicare program by the Dartmouth Atlas Project. Executive summary.* Hanover, NH: Center for the Evaluative Clinical Sciences, Dartmouth Atlas Project.

Wennberg, J., and M. Cooper. 2007. *The Dartmouth atlas of health care 1999. The quality of medical care in the United States: A report on the Medicare program.* Chicago, IL: Dartmouth Medical School.

Wheeler, J. R., N. K. Janz, and J. A. Dodge. 2003. Can a disease self-management program reduce health care costs? The case of older women with heart disease. *Medical Care* 41(6):706-715.

Wood, A. J. 2006. A proposal for radical changes in the drug-approval process. *New England Journal of Medicine* 355(6):618-623.

12

Employers and Employees

Coordinator

Veronica Goff, National Business Group on Health

Other Contributors

Kathy Buto, Johnson & Johnson; Cecily Hall, Microsoft;
Ann Kempski, Service Employees International Union

SECTOR OVERVIEW

Sixty percent of U.S. employers provide health insurance, covering nearly two-thirds of Americans under age 65 years (Stanton, 2004). Companies with more than 200 employees are more likely to offer health benefits (99 percent) than companies with less than 10 employees (45 percent). About 40 percent of the employer market is self-insured, covering about 55 million people.

Over the last 10 years, employer healthcare expenditures rose 140 percent (Mercer Health & Benefits Evolution and Revolution: Benefit Trends, 2007). Large employers spent an average of $8,424 per employee per year on health care in 2006 (Mercer Health & Benefits Evolution and Revolution: Benefit Trends, 2007). Among all employers, the average annual costs for single and family coverage in 2007, including employer and employee contributions, were $4,479 and $12,106, respectively (Claxton et al., 2007).

Over the next decade, healthcare spending is expected to rise 7 percent annually, about twice the rate of overall inflation (CMS, Office of the Actuary, 2007). Corporations report that they cannot drive down business costs and optimize margins enough to keep absorbing these increases (Darling, 2007), and employer-sponsored insurance is eroding as a result. The percentage of workers covered by employer-sponsored healthcare benefits dropped to 59 percent in 2006 from a high of 65 percent in 2001 (The Kaiser Family Foundation and Health Research and Educational Trust,

297

2006). Retiree healthcare coverage was offered by 35 percent of large employers in 2006, down from 66 percent in 1988 (The Kaiser Family Foundation and Health Research and Educational Trust, 2006).

Cost is only part of the problem, however. Wasteful spending and poor outcomes because of the overuse, underuse, and misuse of healthcare services have employers' attention. National business organizations have worked to improve quality and manage costs for more than 30 years. Among them is the National Business Group on Health,[1] established in 1974 at the urging of the Business Roundtable.[2] The National Committee on Evidence-Based Benefit Design is a recent initiative of the National Business Group on Health whose mission is to improve the quality of care and promote value by using benefit designs that encourage and reward the provision of effective care and that discourage the provision of ineffective care.

Regional and community-based coalitions, led by the National Business Coalition on Health,[3] took root in the early 1990s. More recently, several business-led organizations have used combined purchasing leverage to advance quality, safety, and efficiency reforms; most notable among these are the Leapfrog Group,[4] Bridges to Excellence,[5] and Care Focused Purchasing.

Employees bear the cost of the inefficient healthcare system directly.

---

[1]The National Business Group on Health, which represents 272 large employers, including 65 of the Fortune 100, is the nation's only nonprofit organization devoted exclusively to finding innovative and forward-thinking solutions to large employers' most important healthcare and related benefits issues. Business Group members provide healthcare coverage for more than 55 million employees, retirees, and dependents. See http://www.businessgrouphealth. org.

[2]The Business Roundtable is committed to advocating public policies that ensure vigorous economic growth, a dynamic global economy, and the well-trained and productive U.S. workforce essential for future competitiveness. The Business Roundtable believes that its potential for effectiveness is based on the fact that it draws on chief executive officers directly and personally and presents government with reasoned alternatives and positive suggestions. See http://www.businessroundtable.org.

[3]The National Business Coalition on Health (NBCH) is a national, nonprofit, membership organization of nearly 70 employer-led coalitions representing more than 10,000 employers. NBCH and its members are dedicated to the value-based purchasing of healthcare services through the collective action of public and private purchasers. NBCH seeks to accelerate the nation's progress toward safe, efficient, and high-quality health care and the improved health status of the American population. See http://www.nbch.org.

[4]The Leapfrog Group is a voluntary program aimed at mobilizing employer purchasing power to alert America's healthcare industry that big leaps in healthcare safety, quality, and customer value will be recognized and rewarded. Among other initiatives, the Leapfrog Group works with its employer members to encourage transparency and easy access to healthcare information and rewards hospitals that have a proven record of providing high-quality care. See http://www.leapfroggroup.org.

[5]Bridges to Excellence is a not-for-profit organization that designs and creates programs that encourage physicians and physician practices to deliver safer, more effective, and efficient care by giving them financial and other incentives to do so. See http://www.bridgestoexcellence.org.

RAND Corporation researchers found that patients receive the recommended care only about half the time (Asch et al., 2006). Meanwhile, tens of thousands of people die each year in hospitals because of preventable mistakes (Institute of Medicine, 2000).

Employees are also paying more for their health care. Although the share of premiums that employees pay has held relatively steady (in 2007, the average split for employers and employees was 79 and 21 percent, respectively), employees' annual out-of-pocket spending (premium and point-of-care cost sharing) rose 12 percent in 2006 to an average of $3,065 (Hewitt Health Value Initiative, 2006). At the same time, wages are stagnant as employers spend their resources on health care instead.

Employers and employees have much to gain by encouraging evidence-based medicine:

- improved quality of care and improved outcomes by adherence to clinical guidelines and through the appropriate use of services and medications;
- reductions in errors and adverse medical events;
- potential cost savings through reductions in ineffective care, unproven treatments, and interventions that are unnecessarily costly; and
- greater patient satisfaction through informed involvement in health-care decisions.

ACTIVITY CATEGORIES

Many employers are already active in applying medical evidence and use four levers at their disposal:

- *Provider contracting.* Vendor selection and the rewarding of vendors allow the incorporation of evidence-based medical standards into the care that vendors provide employees.
- *Benefit design.* Differential coverage encourages the provision of effective care and discourages the provision of ineffective care.
- *Employee decision support.* Tools and resources assist employees with being more discriminating healthcare consumers and help them make decisions informed by evidence of effectiveness and risk-benefit profiles.
- *Public policy advocacy.* Advocacy helps support comparative effectiveness research, patient safety, and health information technology.

These activities, which are more thoroughly described below, are options that employers and other sponsors of healthcare plans can use.

Large, self-insured employers have more freedom to employ these techniques than small and midsized employers buying insured products. However, the efforts of large employers often result in system changes that benefit small and midsize employers, too.

Not all large employers are alike, however. Some of these approaches fit within an employer's benefits mission, whereas others do not. Experience shows the greatest chance for meaningful, sustainable change comes when employers combine their purchasing power behind specific activities, as noted in the examples in the next section.

Provider Contracting

Provider contracting allows employers to give preferential status to hospitals that meet evidence-based healthcare quality and safety standards. Preferential status might entail an in-network or center of excellence designation, increased reimbursement, or reduced employee cost sharing when an employee chooses a recognized provider.

The Leapfrog Group, the 5 Million Lives Campaign, and the Surgical Care Improvement Project are examples of programs with standards that may be incorporated. For example, the Leapfrog Group began collecting hospital healthcare practice data in 2001. Now, more than 1,300 hospitals in 33 regions participate in the annual survey. In September 2007, 41 hospitals were designated "Leapfrog top hospitals." These hospitals were recognized for their practices in four categories, including evidence-based hospital referral, which assesses how well hospitals perform seven high-risk procedures and how well they care for infants with three high-risk neonatal conditions (The Leapfrog Group, 2007).

Provider contracting also allows employers to give preferential status to physicians and practices that have been recognized for excellence, for example, by the National Center for Quality Assurance (NCQA) Physician Recognition program, the NCQA Physician Practice Connections program, and Bridges to Excellence programs.

For example, Bridges to Excellence programs encourage physicians and physician practices to deliver evidence-based care through the provision of financial and other incentives. Employers work with national insurers, which all have licensed Bridges to Excellence programs, to implement three programs:

- Diabetes Care Link (which offers bonuses for evidence-based diabetes care),
- Cardiac Care Link (which offers bonuses for evidence-based cardiac care), and

- Physician Office Link (which offers bonuses for investments in information technology and automated care management tools).

Another example is the employer and carrier-led Care Focused Purchasing initiative (which has 55 national employers and seven national and regional carriers), which is using existing industry standard provider performance metrics (many of which are based on evidence of effectiveness) to support providers in continual quality and efficiency improvement efforts and educate consumers at the point of need (Care Focused Purchasing Inc., 2007).

Employers may also require insurers or third-party administrators to report on how evidence is applied to treatment decisions and how they align their treatments with the evidence (whenever possible). They should report the following:

- the process that they use to evaluate new treatments;
- the process that they use to apply new evidence to current coverage policies;
- how physicians are encouraged to make evidence-based decisions and to use clinical guidelines;
- how the application of evidence-based medicine leads to quality and efficiency improvements;
- the percentage of providers meeting the patient safety goals of the Joint Commission, the National Quality Forum, and the Leapfrog Group; and
- the percentage of hospitals participating in the 5 Million Lives Campaign.

Employers may also use evidence-based privileging and quality standards whenever possible. For example, an employer may contract only with imaging providers who meet specific standards. If there are not enough providers who meet those standards, employers may pay providers differentially or reduce the administrative requirements for the top performers.

Employers may also stop paying for the most significant "never events," as specified by the National Quality Forum, such as surgery on the wrong body part and healthcare-acquired infections.

Benefit Plan Design

When medical evidence is available, it is incorporated into clinical practice through treatment guidelines, provider profiling, clinical decision support, and value purchasing efforts, such as centers of excellence and pay-for-performance initiatives. However, with the exception of clinical preventive services, it is still rare for sponsors to use benefit design to encourage and reward the provision of effective care and discourage the provision of ineffective care. Leading employers are using benefit design in a variety of ways, as described below.

Employers may link coverage to the determination of effectiveness and the strength of the evidence. For example, there is strong evidence for many clinical preventive services, and many plan sponsors cover a schedule of preventive services at 100 percent and do not subject them to a deductible.

Employers may link coverage to consumer behaviors that support evidence-based care. For example, they may reduce or eliminate copayments for maintenance medications when members participate in disease management programs. This approach is becoming known as a "value-based" pharmacy benefit.

In another example, nonemergency back surgery is covered with 20 percent coinsurance when the following evidence-related criteria are met:

- the patient completes a medically supervised course of intensive multidisciplinary treatment of not less than 8 weeks in duration;
- the patient notifies the plan of his or her intention to undergo surgery and uses company-sponsored medical consultation or decision support services; and
- if the patient smokes, the patient completes a smoking cessation program before spinal fusion is covered.

Employers may link coverage to the use of providers identified as evidence-based performers. For example, employee cost sharing drops to 10 percent from the typical 80 percent-20 percent split when he or she chooses a physician recognized by one of the NCQA physician recognition programs.

Employers may use coverage to promote evidence development through comparative research and observational studies; that is, they may require enrollment in a registry for coverage of new procedures or experimental treatments for which there is evidence of benefit but for which there is a lack of information about the long-term benefits and possible harms.

Employers may offer health improvement programs with incentives to participate. For example, a survey of nearly 3,000 employers found that 53 percent offered a health risk questionnaire in 2006, and many used incentives to encourage participation (Mercer Health & Benefits Evolution and Revolution: Benefit Trends, 2007). Another employer survey found that 28 percent of employers offered premium differentials for participation in health improvement programs in 2007, up from 16 percent in 2006 (National Business Group on Health/Watson Wyatt, 2007).

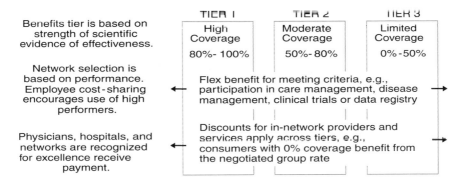

FIGURE 12-1 The National Business Group on Health Benefit Design model.
SOURCE: The National Committee on Evidence-Based Benefit Design publication.

The National Committee on Evidence-Based Benefit Design, established by the National Business Group on Health, proposes a benefit design model that incorporates these approaches (Figure 12-1).

Employee Decision Support

Employers who have provided tools and resources to inform their members about treatment options and the relative benefits and risks of particular options have demonstrated the improved use of evidence-based practices among their employees. For example, one survey of large employers found that 44 percent offer employees access to health coaches, who use evidence-based guidelines when they inform patients about their care options (National Business Group on Health/Watson Wyatt, 2007).

Employers may also provide their employees with educational materials about medical evidence related to specific procedures and treatments that encourage the employees to make informed decisions for healthier lifestyles.

Employer segmenting of the plan population and targeting to each group education and resources on how to use medical evidence and evaluate treatment options can greatly improve their impact on decision making.

Finally, employers can provide their employees tools and information to help them get the most value from their healthcare plan.

Public Policy Advocacy

Policy advocacy and development is also a key activity for employers and employees. Examples of current opportunities to shape public policy relevant to improving evidence development and application include

- initiatives to increase the funding or capacity for comparative effectiveness research;
- encouraging public provider reporting of quality, outcomes, and prices;
- supporting funding of research on consumers and how to most effectively communicate information and engage patients in decision making; and
- signing on to the U.S. Department of Health and Human Services' Value Driven Health Care Initiative, which is aimed at standardizing and expanding healthcare information transparency at the local, state, and federal levels. U.S. Department of Health and Human Services' Secretary Michael Leavitt has encouraged the nation's private-sector employers to support four cornerstone principles for healthcare purchasing: use interoperable health information technology; measure and report healthcare quality; collect and report information on healthcare prices; and implement programs to encourage consumers to use high-quality, cost-effective services (e.g., pay-for-performance reimbursement).

LEADERSHIP COMMITMENTS AND INITIATIVES

Initiatives

Representatives from the employer sector highlighted three initiatives that would be transformational in achieving a healthcare system rooted by medical evidence.

Expand Evidence Base with Clinical Experience and Comparative Effectiveness Research

To better support decision making about the best evidence, both in patient care and in provider coverage, the evidence base needs to be expanded significantly. Information and data capture at the point of care could supplement and refine the current knowledge. The broad application of healthcare information technology tools will be necessary to expand the evidence base with data generated from clinical experience, including data from electronic medical records, registries, and interoperable systems.

Evidence based practice supports will also aid success. An increased emphasis on comparative effectiveness research to determine the effectiveness of various treatments (drugs, devices, surgery, etc.) for a particular condition is also needed to support decision making.

Comparative effectiveness research should

- incorporate cost into effectiveness evaluations;
- incorporate functionality, productivity, and other indirect costs in evaluations;
- address current medical practice as well as new technologies;
- identify the criteria against which the appropriateness of the intervention can be determined; and
- identify health interventions with little or no value.

Use Evidence in Coverage and Payment Policies

There will need to be an agreed-upon process or decision model for the translation of research into coverage and payment policy recommendations. Once recommendations are made, employers can design health benefits and write provider contracts consistent with those recommendations, reinforcing the expectation that evidence-based medicine is the standard and pricing and network steerage will be linked to the practice.

Stimulate Broad Participation in Existing Evidence-Based Medicine Efforts

Many leading employers are already involved in promising evidence-based medicine initiatives through group purchasing efforts and contracts with health plans. Employer groups have driven some of these initiatives, whereas clinicians, health plans, and delivery systems have initiated others. These efforts include the use of agreed-upon standards and measures in quality reporting and pay-for-performance initiatives and the use of health plan-pharmacy benefit plan utilization review and intervention with clinicians and patients.

Cross-Sector Collaboration: Creating Demand for Evidence-Based Medicine

The single most important factor in successfully carrying out the initiatives mentioned above is consumer demand for evidence-based medicine. Today's consumers are largely unaware of the variability in healthcare quality and do not have adequate information with which to make informed healthcare decisions that are based on the evidence and that reflect their values and preferences.

NEXT STEPS

Next steps for expanding the evidence base with comparative effectiveness research include the funding of research and the achievement of agreement on research priorities. The steps necessary for expanding the evidence with clinical experience include the development of standardized clinical tools and practice supports.

Next steps for using evidence in coverage and payment policies are to learn from existing efforts and to develop a transparent methodology for specifying coverage criteria.

Next steps for creating consumer demand include the following:

- Communications research is needed to understand what messages and information resonate with consumers. Research by a variety of stakeholders is already under way. One example, called Communicating about Evidence-Based Health Care Decision Making, is a research project sponsored by the California HealthCare Foundation and conducted by the American Institutes for Research. New research efforts should build on what has already been learned.
- A marketing campaign would pique consumer interest in evidence-based medicine and create demand for decision support information. The campaign should include actions that consumers can take to improve the quality of their health care. The Agency for Healthcare Research and Quality-Ad Council campaign titled Questions Are the Answer is a good example of such an approach.
- Develop standardized transparency and reporting methods and requirements.
- Develop simple, straightforward tools for healthcare consumers. Target groups should include retirees, users of large amounts of health care, and individuals with limited English proficiency or health literacy. Tools should help consumers weigh the risks, benefits, and treatment options and explain the basis of the evidence behind coverage decisions.

Finally, although employers have much to gain from a healthcare system grounded in evidence, the day-to-day responsibilities of benefit managers and human resources executives will keep them at arms length from the Institute of Medicine (IOM) Roundtable process. Some leading employers may participate directly, but most will continue to use their employer associations to represent them and their healthcare vendors to initiate practices deemed appropriate. The more closely that the IOM Roundtable uses initiatives that employers are already engaged in to forward its agenda, the more likely it will be that employers will participate directly in IOM efforts.

REFERENCES

Asch, S. M., E. A. Kerr, J. Keesey, J. L. Adams, C. M. Setodji, S. Malik, and E. A. McGlynn. 2006. Who is at greatest risk for receiving poor-quality health care? *New England Journal of Medicine* 354(11):1147-1156.

Care Focused Purchasing, Inc. 2007. *Brochure 2007.*

Claxton, G., J. Gabel, B. DiJulio, J. Pickreign, H. Whitmore, B. Finder, P. Jacobs, and S. Hawkins. 2007. Health benefits in 2007: Premium increases fall to an eight-year low, while offer rates and enrollment remain stable. *Health Affairs* 26(5):1407-1416.

CMS (Centers for Medicare and Medicaid Services), Office of the Actuary. 2007. *National health expenditures 2006-2016.* Baltimore, MD. http://www.cms.hhs.gov/NationalHealthExpendData/downloads/proj2006.pdf (accessed May 12, 2008).

Darling, H. 2007. *Controlling health care costs through empowerment and partnership, Institute on Health Care Costs and Solutions.* Washington, DC: National Business Group on Health. http://www.businessgrouphealth.org (accessed June 1, 2007).

Hewitt Health Value Initiative™. 2006. Annual Health Care Cost Increases. Lincolnshire, IL: Hewitt Associates, LLC. http://www.hewittassociates.com/_MetaBasicCMAssetCache_/Assets/Press%20Release%20PDFs/2006/10-09-2006.pdf (accessed November 15, 2008).

Institute of Medicine. 2000. *To err is human: Building a safer health system.* Washington, DC: National Academy Press.

The Kaiser Family Foundation and Health Research and Educational Trust. 2006. *Employer health benefits annual survey.* Menlo Park, CA.

The Leapfrog Group. 2007. *41 hospitals are designated Leapfrog top hospitals for 2007.* News release, September 18. Washington, DC.

Mercer Health & Benefits Evolution and Revolution: Benefit Trends. 2007. Paper read at National Business Group on Health, April 18, 2007. Washington, DC: Mercer, LLC.

National Business Group on Health/Watson Wyatt. 2007. Dashboard for Success: How Best Performers Do It. *12th annual National Business Group on Health/Watson Wyatt survey report.* Washington, DC.

National Committee on Evidence-based Benefit Design/National Business Group on Health. 2007. *Evidence-based benefits: A toolkit for employers.* http://www.businessgrouphealth.org/benefitstopics/et_evidencebasedbenefits.cfm (accessed November 15, 2008).

Stanton, M. 2004. *Employer-sponsored health insurance: Trends in cost and access. Research in action: Issue 17, No. 04-0085.* Rockville, MD: Agency for Healthcare Research and Quality.

13

Information Technology

Coordinator

Jim Karkanias, Microsoft

Other Contributors

Michael Gillam, Microsoft, and Nina Schwenk, Mayo Clinic

SECTOR OVERVIEW

Medicine is often viewed as a procedure or intervention-based practice. Although they are often unnoticed by the patient, the information systems used to store relevant patient information work in tandem with providers to deliver appropriate treatment options to patients. Information systems that were initially developed by gathering limited patient demographic and financial data have, in many cases, expanded to include volumes of complex clinical findings, laboratory data, and images. With the significant increase in patient data volume and complexity, healthcare data management is increasingly more challenging. Data management is central to supporting evidence-based medicine. The information technology (IT) sector, a key driver in moving the frontier of evidence-based medicine (EBM), continues to seek opportunities to work with stakeholders to address the complex needs of the healthcare industry.

The IT sector will play a critical role in progressing toward a learning healthcare system that facilitates evidence-based decisions based on experiential clinical data. As a key player in the healthcare arena, the IT sector has evolved from delivering stand-alone, smart medical equipment (e.g., echocardiography systems and radiology systems) to providing increasingly integrated clinical systems and full-function electronic medical records (EMRs) (Table 13-1). The ability to provide clinical decision support at the point of care is a key need in health care, and IT sector solutions for EMRs have resulted in a variety of complex and evolving systems that healthcare

309

TABLE 13-1 Healthcare System IT Functions

Function	Description
Source system	Supports patient data management, administrative and claims data, system of record
EMR	Consolidated and integrated clinical systems provider that supports inpatient and outpatient practices
Administration chain data management	Administrative systems in support of clinical care and research
Personal health record	Provides an interface to providers and hospitals for patients, employers, and insurance companies
Ancillary service management	Systems designed for use in specific functional areas (e.g., laboratory, radiology, outpatient care, and care management)
Decision support	Educational tools, data warehousing, enterprise information management, and data analysis

professionals can use to communicate important information quickly and efficiently.

Despite the significant advances in healthcare IT, work remains to be done to meet the needs of a learning healthcare system. Focused efforts in data warehousing and the development of data analysis tools will enhance the healthcare system's ability to work with large data volumes and images. Allowing patients and providers to search and access data in various forms through the Internet or mass storage will further enhance the delivery of patient care by the use of evidence-based practices.

ACTIVITY CATEGORIES

Evidence-Related Activities Areas for IT Development

The following are evidence-related activities in IT:

- improving consumer access to reliable health and disease management information,
- improving provider access to reliable health and disease management information,
- improving patient-provider communication and interaction,
- improving the application of best practices,
- improving provider operational effectiveness and efficiency,
- improving the ability to manage and analyze large quantities of data, and
- improving research on clinical effectiveness and quality of care.

Priority Areas for IT Development

Seven priority areas will be able to improve the IT sector's ability to support the transformative change implied in the Roundtable's goal. The priority areas range from the development of data standards and a vocabulary that will allow the sector to incorporate data and look at data from different views to developing capabilities to deliver evidence-based medicine at the right time and the right place.

Healthcare IT Standards

The single most transformational step toward achieving the goal of a learning healthcare system is the development and implementation of IT industry standards. This step, more than any other IT initiative, would facilitate the exchange of patient data between clinical IT systems as well as between the spectrum of stakeholders. Even with highly sophisticated clinical systems, the exchange of data between providers and particularly between institutions is complicated by the incompatibilities between proprietary systems and a lack of defined standards in the healthcare IT arena. The impetus to create and standardize data elements will need to come from the IT industry. IT consumers, such as healthcare organizations and providers, will increasingly demand intraoperability between systems as the digitization of clinical information and the use of electronic media in medical offices increases. Beyond individual patient care and data transferability, the accumulating public and population data efficiently necessitate interoperable systems that are suitable for a single-physician practice as well as large multispecialty academic organizations. Anonymous tracking of disease epidemiology, drug interactions, and various complications will facilitate active, concurrent biosurveillance, postmarketing drug reviews, and general public health safety.

Standardized Vocabulary

In conjunction with health IT standards, the healthcare system demands a common vocabulary to facilitate the interoperability of clinical systems and the interpretation of clinical data across multiple sites. The IT sector must collaborate with the medical community to standardize the vocabulary. Precise definitions of medical procedures, events, illnesses, and data parameters and values are mandatory for comparison of information from single patient encounters with different providers as well as encounters with different patient cohorts. Standardization initiatives must be prioritized and approached methodically. For instance, a standardized approach to the medication record and a standardized allergy vocabulary might quickly change the healthcare industry's ability to influence the quality of care, patient safety, and morbidity and mortality from medication administration errors.

Provider Work Flow

Current clinical IT systems often simply duplicate work flows developed and honed in the paper world. The ability to transform the delivery of medical care will require fundamental changes in how providers and clinicians deliver care and communicate with IT. The electronic health records of the future will not only provide a way to collect, view, and communicate patient data but also will transform care delivery workflows to be safer and more effective. A critical piece of this work flow transformation will need to be the seamless movement of data between the various patient care environments. Both virtual and real patient visits will require the same degree of data and information management.

Just-in-Time Evidence Delivery

The volume and complexity of the data requiring aggregation, synthesis, and interpretation in patient care delivery are already beyond the technological capabilities of individual physicians. The ability to put complex data in the context of relevant scientific evidence adds a further dimension to the complexity of safe and appropriate patient care delivery. To continue supporting clinical care, IT will need to deliver the right information at the right time to ensure that the best decisions can be made in partnership with patients. The just-in-time delivery of evidence will ultimately require consumers to be able to gather information on demand about the care provider and his or her level of expertise on any particular topic and for providers to be able to gather information on the potential and real medical condition of the patient, relevant clinical evidence and preformed guidelines, and genomic data and their interpretation. Equally important will be the ability to filter unnecessary data to avoid overwhelming providers with an abundance of information.

Clinical Decision Support

The elements of clinical decision support for providers span the continuum of data collection, aggregation, synthesis, delivery, and interpretation. IT can supply relevant aggregated clinical and experiential evidence data to guide clinicians faced with clinical and biological data from individual patients. Clinical decision support rules are complex and require the flexibility to respond to changing clinical evidence and learning. Any such clinical decision support also needs to be integrated with electronic health records to minimize the number of systems that need to be accessed. A notable function of clinical decision support is alerting providers to a significant patient care event. Alerts can include information on possible drug interactions, medication administration times, and notable events in a patient's history (e.g., history of patient fall precautions, allergies, and details of advance directives). Simplifying alert mechanisms could reduce adverse outcomes and enhance the delivery of evidence-based care. Similar to clinical decision support, alert functions correspondingly require integration with provider work flow and clinical systems.

Flexible Data Views

As the complexity and volume of data increase, simple tables and statistics will not provide an adequate view of the available information. Novel ways of displaying clinical data and their relationship with other data will need to be developed to help users interpret the significance of those relationships and make appropriate and informed patient care decisions. Data visualization needs significant honing and work before the data can be applied to the healthcare arena. Such techniques have already been demonstrated to have value in the financial planning and gaming industries.

Connectivity

Healthcare networks that connect various stakeholders are needed for the seamless transfer of relevant and appropriate information to avoid the duplication of data collection efforts and the recollection of data. Minimizing the sources and the number of data inputs also increases the likelihood of data integrity and reliability. The collection and display of clinical data from all patient care settings are needed for the reliable, consistent, and safe transfer of data. Technology and vocabulary standards will again come in to play if healthcare providers make use of all patient information collected, whether it is through the use of home monitoring devices or in-hospital medical devices.

LEADERSHIP COMMITMENTS AND INITIATIVES

The IT sector can champion three transformational initiatives to facilitate the development of a learning healthcare system. The initiatives provide overlapping benefits to the aforementioned priority areas and are efforts that harness and align existing elements, encourage measured innovation in the near future, and ultimately sustain long-term radical innovation.

Foundational Medical Informatics Ecosystem Initiative

The single most transformational step toward achieving the goal of a learning healthcare system would be enhanced development and implementation of IT industry standards and common vocabularies in the healthcare system. As its goal, this initiative would seek to build and promote the foundational technologies needed to enable healthcare IT-assisted EBM. There are a variety of foundational technologies involving the government and different groups, but deficits remain in those foundational technologies. One of the most important remaining deficits is standards. Standards and a common vocabulary are of absolute importance as building blocks for bringing computational intelligence to aid human cognition as it relates to EBM.

The IT itself can be a barrier to utilization. For example, the National Library of Medicine purchased SNOMED CT (Systematized Nomenclature of Medicine—Clinical Terms) for $25 million and subsequently provided public access. The public access spurred innovation in multiple areas, but difficulties within the SNOMED CT vocabulary prevented full clinical use by healthcare IT firms such as Microsoft and Azyxxi to the extent that SNOMED CT cannot be used commercially. This is illustrated in the following examples of lexical variants and lexical and domain deficits:

- Lasix is sanofi-aventis' trade name for the U.S. generic drug furosemide. In the United Kingdom, where SNOMED CT was developed, the drug is identified as frusemide but not as furosemide or Lasix. Lexical issues such as this are of great clinical frustration to users trying to enter patient medications.
- Clinicians can order skin tests for patients for a variety of different allergies, but many systems omit documentation of test results, which is an easy fix. Unfortunately, this lexical deficit results in an incomplete allergy list. Although patients could be allergic to any medication, not every medication is always included in the allergy list.
- Some natural language-parsing tools (e.g., MetaMap Transfer from the National Library of Medicine) can be used to evaluate unstructured text, look for key words, and then map the text to a particular standard. However, if the key word is "chest pain," these tools will also pick up "no chest pain" and the results will include patients who did not have chest pain or who denied having chest pain.

In light of these gaps, transformation will require an impetus for rectifying deficiencies to create a foundational medical informatics ecosystem.

Ecosystems represent both a community and a technology, creating a virtuous cycle. The more members who join that particular community and use a technology, the more valuable the created technology becomes. eBay is an example in which increasing numbers of people list items and even more people visit the site; it becomes more valuable to put more goods on the site. Such a transformational initiative creates an ecosystem for standards, vocabularies, and tools. Likely, the first area to be targeted would be an evaluation of the technical barriers preventing healthcare IT firms from using the current tools, identification of the barriers, and creation of an impetus for the IT industry to evolve and implement these standards.

IT Core Measures Initiative

Clinical data and an analytic infrastructure are necessary to facilitate the development of EBM. Important to every evidence-based decision is the availability of patient data, collected during consultation and interviews with individual patients. However, the variety of add-on clinical systems almost seems designed to thwart efforts to aggregate patient data and to organize those data for the practice of EBM. Hospitals use multiple documentation, order, billing, and clinical systems; and these often exist as "data islands." The excessive proportion of time that clinicians spend collecting evidence has huge implications for encouraging the practice of EBM.

To illustrate the potential for IT to improve the current situation, imagine a system in which all of those data are stored in one table. This has huge implications for entities aiming to meet the Joint Commission on the Accreditation of Healthcare Organizations and Centers for Medicare and Medicaid Services core measures requirements. In some cases, 15 or 20 different systems will be accessed just to collect the data to confirm compliance with the core measures. In fact, some hospitals have four and five full-time employees who just walk around collecting all these data on paper. The proposed IT Core Measures Initiative could help transform health care by promoting the implementation of an important information infrastructure that would encourage the development of additional measures.

There are a variety of core data essential to supporting the practice of EBM. Identifying specific data elements through Institute of Medicine (IOM)-facilitated initiatives might increase the receptivity of the IT industry to the integration of critical information into clinical systems as well as the demand by clinicians for the information. The development of core analytical tools supporting data analysis and allowing clinicians to draw evidence-supported conclusions will advance the adoption of EBM. IT could provide flexible reporting and enhance the ability to visualize clinical data in a variety of formats, thereby increasing the likelihood of rapid adoption and application to the delivery of care. Furthermore, it will be important to make the data available to other IT systems through data sharing, with the aim of developing additional clinical insights.

Advanced Technical Strategies Innovations Initiative

Finally, innovation needs to be pushed in many of the different priority areas, for example, clinical decision support, just-in-time evidence delivery, alerts, and flexible data views. How can systems currently deemed impossible be developed? How can systems that guide clinical decisions on the basis of individual clinical and biological data with relevant clinical evidence and experiential information gathered from the mining of data on previous patients with similar conditions be developed? To get to these types of innovations that will truly enable the delivery of EBM, the IT sector needs to leapfrog what it is doing today and bring about radical innovation.

Although the Advanced Technical Strategies Innovation Initiative project is oriented around issues related to the IT sector, it will actually require substantial cross-sector collaboration, as, often, the key to radical innovation is diverse participation. To establish an infrastructure to incentivize ongoing innovation in EBM, IOM or other entities could sponsor, support, or establish healthcare IT demonstration projects for advanced, strategic EBM projects that are currently nearly impossible but ultimately extremely valuable. The American Medical Informatics Association or other groups need to be involved to help attract attention; but the core idea is that sponsorship of a contest could lead to multiplicative return on investment, knowledge from doing, diverse participation, and potentially radical innovation.

Opportunities for Cross-Sector Collaboration

On the basis of the perspectives shared by the participants in the different sectors (healthcare delivery organizations, insurers, employers and employees, healthcare product developers, regulators, evaluators and clinical investigators, healthcare professionals, and patients and consumers), the IT sector has identified several areas for potential collaboration. In addition to working with other sectors to develop stronger IT solutions, the IT sector suggests that projects designed to further develop the depth of IT solutions be funded as a critical element of collaboration (Table 13-2).

NEXT STEPS

Foundational Medical Informatics Ecosystem Initiative

In conjunction with other stakeholders, the IT sector can support the establishment of a data and analytical infrastructure to enable the

TABLE 13-2 Areas Identified for IT Collaboration Across Sectors

Elements of IT Use Cases	Healthcare Delivery Organizations	Insurers	Employers/Employees	Healthcare Product Developers	Regulators	Evaluators and Clinical Investigators	Healthcare Professionals	Patients/Consumers
Secure data sharing across multiple platforms to reduce **redundancy** and errors	x	x	x	x	x	x	x	x
Health information exchange/data **warehouse** /aggregated data	x	x		x	x	x	x	x
Standardized data field definitions/terminology	x	x			x		x	x
High **cost** of new technology, lack of cost-effectiveness scrutiny or use in comparative clinical analysis	x	x					x	x
Ready **access** to individual personal health data/EHR for improved quality of care/increased patient participation			x		x		x	x
Incorporates administrative and clinical data and images	x			x	x		x	
New IT must **engage** users, facilitate decision making based on preferences/needs, and fit users' culture				x			x	x
Postclinical trial/postmarket surveillance of interventions, devices, and drugs			x		x			x
Capacity to **analyze** /organize /retrieve/display/disseminate data usefully	x	x				x		
Data **privacy** concerns/IT skepticism slow the adoption of new technology							x	x
Flexible system/software enhancements and upgrades							x	

application of EBM. Through collaborations with the IOM and others, the development of clinical IT standards through a government–industry collaborative ecosystem will foster the continued evolution of EBM. As the clinical standards are developed and adopted, feedback on the standards will increase and the standards can adjust to meet the needs of the users. The virtuous cycle—one that continually feeds outputs back into the cycle as inputs—inherently leads to equilibrium within the medical informatics ecosystem, as seen with eBay, Flickr, and YouTube, and the technology works in harmony with the community. Support for the evaluation of the technical barriers to adopting current publicly supported open-standard vocabularies and tools by healthcare IT providers will enable the IT sector to iteratively address and remove technical barriers. Ultimately, success is measured by technology adoption and use by the healthcare community.

IT Core Measures Initiative

Establishing an infrastructure will create incentives for ongoing innovation in EBM. To accelerate progress, the IOM or others could convene or support initiatives identifying metrics for core measures that address accessibility to core clinical data and core analytical tools, which may include reporting of specifications and the use of data visualization tools to facilitate research in areas such as disease variation and potential evolving drug resistance patterns in particular diseases.

Advanced Technical Strategies Innovations Initiative

Developing cross-sector collaboration through an Advanced Technical Strategies Innovations Initiative sponsored, supported, or established by the IOM could lead to projects that demonstrate advanced, strategic EBM applications. It is through projects with diverse participation by multiple sectors that radical innovation in healthcare IT will grow. As a starting point, key needs for IT development have been drawn from the accompanying strategies of each sector. As illustrated in Table 13-2, the cases are not intended to be comprehensive in nature; however, they provide examples of scenarios in which innovation in healthcare IT can further contribute to systems development.

Patients and Consumers

Representatives from patient and consumer stakeholder groups encourage healthcare IT to increase their access to patient-controlled information sources, including medical records, clinicians, and clinical data, as well as an ability to use IT as a means of communicating and participating in the planning of their care. Specific IT enhancements might include secure data sharing and protection, access to multiple data sources, an ability to access personal medical information, a standardized healthcare data vocabulary, tools for communicating with healthcare professionals, and IT cost containment.

The priority areas identified by the patient and consumer groups include data security and individual patient control of data and data sharing, access to clinicians, and the interconnectivity of healthcare records. Patients and consumers want to designate various levels of medical record access to individuals autonomously, and the security of data storage and transmission are of paramount importance. In addition to using IT to communicate with clinicians on their health status and treatment options, patients and consumers want easy access to a consolidated, user-friendly health record for routine and emergency health needs.

Several transformative initiatives could aid in developing the priority areas identified: advocate for the better capture of clinical data to accelerate evidence development, particularly on late effects and effects on the general population after an initial demonstration of efficacy in controlled clinical trials; collaborate on development in EMRs and IT systems that promote patient safety, patient control and use, secure data sharing that protects patient privacy and that prevents wasteful duplication and avoidable administrative costs; demand interoperable records so that key participants in the delivery of an individual's care can share information (e.g., primary care clinicians, specialists, pharmacies, laboratories, imaging facilities, hospitals, nursing homes, home health agencies); highlight the value that IT provides consumers; and resolve privacy concerns to promote trust in IT and the acceptance and use of IT by consumers.

Healthcare Providers and Healthcare Delivery Organizations

Healthcare providers and healthcare delivery organizations suggest that the healthcare IT sector develop systems that are user-friendly, highly integrated, and interconnected and that allow clinicians to spend more time with patients and access the aggregated clinical information. Specific IT enhancements might include the provision of access to all clinical data sources; a standardized healthcare data vocabulary; tools for communicating with other healthcare professionals; and increased ease of system use, training in system use, user interface development, and system upgrades.

Providers highlight several areas required for the rapid adoption of evidence-based practices. Clinicians want easy access to clinical and research data to aid them with the planning of care. The availability of user interfaces and the facility with which clinicians interact with systems may increase the rate of technology adoption. As healthcare delivery organizations shift toward the use of electronic records, the IT sector should consider how it can support organizations when they want to move to digital formats beyond their financial means.

To advance the application of evidence, clinicians need to remain current on additions to the evidence base. The IT sector could support the endeavor by providing easy and immediate access to Internet-based knowledge repositories. The IT sector might also consider the implementation of multiple pricing structures to ease the burden on small practices, as the perceived initial investment in IT can be significant. Through the development and implementation of a common healthcare IT vocabulary and interoperable technology, patient data can be optimized for the assessment of evidence-based guideline implementation and provide feedback to healthcare professionals. Providers also suggest that the provision of evidence-based guidelines in a format compatible with all forms of EMR, as well as in paper versions for practitioners who do not yet use routinely electronic technology, may speed their adoption and integration into practice.

Clinical Investigators and Evaluators

Clinical investigators and evaluators suggest a need for a healthcare IT system that allows access to data from multiple platforms to support the generation of evidence and the capacity to analyze, organize, display, and disseminate data usefully. Specific IT enhancements might include information from data collected concurrently during the routine delivery of care to assess outcomes, prevention strategies, and treatments; tools designed to aggregate and analyze data efficiently; patient outcomes reporting to empower patients to enter treatment outcomes data; and biobanking initiatives to improve the collection and storage of tissue samples and genetic data. Support for the development of database architectures and governance procedures addressing privacy needs and proprietary interests could support the application of evidence in the research setting.

APPENDIXES

Appendix A

Sectoral Strategies Process

Institute of Medicine
Roundtable on Evidence-Based Medicine

SECTORAL STRATEGIES PROCESS

Charter statement: *The Institute of Medicine's (IOM's) Roundtable on Evidence-Based Medicine has been convened to help transform the way evidence on clinical effectiveness is generated and used to improve health and health care. Participants have set a goal that, by the year 2020, 90 percent of clinical decisions will be supported by accurate, timely, and up-to-date clinical information, and will reflect the best available evidence. Roundtable members will work with their colleagues to identify the issues not being adequately addressed, the nature of the barriers and possible solutions, and the priorities for action, and will marshal the resources of the sectors represented on the Roundtable to work for sustained public–private cooperation for change.*

Issue and aim: To enhance stakeholder focus and effectiveness in activities important to achieve charter goals by outlining specific means by which each sector can contribute. This will entail the engagement of leading organizations within each sector, individually and collaboratively, in coordinated work to develop a sectoral statement that reviews the key issues and opportunities relevant to the sector, identifies a program of activities to address them, and specifies the expected outcomes if implemented. Comments, but not approval, will be sought. These statements will be individually authored, will not represent a formal consensus, and will be presented for discussion at an IOM workshop.

Outcomes sought:
- Identification and action on key sector-specific opportunities to accelerate progress toward a learning healthcare system
- Collaboration within sector to engage those opportunities
- Collaboration across sectors to engage those opportunities
- Ideas for Roundtable action to facilitate

Sample sectoral statement format:
- *Section 1*: Overview profile of the sector and key players, emphasizing elements relevant to improving the generation and application of evidence
- *Section 2*: Specification and description of the key activity categories within the purview of the sector that are most important to the generation and application of evidence
- *Section 3*: Description, by specified category, of the sorts of sectoral initiatives and priorities that could help transform the scene
- *Section 4*: Identification of possible areas for collaboration and cooperation with other sectors
- *Section 5*: Indication of steps necessary to get the sectoral initiatives under way
- *Section 6*: Timetable for expected results if implemented

Approach:
- Each Roundtable member designates a lead staff person to work on the project
- Sectoral cluster coordinator, or designee, convenes initial meeting
- Sectoral group decides on approach and means of engaging participation from sector organizations not on the Roundtable
- Meetings held in whatever fashion deemed most expeditious for task, in coordination with IOM staff
- First draft completed and circulated among participants
- Review draft circulated among Roundtable members represented on sector group
- Revised review drafts assembled into consolidated draft Sectoral Strategies document and circulated for review and comment of all Roundtable members
- Presentation of background papers for public discussion at an IOM Workshop on Sectoral Strategies

Timetable.

- January: initial formation of nine sectoral clusters
- February and March: reach out to other sectoral participants
- April: first draft completed and circulated to sector participants
- May: sector review draft circulated to Roundtable members on each sector group
- June: consolidated draft Sectoral Strategies document sent to all Roundtable members
- July: public discussion at IOM Workshop on Sectoral Strategies

Sectoral clusters: (The lists below are not comprehensive, noting only Roundtable designees.)

Consumer-Patient
- Joyce Dubow, AARP (Coordinator)
- Gail Shearer, Consumers Union
- Ann Kempski, SEIU
- Carolin Hinestorsa, National Breast Cancer Coalition

Health Professionals
- Rae-Ellen Kavey, NHLBI (Coordinator)
- Kimberly Rask, Emory
- Cato Laurencin, University of Virginia
- Nancy Nielsen, AMA

Healthcare Delivery Organizations
- Bob Crane, Laura Tollen, and Kate Myers, Kaiser (Coordinators)
- Denis Cortese, Mayo Clinic
- Benjamin Druss, Emory
- Madhulika Agarwal, VHA
- Jon Perlin, HCA
- Rich Platt, Harvard Pilgrim Health Care

Evaluators/Clinical Researchers
- Rich Platt, Harvard Pilgrim Health Care (Coordinator)
- Carolyn Clancy and Jean Slutsky, AHRQ
- Cato Laurencin, University of Virginia
- Rae-Ellen Kavey, NHLBI
- Don Steinwachs, Johns Hopkins University
- Mark McClellan, Elizabeth Walker, and Elizabeth DuPre, AEI-Brookings

Employees-Employers
- Ronnie Goff, NBGH (Coordinator)
- Kathy Buto, Johnson & Johnson
- Ann Kempski, Service Employees International Union
- Cecily Hall, Microsoft

Information Technology
- Jim Karkanias, Microsoft (Coordinator)
- Adam Bosworth, Google
- Nina Schwenk, Mayo Clinic
- Gail Graham, VHA

Health Care Manufacturers
- Peter Juhn and Christina Farup, Johnson & Johnson (Coordinators)
- Pat Anderson, Stryker
- Cathy Bonuccelli, AstraZeneca

Insurers
- Jack Rowe, Columbia University (Coordinator)
- William Lawrence, North Carolina HHS
- Bob Crane, Kaiser Permanente
- Mark McClellan, Elizabeth Walker, and Elizabeth DuPre, AEI-Brookings
- Liz Goldstein, CMS
- Gerald Penden, Independence Blue Cross

Regulators
- Nancy Derr and Janet Woodcock, FDA (Coordinators)
- Mark Benton, North Carolina HHS
- Mark McClellan, Elizabeth Walker, and Elizabeth DuPre, AEI-Brookings
- Karen Milgate, CMS

Appendix B

Workshop Agenda

**Leadership Commitments to Improve Value in Health Care:
Finding Common Ground**
A Learning Healthcare System Series Workshop
Institute of Medicine Roundtable on Evidence-Based Medicine

Goals:
1. Identify ways that major healthcare stakeholder sectors can contribute to transformative progress toward a learning healthcare system and achievement of the Evidence-Based Medicine Roundtable goal that 90 percent of clinical decisions will, by 2020, reflect and be supported by accurate, timely, and up-to-date evidence.
2. Outline, from the perspective of the major healthcare sectors, some immediate opportunities and steps that can be taken within each sector, as well as among sectors, and propose approaches to taking those steps.
3. Through focused discussion around specific crosscutting issues, develop suggestions for collective efforts—through the Roundtable and beyond—to support the highest-priority transformational initiatives.

Agenda
Day 1: Monday, July 23, 2007

12:45-1:00   **Welcome and Introductory Remarks: Developing a Learning Healthcare System**
Denis Cortese, Chair, Institute of Medicine Roundtable on Evidence-Based Medicine, and Chief Executive Officer, Mayo Clinic

1:00-4:35   **Sector Presentations:** Forty minutes for each sector. The coordinator will take 15 minutes to describe the one to three most important transformative opportunities identified in the group's work, as well as the highest-priority cross-sector collaboration and ways to accomplish it. This will be followed by 2- to 3-minute reactions (to the paper and the highlights) from two workshop participants, selected before the meeting from self-nominees. The last 15 minutes of each sector presentation is reserved for open discussion.

   1:00-1:40   **Healthcare delivery organization sector strategy highlights**
Robert Crane, Kaiser Permanente

   1:40-2:20   **Employer/employee sector strategy highlights**
Veronica Goff, National Business Group on Health

   2:20-3:00   **Insurer sector strategy highlights**
Steven Udvarhelyi, Independence Blue Cross

3:00-3:15   **BREAK**

   3:15-3:55   **Healthcare product developer strategy highlights**
Peter Juhn, Johnson & Johnson

   3:55-4:35   **Regulatory sector strategy highlights**
Janet Woodcock, Food and Drug Administration

4:35-4:50   **Closing Comments**

5:00   **RECEPTION**

Day 2: Tuesday, July 24, 2007

8:45-9:00   **Welcome and Previous Day Highlights**
Michael McGinnis, Senior Scholar, Institute of Medicine

9:00-11:40   **Sector Presentations:** Forty minutes for each sector. The coordinator will take 15 minutes to describe the one to three most important transformative opportunities identified in the group's work, as well as the highest-priority cross-sector collaboration and ways to accomplish it. This will be followed by 2- to 3-minute reactions (to the paper and the highlights) from two workshop participants, selected prior to the meeting from self-nominees. The last 15 minutes of each sector presentation is reserved for open discussion.

   9:00-9:40   **Evaluator/clinical research sector strategy highlights**
Richard Platt, Harvard Medical School and Harvard Pilgrim Health Care

   9:40-10:20   **Health professional sector strategy highlights**
Rae-Ellen Kavey, National Heart, Lung, and Blood Institute

   10:20-11:00 **Patient/consumer sector strategy highlights**
Joyce Dubow, AARP

   11:00-11:40 **Information technology sector strategy highlights**
Michael Gillam, Microsoft

11:40-12:10 **LUNCH**

12:10-2:30   **Crosscutting Issues:** Speakers will spend 20 minutes each sharing a perspective on what might be the ideal experience for the patient or provider or in the approach to producing the needed evidence in a timely fashion, assessing how this ideal stacks up against the current pattern, and identifying the primary barriers to progress. Each presentation will conclude with 15 minutes for follow-up questions.

   12:10-12:45 **Patients**
Margaret C. Kirk, Chair-Elect, National Health Council; Chief Executive Officer Y-ME National Breast Cancer Organization

12:45-1:20   **Providers**
Terry McGeeney, President and Chief Executive Officer, TransforMED

1:20-1:55   **Evidence**
Sean Tunis, Founder and Director, Center for Medical Technology Policy

1:55-2:30   **Sector reactor panel**

2:30-4:00   **Open "Town Hall" Discussion**

4:00-4:30   **Wrap-up and next steps**
Denis Cortese, Chair, Roundtable on Evidence-Based Medicine, and Chief Executive Officer, Mayo Clinic
Michael McGinnis, Senior Scholar, Institute of Medicine

4:30   **ADJOURN**

Appendix C

Biographical Sketches of Participants

Robert Crane, M.B.A., M.P.A., is the senior vice president of research and policy development for Kaiser Foundation Health Plan, Inc., and Kaiser Foundation Hospitals. He also serves as director of the Kaiser Permanente Institute for Health Policy, where he is responsible for its overall operation, as well as for identifying strategic areas of focus. Mr. Crane serves on the boards of several national health policy organizations, including Academy-Health and the Employee Benefit Research Institute. Before joining Kaiser Permanente in 1983, Mr. Crane worked for nearly 4 years with the New York State Department of Health, where he served as the deputy commissioner for program and policy development and the director of its Office of Health Systems Management. This was preceded by 8 years of executive and legislative branch experience at the federal level. Mr. Crane served on the staff of the U.S. House of Representatives Subcommittee on Health and the Environment. Before this position, he held several management positions with the U.S. Department of Health, Education, and Welfare. He holds a master's degree in business and public administration from Cornell University and a bachelor's degree from the College of Wooster.

Joyce Dubow, M.A., is senior advisor in AARP's Office of Policy and Strategy, where she has responsibility for a broad health portfolio related to AARP's healthcare reform initiatives. She has had a special focus on private health plans in the Medicare program, healthcare quality, and consumer decision making. Ms. Dubow serves on numerous standing committees and task forces that address quality improvement and measurement under the auspices of the National Quality Forum, the National Committee for

Quality Assurance, the Joint Commission, the Hospital Quality Alliance, the AQA Alliance, and others. Previously, Ms. Dubow was the executive vice president of the Georgetown University Community Health Plan, a university-sponsored prepaid group practice plan. She was also the director of policy and legislation in the federal Office of Health Maintenance Organizations. Ms. Dubow holds a bachelor's degree in political science from the University of Michigan and a master's degree in urban planning from Hunter College of the University of the City of New York.

Michael Gillam, M.D., is employed by Microsoft Corporation as a computer programmer and is also a board-certified emergency medicine physician who serves as an informatics consultant for the ER One Institutes at MedStar Health in Washington, DC. In his consulting capacity, Dr. Gillam is responsible for designing and deploying technology systems to create an advanced medical care environment. He and the multidisciplinary staff of ER One are currently developing innovative solutions to enable healthcare providers to effectively communicate in the event of a pandemic disease or disaster by using interactive voice response technology and gesture recognition. Dr. Gillam has published several articles in peer-reviewed journals and is a frequent invited lecturer at national conferences. He serves as the research director of the National Institute for Medical Informatics in Washington, DC, and is an instrumental member of the National Biosurveillance Testbed Initiative, a nonprofit effort to enable emergency departments across the nation to coordinate and detect emerging diseases and bioterrorism threats. Before joining Microsoft, Dr. Gillam was the founding director of the Medical Media Lab, a division within the ER One Institutes, and codeveloped the novel Azyxxi information system, the world's fastest and largest real-time comprehensive clinical information system, which was recently acquired by Microsoft. Dr. Gillam previously served as the informatics director for the Division of Emergency Medicine at Evanston Northwestern Healthcare (affiliated with the Northwestern University School of Medicine). He received a medical degree from the Michigan State University College of Human Medicine and completed a residency in emergency medicine at Northwestern University.

Veronica V. Goff, M.S., is senior consultant to the National Business Group on Health (formerly the Washington Business Group on Health [WBGH]), a nonprofit health policy organization representing Fortune 200 companies. She specializes in employer-sponsored health care focusing on healthcare spending and benefit design, evidence-based benefits, consumer decision support, mental health, and pharmacy benefits. Ms. Goff is former vice president for WGBH. As vice president she directed operations and worked with the president and board of directors to position WBGH as the nation's premier business group dedicated to healthcare policy and marketplace innovation. She also led employer initiatives on health and productivity, pharmacy benefit management, mental health, and the uninsured. Before joining WBGH in 1989, Ms. Goff held a faculty position with the University of Virginia Health Sciences Center and supervised an employee health promotion facility for AT&T. Ms. Goff holds a master of science in education degree from Southern Illinois University.

Ada Sue Hinshaw, Ph.D., R.N., F.A.A.N., is a professor in the School of Nursing at the University of Michigan. She was appointed dean of the School of Nursing on July 1, 1994, and stepped out of the position the end of June 2006. Before joining the University of Michigan, Dr. Hinshaw was the first permanent director of the National Center of Nursing Research and the first director of the National Institute of Nursing Research at the National Institutes of Health. Dr. Hinshaw led the institute in its support of valuable research and research training in many areas of nursing science, such as disease prevention, health promotion, acute and chronic illness, and the environments that enhance nursing care patient outcomes. From 1975 to 1987, Dr. Hinshaw served as the director of research and a professor at the University of Arizona College of Nursing and the director of nursing research at the University Medical Center's Department of Nursing. She has also held positions at the University of California, San Francisco, and the University of Kansas. Throughout her career Dr. Hinshaw has conducted nursing research, focusing on quality of care, patient outcomes, measurement of such outcomes, and building positive work environments for nurses because of the impact on patient safety. She is the past president of the American Academy of Nursing. Dr. Hinshaw is a member of the Institute of Medicine (IOM) and a past member of the IOM Council. Dr. Hinshaw received a Ph.D. and an M.A. in sociology from the University of Arizona, an M.S.N. from Yale University, and a B.S. from the University of Kansas.

Peter Juhn, M.D., M.P.H., is responsible for shaping evidence-based medicine policies at the Johnson & Johnson corporate level, especially as payers use evidence-based medicine as a basis for decisions on reimbursement and coverage of pharmaceuticals and medical devices. He works with the various Johnson & Johnson operating companies on a global basis to anticipate the methods and types of evidence needed in this evolving payer environment. He also provides policy coverage for developments in the health information technology initiatives as well as quality-based pay-for-performance activities. Most recently, he was vice president for health improvement resources at WellPoint Health Networks, where he managed the disease management programs for all the operating units. He also held senior positions at Kaiser Permanente, including founding executive director of the Care Management Institute, which is Kaiser's corporate disease management and clinical policy entity, and president and chief executive officer of CareTouch, Inc., an electronic health start-up venture. He has a B.A. from the University of Chicago, an M.D. from Harvard University, and an M.P.H. from the University of Washington, where he was a Robert Wood Johnson Clinical Scholar. He completed his internal medicine residency at the University of Pennsylvania.

Rae-Ellen Kavey, M.D., M.P.H., is responsible for pediatric cardiovascular risk reduction at the National Heart, Lung, and Blood Institute (NHLBI). She is currently coordinating the first evidence-based guideline from NHLBI, an integrated approach to cardiovascular risk reduction for pediatric healthcare providers. In addition, she is a clinical professor of pediatrics at the Center for Heart and Kidney Disease at Children's National Medical Center in Washington, DC. Most recently, she was the Getz Endowed Professor of Pediatrics and the chief of pediatric cardiology at Children's National Medical Center in Chicago. She is past chair of the Council for Cardiovascular Disease in the Young of the American Heart Association and is currently president of Alpha Omega Alpha. She has a bachelor of science degree from McGill University, an M.D. from McGill University and the State University of New York, Downstate, and an M.P.H. from the University of Rochester. She completed residency training in pediatrics at the New York Hospital–Cornell Medical Center and fellowship training in pediatric cardiology at Montreal Children's Hospital and Columbia Presbyterian Medical Center.

Margaret C. Kirk joined the staff of Y-ME National Breast Cancer Organization as chief executive officer on July 9, 2001. Although she has not personally experienced breast cancer firsthand, she has lost several close friends to the disease and has supported others who are survivors. It was partly this experience that resulted in her interest in joining the staff of Y-ME. Ms. Kirk has nearly 30 years of experience with not-for-profit organizations, including academic, arts, and healthcare organizations, on the local, regional, and national levels. Her experience includes management, fundraising, and affiliate relations. Most recently, she worked for the Alzheimer's Association for 10 years, starting as the first executive director of a small chapter. Ms. Kirk later served as the executive director of a second chapter and held several positions on the national staff, including vice president of chapter services and vice president of development. During her 4-year tenure as vice president of development, the contributed income of the association increased from $22 million to $52 million. A native of

Tennessee, Ms. Kirk holds a bachelor of science degree from East Tennessee State University and a master of arts degree from Indiana University.

Terry McGeeney, M.D., M.B.A., is president and chief executive officer of TransforMED, a subsidiary of the American Academy of Family Physicians that provides ongoing consultation and support to physicians looking to transform their practices to a new model of care that is based on the concept of a relationship-centered personal medical home. Dr. McGeeney has nearly 30 years of experience as a board-certified family physician, including more than a decade in rural solo practice, where he practiced the full spectrum of family medicine, including obstetrics and extensive emergency room experience, and nearly 15 years of experience in a large multispecialty group, where he served as medical director. Dr. McGeeney earned an undergraduate degree from Benedictine College, Atchison, Kansas, and a medical degree from the University of Kansas School of Medicine, Kansas City. He completed his residency at the University of Kansas Medical Center. He later received an M.B.A. in healthcare administration from the University of Colorado. He is a member of the American College of Physician Executives, the Kansas City Southwest Clinical Society, and the Iowa Medical Society. He also is a fellow of the American Academy of Family Physicians, an earned degree awarded to family physicians for distinguished service and continuing medical education, and recently accepted an appointment from the University of Kansas School of Medicine as an assistant professor of family medicine.

Richard Platt, M.D., M.S., is professor and chair of the Department of Ambulatory Care and Prevention at Harvard Medical School and Harvard Pilgrim Health Care, a New England health maintenance organization that supports research and teaching. He is an internist trained in infectious disease and epidemiology and is also a professor of medicine at Harvard Medical School and the Brigham and Women's Hospital, where he is hospital epidemiologist. He is a member of the Food and Drug Administration Drug Safety and Risk Management Advisory Committee, the American Association of Medical Colleges' Advisory Panel on Research, and the national steering committee for AHRQ's Centers for Education and Research in Therapeutics. He is the former chair of the National Institutes of Health study section Epidemiology and Disease Control 2, former chair of the Centers for Disease Control and Prevention's (CDC's) Office of Health Care Partnerships' steering committee, former cochair of the Board of Scientific Counselors of CDC's Center for Infectious Diseases, and former chair of the executive committee of the HMO Research Network. His research focuses on developing multi-institution automated record linkage systems for use in pharmacoepidemiology and for population-based surveillance, reporting, and control of both hospital- and community-acquired infections, including bioterrorism events. He is principal investigator of the CDC-sponsored Center of Excellence in Public Health Informatics, the Agency for Healthcare Research and Quality-sponsored HMO Research Network Center for Education and Research in Therapeutics, and co-principal investigator of the Modeling Infectious Disease Agent Study and the CDC-sponsored Eastern Massachusetts Prevention Epicenter.

Sean Tunis, M.D., M.Sc., is the founder and director of the Center for Medical Technology Policy (CMTP). Before joining CMTP, he was senior fellow at the Health Technology Center in San Francisco, where he worked with healthcare decision makers to design and implement real-world studies of new healthcare technologies. Through September 2005, Dr. Tunis was director of the Office of Clinical Standards and Quality and chief medical officer at the Centers for Medicare and Medicaid Services (CMS). In this role, he had lead responsibility for clinical policy and quality for the Medicare and Medicaid programs. As chief medical officer, Dr. Tunis served as the senior advisor to the CMS administrator on clinical and scientific policy. He also cochaired the CMS Council on Technology and Innovation. Before joining CMS, Dr. Tunis served as the director of the Health Program at the Congressional Office of Technology Assessment and as a health policy advisor to the U.S. Senate. He received a B.S. degree in the history of science from Cornell University and an M.D. from Stanford University and did his residency training in emergency medicine and internal medicine at the University of California, Los Angeles, and the University of Maryland. He is board certified in internal medicine and holds adjunct faculty positions at the Schools of Medicine of Johns Hopkins and Stanford Universities.

I. Steven Udvarhelyi, M.D., S.M., is senior vice president and chief medical officer for Independence Blue Cross and its affiliated companies, Keystone Health Plan East and AmeriHealth. In his role as chief medical officer, Dr. Udvarhelyi has overall responsibility for medical management programs and policies, provider contracting and provider relations, pharmacy operations, and informatics. He also serves as the chief medical spokesperson for the company. Specific areas of responsibility include utilization management; case management; disease management; quality management; pharmacy operations; prevention and wellness; research and evaluation activities; claim payment policy; hospital, physician, and ancillary provider contracting; and provider relations. In his role of overseeing informatics, Dr. Udvarhelyi is responsible for the corporate data warehouse initiative and other corporate-wide information management activities. Dr. Udvarhelyi is a board-certified internist and has 15 years of experience in the managed care industry. He currently serves on the board of directors of the National Committee for Quality Assurance, the National Council of Physician Executives of the Blue Cross Blue Shield Association, and on the Chief Medical Officers' Committee of America's Health Insurance Plans.

Appendix D

Workshop Attendees

Patricia Adams
National Pharmaceutical Council

Madhu Agarwal
Veterans Health Administration

John Agos
sanofi-aventis

Shilpa Amin
Agency for Healthcare Research
  and Quality

Mara Baer
BlueCross BlueShield Association

Annette Bar-Cohen
National Breast Cancer Coalition

Mercedes Barrs
Amylin Pharmaceuticals, Inc.

Rachel Behrman
Food and Drug Administration

Carmella Bocchino
America's Health Insurance Plans

Douglas Boenning
Children's National Medical Center

Marilyn Sue Bogner
Institute for the Study of Human
  Error, LLC

William Bornstein
Emory Healthcare

Kelly Brantley
Health Assistance Partnership

Patti Brennan
University of Wisconsin-Madison

Jennifer Bright
Mental Health America

Kristin Brinner
U.S. Department of Health and
  Human Services

Robert Browne
Eli Lilly & Company

Lynda Bryant-Comstock
GlaxoSmithKline

Ted Buckley
Biotechnology Industry
    Organization

Randy Burkholder
Pharmaceutical Research and
    Manufacturers of America

Jeffrey Bush
Becton, Dickinson and Company

Guia Calicdan-Apostle
Social Policy and Practice

Sarah Callahan
National Association of State
    Mental Health Program
    Directors

Tanisha Carino
Avalere Health, LLC

Linda Carter
Johnson & Johnson

Margaret Cary
Veterans Health Administration

Kalipso Chalkidou
National Institute for Clinical
    Excellence, United Kingdom

Richard Chapell
Merck & Co., Inc.

Nancy Chockley
National Institute for Health Care
    Management

Alex Clyde
Medtronic, Inc.

Perry D. Cohen
Parkinson Pipeline Project

Rebecca Singer Cohen
United BioSource Corporation

Robert Connors
Telemedicine and Advanced
    Technology Research Center
U.S. Army

Garen Corbett
Health Industry Forum

Denis Cortese
Mayo Clinic

Sidney Coupet
American Osteopathic Association

Robert M. Crane
Kaiser Foundation Health Plan,
    Inc.

Robert Cunningham
Health Affairs

Helen Darling
National Business Group on
    Health

Nancy Derr
Food and Drug Administration

Don Detmer
American Medical Informatics
　Association

Deirdre DeVine
Tufts-New England Medical
　Center

Christopher M. Dezii
Bristol-Myers Squibb Co.

Louis Diamond
Thomson Healthcare

Rebecca Diekemper
BJC HealthCare

David E. Domann
Ortho-McNeil Janssen Scientific
　Affairs, LLC

Mara Krause Donohue
Association of State and Territorial
　Health Officials

Stan Dorn
Urban Institute

Denise Dougherty
Agency for Healthcare Research
　and Quality

Andrea Douglas
Pharmaceutical Research and
　Manufacturers of America

Michael Dribbon
Children's Specialized Hospital

Joyce Dubow
AARP

Jill Eden
Institute of Medicine

Christine Eickhoff
Medtronic, Inc.

Lynn Etheredge
George Washington University

Jeff Farkas
Medtronic, Inc.

Nancy Featherstone
AstraZeneca LP

Alexandra Federer
Institute for the Advancement of
　Social Work Research

Shamiram Feinglass
Centers for Medicare and
　Medicaid Services

Reuven Ferziger
Johnson & Johnson

Shelley Fichtner
Pharmaceutical Research and
　Manufacturers of America

Daniel Fox
Milbank Memorial Fund

Susan Friedman
American Osteopathic Association

Richard Fry
Foundation for Managed Care
　Phamacy

Jean Paul Gagnon
sanofi-aventis

Janice Genevro
Agency for Healthcare Research
    and Quality

Barry Gershon
Wyeth Pharmaceuticals

Kim Gilchrist
AstraZeneca, LP

Michael Gillam
Microsoft

Ron Goetzel
Cornell University/Thomson
    Healthcare

Veronica Goff
National Business Group on
    Health

David Gollaher
California Healthcare Institute

Alex Goolsby
Independent consultant

Merrill Goozner
Center for Science in the Public
    Interest

Mary Grealy
Healthcare Leadership Council

Carmen Green
Institute of Medicine

Lea Greenstein
Institute of Medicine

Jim Guest
Consumers Union

Jenissa Haidari
American Academy of
    Otolaryngology

Nancy Hardt
Office of Speaker of the House of
    Representatives Nancy Pelosi

Alex Hathaway
GlaxoSmithKline

Robert Henry
Glendalough Productions, Inc.

Alejandra Herr
Avalere Health, LLC

Dorothy Hoffman
Eli Lilly & Company

Carmen Hooker Odom
State of North Carolina
    Department of Health and
    Human Services

Jane Horvath
Merck & Co., Inc.

Julianne Howell
Centers for Medicare and
    Medicaid Services

Belinda Ireland
BJC HealthCare

Christine M. Jackson
Medtronic, Inc.

Ellen Jaffe
American Psychiatric Association

Bonnie Jennings
American Academy of Nursing

Michael Johns
Emory Healthcare

Roger Johns
Johns Hopkins University School
of Medicine

Stephanie Johnson
American Psychological
Association

Rima Jolivet
Childbirth Connection

Peter Juhn
Johnson & Johnson

Douglas Kamerow
RTI International

Rae-Ellen Kavey
National Heart, Lung, and Blood
Institute

Amelia Kaye
RESULTS

Marcia Kean
Feinstein Kean Healthcare

Bruce Kelly
Mayo Clinic

Margaret C. Kirk
Y-ME National Breast Cancer
Organization

Jim Knutson
Aircraft Gear Corp

Harry Kotlarz
DePuy Orthopaedics, Inc.
(Johnson & Johnson)

John Kraemer
Office of Management and Budget

Page Kranbuhl
Stryker

Philip Kroth
University of New Mexico

Tara Larson
Division of Medical Assistance
U.S. Department of Health and
Human Services

Cato Laurencin
University of Virginia

William Lawrence
U.S. Department of Health and
Human Services

Bill Leinweber
Research!America

Jeffrey Lerner
ECRI Institute

Elana Leventhal
Academy Health

Arthur Levin
Center for Medical Consumers

Douglas Levine
AstraZeneca, LP

Jenifer Levinson
Schering-Plough

Kenneth Lin
Agency for Healthcare Research
and Quality

Susan Lin
National Center for Health
 Statistics

Bryan Luce
United BioSource Corporation

Iris Mabry-Hernandez
Agency for Healthcare Research
 and Quality

Norman Marks
Food and Drug Administration

Robyn Martin
Service Employees Internation
 Union

Karen Matsuoka
Office of Management and Budget

Lee McCabe
Johns Hopkins School of Public
 Health

Melissa McCreery
FasterCures

Newell McElwee
Pfizer, Inc.

Terry McGeeney
TransforMED

Scott McKenzie
Ortho Biotech Clinical Affairs

Kathryn McLaughlin
America's Health Insurance Plans

Robert Mechanic
Brandeis University

Erik Mettler
Food and Drug Administration

Creagh Milford
Centers for Medicare and
 Medicaid Services

Karen Milgate
Centers for Medicare and
 Medicaid Services

Amy Miller
Personalized Medicine Coalition

Tom Miller
American Enterprise Institute

Hazel Moran
Mental Health America

Tom Mowbray
CPHIMS Program
Member, National Press Club

Anne Mueller
AstraZeneca, LP

Alexandra Mugge
Centers for Medicare and
 Medicaid Services

Barbara Myklebust
George Washington University

Chalapathy Neti
IBM Research

Georginah Anne Nyambura
 Munene
Umoja Women Health Care
 Mobile-Clinics and Centres

Liz Parry
American Academy of Nursing

Avinash Patwardhan
URAC

Ronald Paulus
Geisinger Health System

Steven Pearson
America's Health Insurance Plans

Gerald Peden
Independence Blue Cross

Eleanor M. Perfetto
Pfizer, Inc.

Gary Persinger
National Pharmaceutical Council

Brittney Petersen
Association of State and Territorial
    Health Officials

Robert Phillips
American Academy of Family
    Physicians

William Pilkington
Public Health Authority of
    Cabarrus County

Sarah Pitluck
Genentech, Inc.

Rich Platt
Harvard Medical School and
    Harvard Pilgrim Health Care

Jonathan Profili
AstraZeneca, LP

Greg Raab
Raab & Associates, Inc.

Eric Racine
sanofi-aventis

John Rausch
CIGNA HealthCare

Wayne Rosenkrans
AstraZeneca Pharmaceuticals

Murray Ross
Kaiser Permanente Institute for
    Health Policy

Eileen Salinsky
Grantmakers in Health

Karen Sanders
American Psychiatric Association

Phil Sarocco
Boston Scientific

Karen Schoelles
ECRI Institute

David Schulke
The American Health Quality
    Association

Nina Schwenk
Mayo Clinic

Art Sedrakyan
Agency for Healthcare Research
    and Quality

Sven Seyffert
Medtronic, Inc.

Hemal Shah
Boehringer Ingelheim
    Pharmaceuticals, Inc.

Gail Shearer
Consumers Union

Kathleen Shoemaker
Eil Lilly & Company

Susan Shurin
National Heart, Lung, and Blood
    Institute

Dee Simo
Biogen Idec

John Siracusa
Biotechnology Industry
    Organization

Peter Slone
Medtronic, Inc.

Cynthia Smith
Merck & Co., Inc.

Fran Spigai
Chronic Care Comm. Lincoln
    County Oregon

Melissa Stegun
George Washington University

Mark Stewart
American College of Cardiology

Lisa Summers
American College of
    Nurse-Midwives

Patrick Terry
Genomic Health, Inc.

Valerie Tully
Eli Lilly & Company

Sean Tunis
Center for Medical Technology
    Policy

I. Steven Udvarhelyi
Independence Blue Cross

Steve Vinter
Google, Inc.

Andrew Wallace
U.S. Department of Health and
    Human Services

Marc Walton
Food and Drug Administration

Jeff Weinfeld
Office of Health Information
    Technology

Kathleen Weis
Pfizer, Inc.

Harlan Weisman
Johnson & Johnson

Lynda Welage
University of Michigan College of
    Pharmacy

Brandon Welch
Personalized Healthcare Initiative

Bill Weldon
Johnson & Johnson

Ben Wheatley
Institute of Medicine

Karen Williams
National Pharmaceutical Council

Lorie Williams
Division of Medical Assistance

Mark Williams
Society of Hospital Medicine

Reginald Williams
Avalere Health

Janet Woodcock
Food and Drug Administration

Brett Youngerman
Finance Committee, U.S. Senate

Jason Zielonka
Ortho-McNeill Janssen Scientific
Affairs